To Jeff, who is finally learning to be a mensch

To Jenn, the path to knowledge is hard work. Continue on this path and you will find happiness and fulfillment.

To Aunt Ronnie, who has always been there for us

To Reg, the glue that makes us a family

And finally

To the late, great Hymie Pike (ask me and I'll tell you)

About the Author

Dr. Howard D. Schwartz has been working as a speech–language pathologist since 1974. Dr. Schwartz has clinical experiences in the public schools, hospitals, university clinics, and private practice. He received his BA degree from SUNY College at New Paltz, Masters Degree from Michigan State University, and PhD from Syracuse University. Since 1986, Dr. Schwartz has been a member of the graduate faculty at Northern Illinois University. Dr. Schwartz has served as the Coordinator of speech–language pathology, Institutional Review Board Chair, and Membership Chair for the International Fluency Association. Dr. Schwartz has specialized in the area of stuttering and has taught, supervised, and provided therapy in this area in addition to authoring the book and video, *A Primer on Stuttering Therapy* (Allyn & Bacon, 1999). Dr. Schwartz's first love continues to be teaching. As a result, he has been teaching the introductory course in Communicative Disorders since he began teaching at Northern Illinois University and continues to refine his course to best meet the needs of his students. When not fulfilling university obligations, Dr. Schwartz enjoys fly fishing, photography, and collecting tattoos.

A Primer on Communication and Communicative Disorders

Howard D. Schwartz

Northern Illinois University

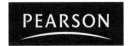

Boston   Columbus   Indianapolis   New York   San Francisco   Upper Saddle River
Amsterdam   Cape Town   Dubai   London   Madrid   Milan   Munich   Paris   Montreal   Toronto
Delhi   Mexico City   São Paulo   Sydney   Hong Kong   Seoul   Singapore   Taipei   Tokyo

Vice President and Editor in Chief: Jeffery W. Johnston
Executive Editor and Publisher: Stephen D. Dragin
Editorial Assistant: Jamie Bushell
Vice President, Director of Marketing: Margaret Waples
Marketing Manager: Weslie Sellinger
Senior Managing Editor: Pamela D. Bennett
Senior Project Manager: Linda Hillis Bayma
Senior Operations Supervisor: Matthew Ottenweller
Senior Art Director: Diane C. Lorenzo
Cover Designer: Candace Rowley
Cover Photos: Howard D. Schwartz
Full-Service Project Management: Michael B. Kopf, S4Carlisle Publishing Services, Inc.
Composition: S4Carlisle Publishing Services, Inc.
Printer/Binder: Edwards Brothers
Cover Printer: Lehigh-Phoenix Color/Hagerstown
Text Font: Helvetica

Credits and acknowledgments for material borrowed from other sources and reproduced, with permission, in this textbook appear on the appropriate page within the text.

Every effort has been made to provide accurate and current Internet information in this book. However, the Internet and information posted on it are constantly changing, so it is inevitable that some of the Internet addresses listed in this textbook will change.

Photo Credits: Images supplied by vendors are credited on the page with the photo; all other photos by Howard D. Schwartz.

Library of Congress Cataloging-in-Publication Data

Schwartz, Howard D.
  A primer on communication and communicative disorders / Howard D. Schwartz, Northern Illinois University.
      p. cm.
  Includes bibliographical references and index.
  ISBN-13: 978-0-205-49636-5
  ISBN-10: 0-205-49636-9
  1. Communicative disorders.   2. Speech therapy.   3. Audiology.   I. Title.
[DNLM: 1. Communication Disorders.   2. Communication. WL 340.2]
  RC423.S258 2012
  362.196'855—dc22
                                                        2010050452

10 9 8 7 6 5 4 3 2 1

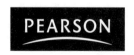

www.pearsonhighered.com

ISBN-10:   0-205-49636-9
ISBN-13: 978-0-205-49636-5

PREFACE

Why do we need another intro text? It seems like a lot of authors have written introductory texts, so why another one? I wrote this text to provide an easy-to-read, comprehensive view of normal and disordered communication. Students considering a variety of different professions will gain a firm foundation of information that will be valuable for future careers as classroom teachers, special educators, rehabilitation counselors, administrators, and of course speech–language pathologists and audiologists. This information will be a resource even for those readers who go on to become parents.

Many of the chapters have been "field tested" in my Introduction to Communicative Disorders course since I began teaching it in 1984. During the past few years, I have used these chapters with my students and received positive comments regarding the readability of the material. The material is presented so that freshmen and sophomores can get excited about this material and continue to ask questions. I have also tried to provide enough science and detail for those students looking to build their knowledge base for future courses in communication sciences and disorders.

I believe that I understand what information a student is seeking. I have included features like "Quiz on the Fly" so that as a student progresses through a chapter, he or she can quickly review some important facts and find the answers later on in the chapter. I have also included real-life stories from professionals and clients to give a student some practical reference for the more theoretical facts that are being presented. We call these stories "Making a Difference," "I Can't Do This Alone," and "In the Clinic." Take time to read these and recognize that a lot of the information we discuss has practical, real-world application. To help students with the italicized vocabulary words throughout the chapters, we have developed crossword puzzles that can serve as study guides. These crossword puzzles can be found on the Companion Website for this text (www.pearsonhighered.com/schwartz).

My goal in teaching is to get students excited about normal and disordered communication. Although I have specialized for more than 25 years in working with children and adults who stutter, I see myself as a recruiter for speech–language pathology and audiology. Let me tell you, there is no better feeling than having a student tell you, "I changed my major because of your class."

NEW! COURSESMART eTEXTBOOK AVAILABLE

CourseSmart is an exciting new choice for students looking to save money. As an alternative to purchasing the printed textbook, students can purchase an electronic version of the same content. With a CourseSmart eTextbook, students can search the text, make notes online, print out reading assignments that incorporate lecture notes, and bookmark important passages for later review. For more information, or to purchase access to the CourseSmart eTextbook, visit www.coursesmart.com.

SUPPLEMENTAL MATERIALS

For the instructor, to help with preparation of the course, we have provided an Instructor's Resource Manual and PowerPoint Slides. Both supplements are available online or you can contact your Pearson sales representative. To download and print the supplement files, go to www.pearsonhighered.com and then click on "Educators." For the student, a Companion Website (www.pearsonhighered.com/schwartz) is available that provides additional interesting content by chapter, along with study questions that will help ensure subject mastery.

ACKNOWLEDGMENTS

There are many people to thank for their love and support during a long book-writing process. I would first like to acknowledge my family, Reg, Jenn, Jeff, Aunt Ronnie, Susan, Paul, and of course Dr. Teddy, for their encouragement and patience throughout the process. As you might imagine, Jeff was always asking, "Aren't you done yet?"—there's always one in the crowd. Throughout all of the writing, Dr. Teddy (he's a Newfoundland) was patiently guarding the floor under my desk.

I would especially like to thank Executive Editor Steve Dragin for his friendship, encouragement, and willingness to share the *michigas* of publishing and listen to the craziness of university politics. Jamie Bushell, Linda Bayma, and Carol Sykes of Pearson were great with their nonthreatening nudges and encouragement to get the process finished, and they were always there to provide support and answers to my numerous questions. During the final stages of production, project editor Michael Kopf and copyeditor Michael Toporek of S4Carlisle Publishing Services helped to put this manuscript into the final form that you are currently reading. Thank you all!

Special thanks to four colleagues who helped to fill in my knowledge gaps and provided outstanding information for the reader in the chapters they wrote. The authors were Bernard Grela at the University of Connecticut, Nina Capone at Seton Hall University, Amy Weiss at the University of Rhode Island, and Cindy Hildner at Northern Illinois University. Without your help, the book would lack some important information.

Many thanks to my colleague Sherrill Morris, who was willing to read chapters, provide editorial comments, serve as a photographic model, and listen to me complain. Thanks to all of my colleagues at Northern Illinois University and beyond who were willing to give up some time to provide the clinical anecdotes used throughout the book. Thanks to Diane Schecklong, Heidi Kluga, Elia Olivares, Susan Major, Cindy Hildner, Sarah Meyers, Mike Karnell, Chookie Aron, Bubba, Corey Emert, Jennifer Heinisch, and Karen Munoz. Thanks also to the many colleagues who provided clinical anecdotes that couldn't fit into the text. Your willingness to share these stories with me will always be remembered.

Former students and current students really stepped up when I asked for editorial assistance, and I would like to acknowledge their participation in no particular order: Emily Block, Jenny Salvesen, Elizabeth Glyda, Gracie Wybourn, Erin Kowalczyk, Laura Zalnis, and Lauren Staub.

To the students, clients, and friends who willingly served as photographic models, I say thank you.

My thanks also go to the following reviewers: Amy Booth, University of Maine; Kathryn Chezik, Marshall University; John Greer Clark, University of Cincinnati; Thallia Coleman, Appalachian State University; Janet Ford, State University of New York at Cortland; Dorothy Fulton, Fort Hays State University; Yvonne Gillette, University of Akron; Beverly Goldfield, Rhode Island College; Diane Gonzales, Texas State University–San Marco; Heidi Harbors, Illinois State University; Michael D. Z. Kimelman, Duquesne University; James McCartney, California State University–Sacramento; Gary McCullough, University of Central Arkansas; Patricia Mercaitis, University of Massachusetts–Amherst; Renee Miller, California State University–Fullerton; Benjamin Munson, University of Minnesota–Twin Cities; Nan Bernstein Ratner, University of Maryland; Carolyn Sotto, University of Cincinnati; and Laura Ann Wilber, Northwestern University.

Finally, warm thanks to Dan, Josie, and Wooly Owen and the families of Tatitlek, Alaska, in Prince William Sound, who allowed me to take some of the photographs for the book.

BRIEF CONTENTS

CONTENTS

7 NEUROLOGICAL IMPAIRMENT: SPEECH AND LANGUAGE DISORDERS IN ADULTS   140

8 *VOICE DISORDERS   164*

10 *FLUENCY DISORDERS*   *212*

11 *ANATOMY AND PHYSIOLOGY OF HEARING AND HEARING DISORDERS*   *236*

12 *HEARING TESTING AND MANAGEMENT OF HEARING DISORDERS   254*

A Primer on Communication and Communicative Disorders

1

Communication and Communicative Disorders

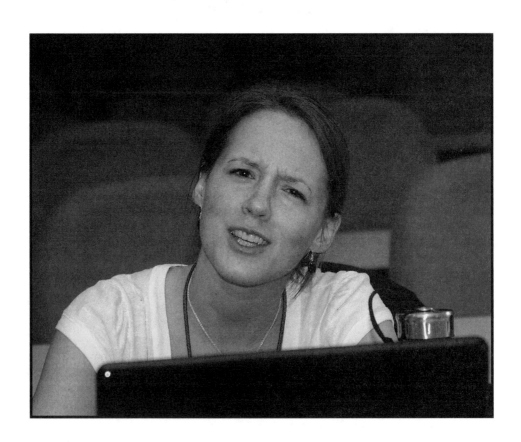

Understanding communicative disorders requires more than an ability to observe and note differences when people are communicating. Fundamental to our ability to identify a communicative disorder is our understanding of typical human communication. When we understand how people communicate and what people communicate, we will have a better appreciation for the physiological breakdowns and cognitive and emotional difficulties associated with the person's problem. In the following section we will discuss what is actually communicated.

COMMUNICATION

It is best that we start our discussion by examining a definition of communication. According to the online Merriam-Webster dictionary (2010), communication is a process by which information is exchanged between individuals through a common system of symbols, signs, or behavior. As we can note from the definition, at least two individuals are involved during this communication process. The next question to ask is, "What do we communicate?" In the above definition we noted that information is exchanged between individuals. This information can be a person's feelings, thoughts, or ideas. If we examine the following sentence, we note that verbal exchanges often contain a variety of different types of information. You are sitting in your favorite coffee shop, drinking an espresso, and overhear the couple at the adjacent table, "Contrary to what your parents may think (*thought*), I love you (*feeling*) and believe we should elope and go to Paris (*idea*)." This type of situation, a verbal exchange between two individuals, is probably what first comes to mind when the reader thinks about communication. For the majority of readers, verbal communication is probably their primary form of communication.

In addition to verbal communication, we also recognize the importance of writing and reading as important means of communicating. Can you think of any part of your day-to-day activities that doesn't involve reading and writing? Suppose you need to use the bathroom when you are in a public place. You need to look for the sign indicating the men's or women's restroom. Perhaps you need to exit the highway at the correct location, take the train to the correct stop, text a friend to meet for coffee, wear a tee shirt to announce your school allegiance, or send your spouse a love note. These are all examples of routine activities that we take for granted but are important forms of communication using reading and writing. We quickly learn that reading and writing are the tools of learning in school. We write essays, read directions, and improve our writing skills so that we are better able to share information. Recognize that each of these activities involves an exchange of information.

How does a classroom teacher know that her students do not understand her lecture? How does the stand-up comedian know that his jokes have bombed? How does an airport screener know that a specific passenger is atypical? One explanation is the ability to observe and understand facial expressions. There is no question that facial expressions can be used as a form of communication in which one person produces an expression and the second person is able to interpret the reaction.

Research on facial expressions has shown that the movements of the muscles of the face reflect the internal emotional reactions of the individual. While these facial expressions can be voluntary, the majority of facial expressions are involuntary. Investigators have noted six universal facial expressions: disgust, sadness, happiness, fear, anger, and surprise. Through experimentation, investigators have noted that cultures around the world, including those with limited cross-cultural contacts, were able to identify these facial expressions when presented during experimental tasks. During the 1970s, Paul Ekman and Wallace Friesen developed the Facial Action Coding System (Ekman & Friesen, 1978) to train individuals to recognize facial expressions. More recently this work has evolved toward the detection of microexpressions that have been described as involuntary, brief facial expressions that are used by individuals during situations where the person is stressed and recognizes that something might be gained or lost during the interaction. Psychologists have used these microexpressions during marital therapy, jury selection, and training sessions for law enforcement officers and security screeners to detect potentially problematic situations.

Another form of communication that does not require verbalization is gestural communication. For those individuals who are unable to verbally communicate, such as those persons with a profound hearing loss, manual communication, sign language, and finger spelling are the primary methods used for communicating. In the United States, *American Sign Language* (ASL) is the natural language within the Deaf community (see Figure 1.1). ASL is defined as a conceptual language with its own structure and rules. It is important to note that ASL does not follow the rules of English grammar and, when used, involves the hands, head, and body to best facilitate communication.

Do you use other types of gestures to communicate? Do you remember the last time you were driving your car and someone cut you off? Was there an obscene hand gesture that you used? Do you think this effectively communicated your feelings toward the other individual? How about the Hawaiian Shaka sign (see Figure 1.2). This sign has been used in a variety of contexts to signify "Hello," "Cool," "What's up," and "Hurray," and now appears to be a gesture used throughout the United States. However, be aware that if this sign is used in Venezuela, it is an indicator for sexual intercourse. In a similar manner, we gesture with our thumb and first finger to make a circle while extending our remaining fingers

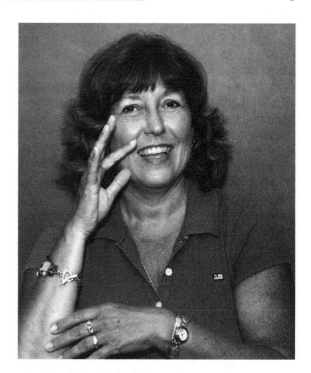

FIGURE 1.1
Gestural communication using
American Sign Language.

(see Figure 1.3). Most people recognize this gesture as "OK." However, in France this gesture means zero, in Japan it means "I like my change in coins," and in Brazil, Germany, and Russia it is seen as obscene.

We end our discussion by examining touch as a form of communication. Do you think of touch as a form of communication? Have you ever encountered a serious

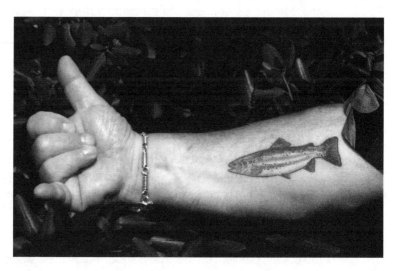

FIGURE 1.2
Hawaiian Shaka sign saying "It's cool" or "Way to go" or "Aloha."

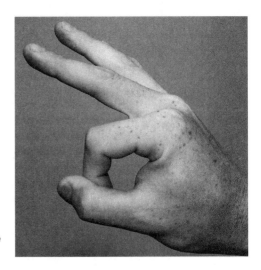

FIGURE 1.3
American gesture for "OK" but an obscene
gesture in Brazil, Germany, and Russia.

emotional trauma and it was not the words of the individual with whom you were talking but their touch that finally helped you to deal with the situation? We know that infants who are deprived of touch and parental contact may develop emotional problems, stunted growth, personality disorders, and in some extreme cases may develop failure to thrive, a condition that can lead to death. For adults, environment and gender appear to play a role in how touch is used as a form of communication. Within the workplace, a handshake appears to be the most common form of touch. However, not all handshakes are the same and the nature in which a handshake occurs (firm grasp versus weak, limp grasp) often transmits additional information. Touches between bosses and subordinates are very often uncomfortable situations and sometimes suggest the perception of power between the two. During social interactions it has been noted that, during same-sex interactions, men are more comfortable being touched on the shoulder or arm and women are more comfortable being touched on the arm. Interestingly, when a stranger of the opposite sex touches a man, he generally enjoys the interaction, but for a woman, being touched by a strange man is generally an uncomfortable situation. In retrospect we can see that communication goes well beyond just speaking with another individual.

COMMUNICATIVE DISORDERS

The question now arises as to what happens when communication fails to develop, or breakdowns in communication are perceived to characterize the personality of the individual, or when an individual has been able to communicate for his or her entire life and then loses that ability. We might consider a child whose speech and language are slow to develop when compared with his peers. What is the impact of this communication problem on the child's social interactions with other children? How will the child's parents react to this delay and what are the potential consequences of not seeking treatment and "hoping for the best"? In another scenario we have a child whose speech and language has been developing in a typical manner and sometimes appears to be more advanced. However, by the time this child reaches 3 years of age, he is repeating and prolonging sounds. What is the impact of these breakdowns on the child's perception of communication? Do these breakdowns affect the manner in which the child enters into communicative situations? Additionally, do listeners alter their perception of this child as a result of his repetitions and prolongations? Is the child seen as being more nervous, less intelligent, and less likely to be successful? In our final scenario we see a very successful corporate executive who is used to being an effective communicator, can conduct large meetings, and is used to being in total control of most situations. While getting ready for work one day, the individual attempts to call to his wife as he perceives a weakness on the right of his body and falls to the floor, losing consciousness. When this man awakens in his hospital bed, his speech is slurred, he has difficulty swallowing, and he is unable to say his name or identify simple objects. How will these events affect the future of this person? Will his family need to make decisions about the man's future? Will the man be able to make his own decisions? Will this man ever be the communicator that he was prior to getting sick? These types of descriptions lead us to a brief overview of communicative disorders in the section to follow and, more important, an examination of communicative disorders and their potential impact on individuals and families.

In the chapters to follow, we are going to discuss typical communicative development in children and adults, and follow this with an exploration of the disorders associated with these breakdowns. Our discussion of communicative disorders will begin with an exploration of four concepts that help to identify the nature of communicative breakdown. These concepts are *formulating*, *transmitting*, *receiving*, and *comprehending*. By understanding where a breakdown occurs we can better understand the nature of communicative disorders.

When an individual is getting ready to communicate, he or she must come up with the message to communicate. This message might be a group of words or an idea that is going to be shared with another individual. A child might be asked to name the color of a block. The child looks at the block and says "I don't know" or "Blue" when the block is red. An adult is asked to identify the timepiece on his wrist and he says "It's a . . . , It's a. . . . Something you use to tell time." This individual was unable to formulate the word *watch*. *Formulation* is the ability to put thoughts and ideas into words or signs or symbols.

Have you been introduced to an individual who said "Hi, I'm DDDD Don"? Perhaps you've spoken with a child who said "I thee the three planes." You recognize that these individuals know what they want to communicate but in their attempts at *transmitting,* their systems break down. Transmitting involves organizing and coordinating speech muscles or limbs (signing) with thoughts and ideas.

Sarah was born deaf. Although she has tried wearing hearing aids, Sarah must rely on sign language to communicate. In terms of spoken speech and language, Sarah has difficulty *receiving* information. Receiving information is our ability to use our sensory systems (e.g., hearing, vision, touch receptors) to transmit information to the brain.

Steve has taken a trip to Japan. All of Steve's sensory systems are intact. Steve is asked a question in Japanese by the immigration officer, and although

Steve receives this information, he is unable to understand the nature of the question. Benny was in a motorcycle accident and attends speech therapy. During therapy, Benny is asked to read aloud from the newspaper. Benny is able to read the newspaper, but when questioned about the content, Benny explains that he doesn't know. Both of these individuals have *comprehension* problems, that is, decoding and understanding the message that was sent.

Examples of Communicative Disorders

When we encounter a child who has problems producing a specific sound, we recognize this as an *articulation* problem. It is interesting to note that a number of Warner Brothers' cartoons often feature characters with articulation problems. For example, Elmer Fudd says "You wascally wabbit" instead of "You rascally rabbit," where he substitutes a *w* sound for an *r* sound. In addition, we may know an individual who has had a stroke or was in a motorcycle accident, and when we visit him in the hospital, the first thing we note is that his speech is slurred and it sounds like his words are coming up through his nose. Brain damage that results in weakness of the speech muscles is called *dysarthria.*

Perhaps you've encountered a child in your early intervention classroom who was unable to name common objects although many of the other children had little problem completing this task. You may have noticed a child who was able to follow simple directions, but when these directions included two or three tasks, the child was unable to complete the task. How about the child who fails to use the pronoun *I* and often produces sentences like "Me no want do that." Do you know an adult who during social situations cannot maintain a conversation and frequently refers to his work tasks because he is unable to produce social language? Have you visited a family member in the hospital who has had a brain injury and cannot tell you his name, identify his wife, and speak distinctly, instead producing long strings of speech that sound like something you should understand but you cannot understand? In all of these cases we are discussing *language problems.*

Renaldo knows what he wants to say and is an honor student at Stuyvesant High School in New York. When called upon in class, Renaldo will often tell his teacher that he doesn't know the answer or provide the wrong answer, because he can say those specific words but not the correct answer. When Renaldo is talking with his friends, he often produces sound and syllable repetitions, and sometimes, his entire mouth freezes and nothing comes out. Renaldo has a fluency problem known as *stuttering.*

Jenna is a singer with her band "If Anyone Can, Yukon." Jenna also works part time as a bartender to make some extra cash. When Jenna first started singing, she noted that she would occasionally lose her voice but it would return within a day. At times, Jenna's voice is hoarse and breathy, and while some of the male customers like the way her voice sounds, this hoarseness is starting to impact her singing. After seeing an ear, nose, and throat (ENT) specialist, Jenna is told that her singing and working in a bar have resulted in changes to her vocal mechanism. Jenna has a *voice disorder,* and if she doesn't make some lifestyle changes, Jenna might develop a more serious problem.

At 6 months of age, Jeff was diagnosed with a profound hearing loss and recommendations were made for Jeff to wear hearing aids. By 1 year of age, Jeff did not appear to benefit from these hearing aids and was considered for a cochlear implant. After meeting with a number of professionals, Jeff's parents decided that a cochlear implant was his best chance for successfully learning speech and language. Following Jeff's surgery, it was recommended that Jeff receive regular and consistent therapy to maximize his ability to use his cochlear implant. By the time Jeff reached fourth grade, he was integrated into a regular classroom environment, and Jeff has become an effective communicator.

At age 50, Larry began to wonder why he was having difficulty hearing people on the telephone. Larry's wife was always complaining that the volume of the television was too loud. Larry noticed that he had started to avoid social situations because he had problems understanding what people were saying. With some encouragement, Larry went to have his hearing tested and learned that he could wear hearing aids to help him to hear better in situations that had become a problem.

Given our previous discussions of different types of communicative disorders, the question arises regarding the people who are specially trained to work with problems like articulation, language, fluency, voice, and deafness. In the section to follow we will discuss the professionals who work with persons who exhibit communicative disorders, explore the necessary training and requirements, and identify the places where these professionals work.

PROFESSIONALS WHO WORK WITH DISORDERED COMMUNICATION

Speech–Language Pathologists

Speech–language pathologists (SLPs) are professionals trained to identify, diagnose, treat, and help to prevent communicative disorders. In addition to working with individuals who exhibit articulation, language, fluency, voice, and hearing problems, SLPs also work with individuals who have swallowing disorders as a result of some type of medical condition. A licensed SLP is an independent professional who does not require a prescription to work with individuals with communicative disorders.

Training, Certification, and Licensure

The typical path for training to become an SLP involves obtaining a master's degree from a graduate program that is accredited by the American Speech-Language-Hearing Association (ASHA, http://www.asha.org). In 2009, approximately 240 colleges and universities provided accredited graduate programs in speech–language pathology (Bureau of Labor Statistics, 2010a). As part of the graduate program, a student must complete a minimum of 36 hours of graduate work and 400 hours of client contact (25 hours of observation and 375 hours of direct client contact). After a student completes the graduate program, the student will take his or her first job in speech–language pathology and complete

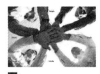

I CAN'T DO THIS ALONE

Throughout my career as a speech–language pathologist, I have always been fortunate to work very closely with other professionals who have embraced an interdisciplinary approach to treatment. My first job was in a pediatric outpatient rehabilitation setting. I had the opportunity to cotreat children who were also being treated by occupational therapists, physical therapists, and developmental specialists. This interdisciplinary approach toward treatment increased my appreciation for treating the whole child (rather than just treating the disorder) as well as addressing the needs of the family as it related to the child's other therapies and my speech and language program.

For many years, I worked in the Early Intervention Program providing services to children and their families within their home environments. I provided diagnostic and therapeutic services in conjunction with a team of professionals including developmental therapists, physical therapists, nutritionists, and social–emotional specialists. These experiences have shaped who I am as a therapist and the treatment I provide to my clients and their families. I have learned a tremendous amount from the other therapists I have worked with, but, most important, I have learned how to listen and be compassionate towards a family who wants to see their child reach his or her highest potential. I have been able to carry these experiences with me as I changed jobs, and, most important, I continue to recognize the importance of working with both the child and his or her family to make a difference in the child's communication.

Contributed by Susan Major, MA, CCC-SLP, clinical faculty member, Northern Illinois University.

the speech–language pathology clinical fellowship. This fellowship consists of 36 weeks of mentored practice that includes diagnosis, treatment, record keeping, and regularly scheduled meetings with the fellowship mentor. The fellowship mentor is certified by ASHA and provides guidance and assessment during the 36-week fellowship period.

In addition to completing the clinical fellowship, an SLP must pass a national examination that is administered by ASHA. This exam is viewed as a summative assessment of learning outcomes following a student's graduate experience. When an individual completes the graduate program, clinical fellowship, and passes the national exam, the person is awarded the Certificate of Clinical Competence in SLP (CCC-SLP). This certificate is viewed as the seal of approval from ASHA and indicates that this person is qualified to provide services in any work setting, according to ASHA standards. In the majority of states across the country, licensure is required to work as an SLP. For some states, certification from ASHA meets some or all of the requirements for the state license. In other states, additional course work or other requirements may be necessary to meet state licensure laws. As with most professions, ASHA always requires and states often require a regular program of continuing education to maintain certification and licensure.

Employment

Where do you think an SLP might work? To most readers, schools and hospitals will come to mind first. It appears that about half of the SLPs work in educational settings, and the remaining half work in hospitals, nursing homes, long-term care facilities, private clinics, not-for-profit clinics, home health care, university clinics, and as consultants to industry.

Audiologists

Audiologists are specialists trained in the nonmedical treatment of hearing, balance, and other related ear problems. An audiologist is trained to evaluate individuals who exhibit symptoms of hearing loss, balance disorders, and other auditory-related problems. Using specialized equipment, an audiologist can help to determine the levels at which a person is hearing and make recommendations regarding the best methods for managing the individual's problem. In some cases, audiologists will recommend amplification for the individual and then counsel these individuals on methods for maximizing hearing. When working with infants who have been identified with hearing loss, audiologists will work closely with the parents and an ENT physician (otolaryngologist) to determine the benefits of early amplification and the child's potential for a cochlear implant. For patients with balance problems, the audiologist will also consult with the ENT regarding testing and test results to best meet the needs of the individual.

Training, Certification, and Licensure

The typical path for training to become an audiologist involves obtaining a doctoral degree from a graduate program that is accredited by ASHA. While a student may obtain a PhD or EdD to satisfy this requirement, the majority of graduate programs are offering a clinical doctorate in audiology, with the designation AuD. In 2009, 70 colleges and universities provided accredited graduate programs in audiology (Bureau of Labor Statistics, 2010b). The AuD degree requires that a student complete 75 hours of course work that includes courses in physics, statistics, and biology, as well as graduate course work in anatomy and physiology of the ear, balance, neuroanatomy, and ethics. The AuD degree typically takes 3 to 4 years to complete and includes a requirement of 52 work weeks (35 hours per week) of supervised clinical practicum experience by an ASHA-certified audiologist. To obtain ASHA certification, the audiology graduate must pass the national certification exam to receive the Certificate of Clinical Competence in Audiology (CCC-A). In addition, another type of certification is also available through an independent organization of audiologists, the American Board of Audiology (http://www.americanboardofaudiology.org/). Audiology licensure is required in all states.

MAKING A DIFFERENCE

Heidi Kluga, a clinical faculty member in audiology at a large university, worked for a number of years as an educational audiologist. Heidi related the following interaction regarding her work in the schools:

I met Clinton when he was in the fourth grade and his father brought him in for a hearing evaluation. Clinton's dad reported that Clinton had been placed in a behavior disorder (BD) classroom at the end of second grade because he would not listen. Clinton spent the entire third grade in this classroom. This placement seemed to be a simple remedy, according to school personnel.

During the early part of the fourth grade, Clinton's hearing was evaluated and it was determined that he exhibited a bilateral, moderate sensorineural hearing loss. He had just enough hearing to know that people were talking, but could not interact during conversation unless he was looking directly at the speaker. It was obvious that Clinton was skilled at reading lips. When the school was informed that Clinton had a hearing loss and this may have accounted for his behavioral issues, the school personnel insisted that there would be no changes for Clinton, as this was the only classroom where his behavior problems could be managed.

In view of Clinton's documented hearing loss, the school speech–language pathologist agreed to reevaluate Clinton. She was able to document significant differences in his preamplification and postamplification performances. An itinerant teacher of the hearing impaired observed Clinton in his classroom and also noted significant differences between his preamplification and postamplification performances, and recognized that many of his previous "behavior" problems were associated with his frustration at not being able to understand speech and language. An independent counselor of the hearing impaired was also asked to observe and evaluate Clinton regarding specific placements for him to maximize his academic performance.

When all of the observing and testing was completed, a meeting was held at Clinton's school to share the recommendations of the educational audiologist, school speech–language pathologist, itinerant teacher of the hearing impaired, and counselor of the hearing impaired, and then he successfully returned to a regular education setting.

Contributed by Heidi Kluga, MA, clinical faculty member at Northern Illinois University.

A number of states require the doctoral degree to qualify for licensing and other states are moving in that direction. Because a number of audiologists also dispense hearing aids, some states require additional certification and licensing to provide hearing aid services to the public. To maintain certification and licensure, continuing education is a requirement.

Quiz on the Fly 1.1

1. _____ is a process by which information is exchanged between individuals through a common system of symbols, signs, or behavior.

2. In addition to verbal communication, we can communicate using _____, _____, _____, _____, and _____.

3. An individual who exhibits problems making speech sounds has an _____ problem.

4. A professional trained to identify, diagnose, treat, and help to prevent communicative disorders is called a _____.

5. Specialists trained in the nonmedical treatment of hearing, balance, and other related ear problems are called _____.

Employment

Most typically, audiologists are employed in some type of health care facility. Many audiologists work in hospitals or are affiliated with ENT offices. Audiologists also work in outpatient care facilities and university clinics. Within university clinics, audiologists will provide hearing services to the public while at the same time training graduate students working toward their doctoral degrees. A number of audiologists are employed by hearing aid manufacturers to help in the research and development of new technologies and the education and dissemination of new information regarding these products. In some rare cases, audiologists might also serve as expert witnesses in legal cases that might relate to causes of hearing loss within the workplace or the ability of residents in a home to hear a smoke alarm during a fire.

PROFESSIONAL ORGANIZATIONS

American Speech-Language-Hearing Association

ASHA is the professional organization representing SLPs, audiologists, and speech–language and hearing scientists. As previously mentioned, ASHA provides the credentialing of professionals and lists 140,000 members within the United States and around the world. According to the ASHA Web site (http://www.asha.org), "ASHA helps to advocate on behalf of persons with communicative disorders, advances communicative science, and promotes 'effective human communication'."

At the end of 2009, ASHA was composed of 18% male audiologists and 6% male SLPs. In addition, approximately 7% of the ASHA membership are members of a racial minority and approximately 23% of the members are 55 years old or older. Given these numbers it is not surprising that within the past few years ASHA has been working very hard to increase interest in careers in speech–language pathology and audiology among the underrepresented groups.

How does an organization ensure that its membership follows a set of moral and ethical principles so that the public, the clients, other professionals, and colleagues are treated in the best possible manner? ASHA has developed a code of ethics (2010b) that focuses on the importance of the welfare of the client being treated, as well as the member's responsibility to maintain professional competence, provide accurate and honest information to the public, and monitor the professional standards of colleagues. By maintaining and enforcing this code of ethics, ASHA is able to set a standard of performance for all of its members.

ADDITIONAL PROFESSIONAL ORGANIZATIONS

Although ASHA is the primary organization associated with certification of SLPs and audiologists, there are a variety of other professional organizations that enable practicing professionals to interact with colleagues who have professional interests that are more specialized than the entire field of speech or hearing. For example, the International Fluency Association is an organization "devoted to the understanding and management of fluency disorders, and to the improvement in the quality of life for persons with fluency disorders" (http://www.theifa.org). The American Academy of Audiology is self-described as the largest professional organization for audiologists, with an active membership greater than 10,000 members. This organization is "dedicated to providing quality hearing care services through professional development, education, research, and increased public awareness of hearing and balance disorders" (http://www.audiology.org). For those audiologists who are independent practitioners, there is the Academy of Doctors of Audiology (http://www.audiologist.org), and for those SLPs who work with persons with neurological problems, there's the Academy of Neurologic Communication Disorders and Sciences (http://www.ancds.org). There is no question that there are a number of organizations that can meet the professional and educational needs of practicing SLPs and audiologists.

Quiz on the Fly 1.1 Answers

1. Communication is a process by which information is exchanged between individuals through a common system of symbols, signs, or behavior. **2.** In addition to verbal communication, we can communicate using **writing, reading, facial expressions, gestures,** and **touch. 3.** An individual who exhibits problems making speech sounds has an **articulation** problem. **4.** A professional trained to identify, diagnose, treat, and help to prevent communicative disorders is called a **speech–language pathologist. 5.** Specialists trained in the nonmedical treatment of hearing, balance, and other related ear problems are called **audiologists**.

SUMMARY AND REVIEW

We began this chapter by defining communication and exploring the many ways we have of sharing information. While we typically think of verbal communication, we realize that we can communicate through writing, facial expressions, gestures, and touch. Discussion then focused on breakdowns in communication that might originate with formulating, transmitting, receiving, or comprehending information. We then presented a brief introduction to communicative disorders, noting that more expansive descriptions would make up the majority of this text. The professions of speech–language pathology and audiology were described as well as the training and certification processes required to become a practicing professional. The chapter ended with a description of ASHA and other professional organizations.

Communication

What is communication?

Communication is a process by which information is exchanged between individuals through a common system of symbols, signs, or behavior.

Communicative Disorders

How do the concepts of formulation, transmission, receiving, and comprehending relate to communication and communicative disorders?

In order for two people to communicate, it is necessary to first put thoughts into words or signs (formulation), and then organize and coordinate the speech muscles or limbs to transmit the words. Next, the second person must be able to receive this information through sensory organs like the ears or eyes, and finally the signal must reach the brain where it is understood or comprehended.

Professionals Who Work with Disordered Communication

Who are the professionals who work with people who exhibit communicative disorders?

Speech–language pathologists (SLPs) are professionals trained to identify, diagnose, treat, and help to prevent communicative disorders, and audiologists are specialists trained in the nonmedical treatment of hearing, balance, and other related ear problems.

Professional Organizations

What is the organization that certifies SLPs and audiologists?

The American Speech-Language-Hearing Association (ASHA) is the professional organization representing SLPs and audiologists. ASHA provides the credentialing of professionals and lists 140,000 members within the United States and around the world.

Additional Professional Organizations

What other organizations might an SLP or audiologist join?

In addition to being members of ASHA, SLPs and audiologists will typically be members of other organizations that support specialty interests in their profession.

WEB SITES OF INTEREST

Academy of Neurologic Communication Disorders and Sciences
http://www.ancds.org

American Academy of Audiology
http://www.audiology.com/

American Board of Audiology
http://www.americanboardofaudiology.org/

American Speech-Language-Hearing Association
http://www.asha.org/

Handspeak.com
http://www.handspeak.com/

The International Fluency Association
http://www.theifa.org/

2

Anatomy and Physiology of Speech, Language, and Voice Production

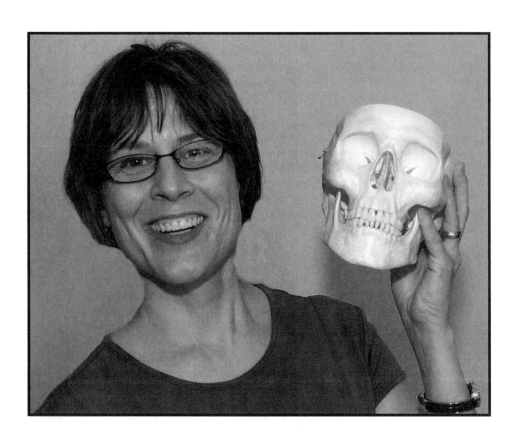

The focus of this chapter is the anatomy and physiology of speech, language, and voice production. We are interested in how our brain interacts with our lungs, voice box, lips, teeth, and tongue to enable us to communicate. Our understanding of disordered communication is best facilitated by understanding how the normal system works.

CENTRAL NERVOUS SYSTEM

To best understand how humans are able to communicate, we have to begin with an exploration of our nervous system. Our examination of the nervous system will focus on the central nervous system, a system for receiving sensory information, integrating these signals with thoughts and memories, and organizing these thoughts to complete some action. The central nervous system is comprised of the brain and the spinal cord (see Figure 2.1). Both the brain and the spinal cord are protected by a bony covering. The brain is protected by the skull, and the spinal cord is protected by the spinal column. In addition to this bony covering, both the brain and spinal cord are covered by three membranous layers called the *meninges* that also serve as protection. The outermost layer of the meninges is the dura mater. The dura mater is the tough and fibrous outer covering of the brain. The second layer of the meninges is the arachnoid mater, which is weblike and sends projections into the third layer of the meninges, the pia mater. The pia mater is described as a delicate fibrous membrane. These three layers compose the meninges and cover both the brain and spinal cord.

Brain

The wrinkled and convoluted structure that we typically refer to as the brain is actually the topmost portion of the brain that is called the *cerebrum*. The cerebrum can be examined on a number of structural levels. The brain is divided into two hemispheres, the left and right hemisphere. These two hemispheres are connected via a band of communication fibers known as the *corpus callosum* (see Figure 2.2). The corpus callosum enables the two cerebral hemispheres to communicate with one another. The two hemispheres are organized into lobes. The structure of the lobes can be noted by examining the hills or ridges called *gyri* and the indentations called *sulci*. A deeper indentation is referred to as a *fissure*. The two cerebral

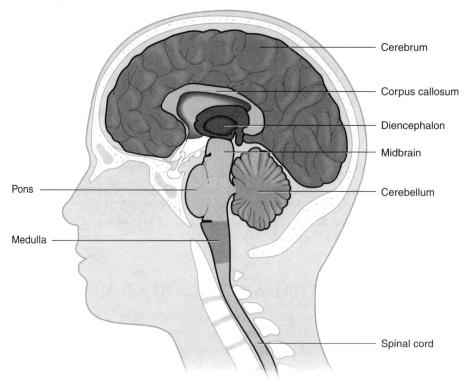

FIGURE 2.1
Central nervous system: brain and spinal cord.

hemispheres are divided by the *longitudinal fissure* (see Figure 2.2). Each of the cerebral hemispheres (left and right) can be divided into four lobes. These are the frontal lobe, parietal lobe, temporal lobe, and occipital lobe (see Figure 2.3).

The *frontal lobe* contains the primary motor area, or motor cortex. Within this area, the muscles of the body are represented along the motor strip. Research has shown that electrical stimulation of a specific point on this motor strip elicits a discrete movement in a specific muscle on the opposite side of the body. When the cells of the motor strip are activated in the left frontal lobe, the person's muscles in his or her right arm or leg are activated. This transmission of a motor signal to move a limb, such as an arm or leg, is called an *efferent* signal. It has been determined that the areas of the body that require greater muscular coordination are represented by larger areas within the motor strip. This representation of muscle function has been called the *motor homunculus* and can be seen in Figure 2.4. As the reader will note, the areas of the face, mouth, and tongue have larger representations, suggesting more complex motor control functions. The frontal lobe plays a role in motor planning, emotional control, judgment, problem solving, and socialization.

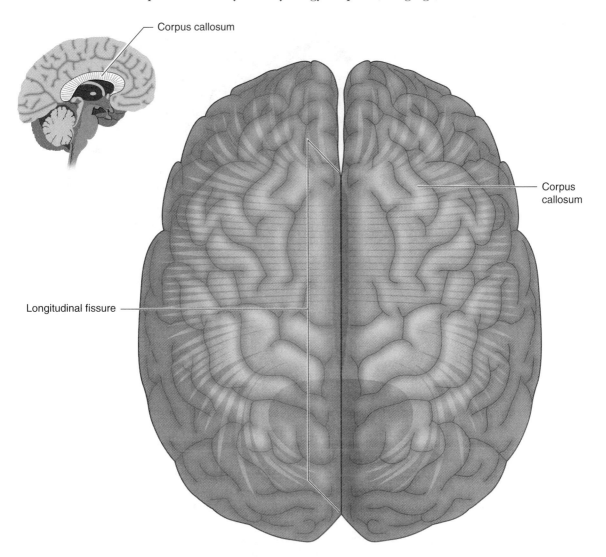

FIGURE 2.2
Brain with longitudinal fissure and corpus callosum.

One such area for speech motor planning has been named *Broca's area* (see Figure 2.5), following its discovery by the French physician Pierre Paul Broca who completed an autopsy on a speech-impaired patient in 1861. The *parietal lobe* contains the primary sensory area, or sensory cortex. In a manner similar to the frontal lobe and the motor strip, the sensory areas of the body are represented along the sensory strip. Pain, temperature, and touch information is received in the brain from the opposite side of the body. The sensory information that is received

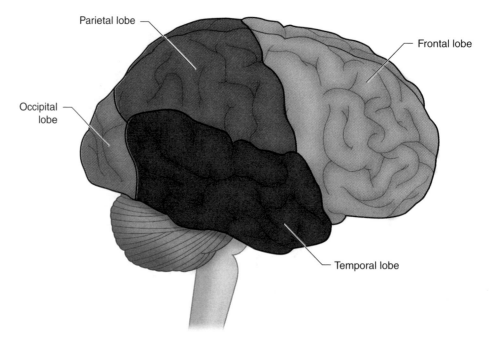

FIGURE 2.3
Lobes of the brain.

IN THE CLINIC

Robin is a speech–language pathologist working at a large metropolitan hospital in the acute-care wing (patients who were just admitted to the hospital). In this acute-care wing is a patient named Jeff who is 65 years old and has had a stroke. Robin received a referral to evaluate Jeff because he is having difficulty communicating. At this time, Robin has no additional information and must consult the patient's chart. When Robin is unable to find the patient's chart, she visits the patient at bedside and begins her evaluation. Robin notes that Jeff is unable to move his right arm, his mouth is drooping on the right side, and when he sticks out his tongue, it moves to the right. Despite the fact that Robin was unable to find the patient's chart, she is able to draw some initial conclusions because of her familiarity with normal neurological functioning. Robin concludes that Jeff appears to have experienced some damage to the left side of his brain, which controls the muscle movements (e.g., arm muscles, lip muscles, and tongue muscles) on the right side of his body. Understanding how the brain works in conjunction with speech and motor systems enables Robin to plan additional testing. Robin further concludes that she needs to find Jeff's chart to share her speech and language findings with other medical staff working with the patient.

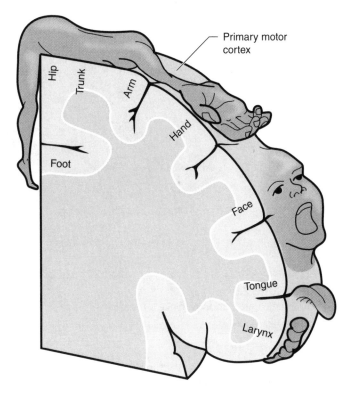

FIGURE 2.4
Motor homunculus.

on the periphery and transmitted toward the brain is called *afferent* information. The sensory area is a mirror image of the motor area in the frontal lobe. In a manner similar to the motor homunculus, areas with greater amounts of sensory receptors (e.g., fingers, lips, tongue) are represented by a larger area of the sensory strip. The *temporal lobe* contains the primary auditory cortex, responsible for the processing of sound and the location of the brain's language center called *Wernicke's area* (see Figure 2.5). It is interesting to note that for 95% of right-handed people, the dominant language area can be found in the left cerebral hemisphere. However, for left-handed individuals, only about 19% have language dominance in their right cerebral hemisphere and about 20% exhibit language functions in both hemispheres. The *occipital lobe* receives and helps to interpret visual information.

Below the cerebrum we find two areas of the brain that are also important. These include the *cerebellum* and the *brain stem*. The cerebellum is located below and to the back of the cerebrum. Historically the cerebellum was thought to only be involved with motor coordination, balance, and movement. However, more recently, studies have implicated the cerebellum in disorders such as stuttering and autism (Ingham et al., 2004; Allen, 2006). The second structure to discuss is the brain stem. The brain stem is viewed to be the more primitive part of the brain and the portion of the brain that humans have most in common with reptiles and other less

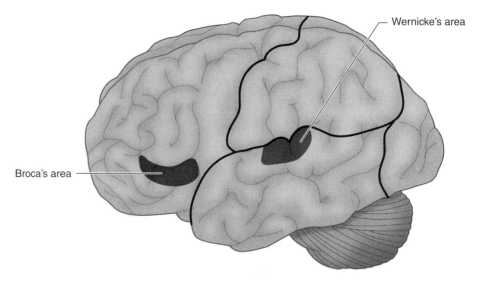

FIGURE 2.5
Broca's area and Wernicke's area.

developed animals. Within the brain stem, bodily functions such as breathing and heart rate are controlled. Within the structures of the brain stem, pathways from the cerebral cortex pass on their way to the lower portions of the body, while at the same time, sensory information that was received by our hands, feet, and body is also passing through the brain stem on its way to the cerebral cortex. The brain stem includes such structures as the *midbrain, pons,* and *medulla.* It is important to note that the majority of motor fibers that originate in our cerebral cortex cross over at the medulla to send information to the opposite side of our body. Thus, motor or muscular information that originates on the left side of our brain controls the movements on the right side of our body. When we see a relative who has had a stroke or brain damage and exhibits weakness on the right side of his or her body, we can probably conclude that the left side of his or her brain was affected. In a similar manner, weakness or damage of the left side of the body was probably due to damage in the opposite (right) side of the brain.

Spinal Cord

The second major component of the central nervous system is the spinal cord. The spinal cord is an extension of the brain stem as it passes through an opening in the skull and continues through a channel in the bony *spinal column.* Like the brain, the spinal cord is also protected by the meninges. The spinal column is divided into segments, and the segments of the spinal cord are often associated with these same anatomical locations. These segments are the *cervical, thoracic, lumbar, sacral,* and *coccygeal* segments (see Figure 2.6).

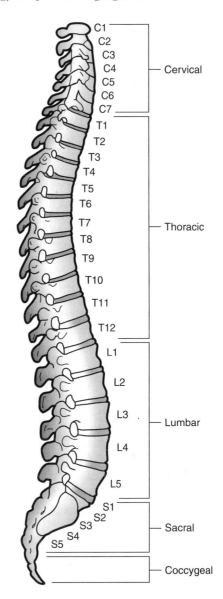

FIGURE 2.6
The anatomical segments
of the spinal column.

Quiz on the Fly 2.1

1. The brain is covered by the _____.
2. The central nervous system is comprised of the _____ and the
   _____.
3. The lobe of the brain where motor functions originate is the _____.

4. Sensory signals that travel toward the brain are called _____ information.

5. The primary language area of the brain is called _____ area.

PERIPHERAL NERVOUS SYSTEM

The *peripheral nervous system* by definition is all neural tissue outside of the brain and the spinal cord. We are most concerned with the spinal nerves and cranial nerves. The identification of these nerves indicates their location and point of origin. The spinal nerves originate in the spinal cord and exit through the spinal column. The spinal cord sends out 31 pairs (one left and one right) of spinal nerves to various parts of the body. It is through these spinal nerves that motor information is transmitted for bodily action and sensory information is received and transmitted to the brain.

Cranial Nerves

The *cranial nerves* originate in the brain stem and exit at the base of the skull. The 12 cranial nerves (see Table 2.1) serve two functions. They transmit

TABLE 2.1
Cranial nerves

Number	Name	Function
I	Olfactory Nerve	Smell
II	Optic Nerve	Vision
III	Oculomotor Nerve	Eye movement
IV	Troclear	Eye movement, pupillary constriction
V	**Trigeminal**	**Muscles for chewing, eardrum tension**
		Sensory: face and head
VI	Abducens	Eye movement
VII	**Facial**	**Muscles of facial expression**
		Sensory: tongue and pharynx
VIII	**Acoustic**	**Hearing and balance**
IX	**Glossopharyngeal**	**Motor: pharynx, swallowing**
		Sensory: tongue and pharynx
X	**Vagus**	**Motor: swallowing, laryngeal control**
		Respiratory, cardiac, and gastrointestinal systems
XI	**Accessory**	**Shoulder, arm, and throat movement**
XII	**Hypoglossal**	**Tongue movement**

Highlighted nerves serve a more important role in communication.

smell, vision, hearing, and taste information from bodily structures to the brain. In addition, these same cranial nerves transmit information from the brain to perform voluntary movements of the eyes, mouth, lips, tongue, and larynx. While all of the cranial nerves are important, some of them are more important for communication. Examination of Table 2.1 will highlight those cranial nerves associated with communication.

Autonomic Nervous System

The autonomic nervous system (ANS) helps us to maintain our internal equilibrium through its two branches, the *sympathetic* and *parasympathetic* nervous systems. While this system is not directly responsible for speech or language production, changes in our internal emotional state can certainly have an impact on our speech and language. The sympathetic branch of the ANS helps to protect our bodies against emergencies. When faced with some type of emotionally demanding situation, our ANS prepares our body for action by increasing our heart rate, increasing the speed of our breathing, increasing secretions such as perspiration, and redirecting activity away from digestion. In this manner, our bodies are prepared to act. When the emergency has passed, our parasympathetic nervous system activates, and our bodily systems return to a state of equilibrium.

ANATOMY AND PHYSIOLOGY OF SPEECH PRODUCTION

Recognizing that the nervous system provides the necessary signals from the brain to initiate communication, we need to examine the complex interactions between the respiratory, laryngeal/phonatory, and articulatory systems that enable us to produce speech. The respiratory system provides the necessary energy to set the system in motion. The laryngeal system, driven by the air of the respiratory system, produces the acoustic vibration that is ultimately converted by the articulatory system into sounds that we are able to perceive and recognize as speech. An examination of the individual components of the system will enable us to better understand this process.

Respiratory System

The respiratory system serves two important functions. The primary function of the respiratory system is breathing. To sustain life, we need to be able to take in oxygen and exchange it with the carbon dioxide that is produced by our bodies. The second function of this system is to provide the power source for the production of speech. To best understand the respiratory system, we need to examine how it is packaged.

Anatomy of Breathing

To best envision the respiratory system, we need to think about a bony cage surrounding the internal structures for breathing. The thorax, or chest, is a large container that is formed by the spinal column in the back (see Figure 2.7B), the ribs

Anterior View   **Posterior View**

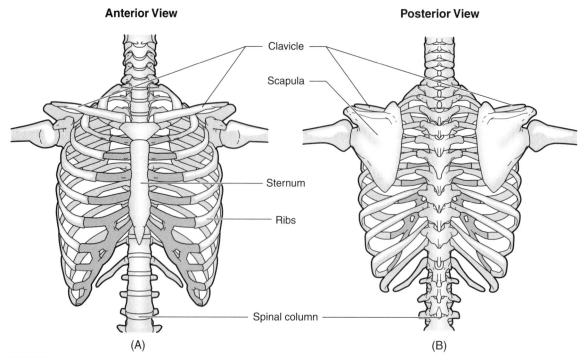

Clavicle

Scapula

Sternum

Ribs

Spinal column

(A)   (B)

FIGURE 2.7
The bony thorax (A) front view and (B) rear view.

to the sides, and the sternum, or breastbone, in the front (see Figure 2.7A). The upper border of the thorax is formed by the clavicle, or collarbone, and the scapulae, or shoulder blades. The thorax is an airtight cavity lined with membranes that link the movements of lungs with movements of the ribs. This linkage will have implications for our discussions of the breathing process. Within this bony case, we find the lungs and the airways leading to the lungs.

The lungs and the airways leading to the lungs are called the *pulmonary system* (see Figure 2.8). The term *pulmonary* relates to lung function. The respiratory system is divided into two sections, and this division occurs at the vocal folds in the larynx. The upper respiratory system includes the airways found within the nose, mouth, and throat above the vocal folds. In practical terms, when we experience a cold and sore throat, we are experiencing an upper respiratory infection. The lower respiratory system begins just below the vocal folds in the trachea, or windpipe, and continues into the lungs.

Quiz on the Fly 2.1 Answers

1. The brain is covered by the **meninges**. **2.** The central nervous system is comprised of the **brain** and the **spinal cord**. **3.** The lobe of the brain where motor functions originate is the **frontal lobe**. **4.** Sensory signals that travel toward the brain are called **afferent** information. **5.** The primary language area of the brain is called **Wernicke's** area.

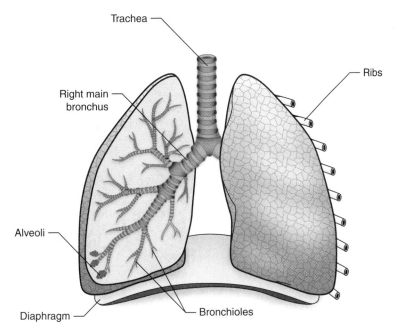

FIGURE 2.8
The pulmonary system.

The *trachea* is a series of 20 C-shaped cartilaginous rings that are connected to form a somewhat rigid but flexible tube. The trachea branches into two bronchi, and the bronchi subdivide into bronchioles within the lungs. Although the non-professional thinks of the lungs as an open air-filled sac or balloon, Kent (1997) has suggested that we think of the lungs as a treelike structure with multiple air-filled branches (bronchioles) that terminate in tiny elastic sacs called *alveoli*. The branching occurs 20 to 28 times within the lungs, and ultimately the bronchioles become alveolar ducts that connect with the alveolar sacs. There are approximately 300 million alveolar sacs where oxygen is exchanged for carbon dioxide.

At the bottom of the thoracic cavity we find a dome-shaped, or parachute-shaped, muscle called the *diaphragm* (see Figure 2.9). When the diaphragm contracts, it flattens out and increases the size, or volume, of the chest cavity. This flattening of the diaphragm is the first step in the process of breathing.

Physiology of Breathing

To best understand the process of breathing, we first have to examine a law in physics known as *Boyle's law*. Boyle's law states that Energy = Pressure × Volume. When Boyle's law is applied to the respiratory system, we know that energy in this closed system is a constant. As a result, if energy remains a constant, then pressure and volume are reciprocals. As one goes up, the other goes down. If we increase the volume, we decrease the pressure and vice versa. This law will be very important during our discussion of breathing.

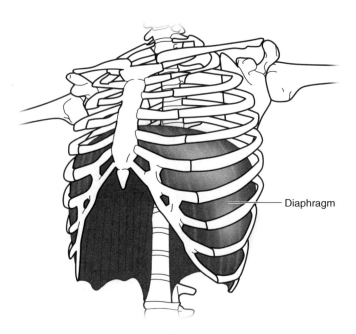

Diaphragm

FIGURE 2.9
The diaphragm.

As we discussed previously, the lungs and attached airways are all linked within the thoracic cavity. To begin the process of breathing, we first contract and flatten the diaphragm. The flattening of the diaphragm results in increased volume in the thoracic cavity as the size of the cavity is increased. According to Boyle's law, as we increase the volume of the thoracic cavity, we are also lowering the pressure within this cavity. Because we have lowered the pressure within the thoracic cavity, the air pressure outside of the body is now greater than the air pressure within the body, and as a result, the air flows from an area of high pressure to an area of low pressure, filling the lungs with air. This process is referred to as inhalation. As the lungs fill up with air, the pressure in the lungs increases while the volume of the thoracic cavity decreases. When the air pressure within the lungs is greater than the air pressure outside of the body, the air rushes out; this is called exhalation. When an individual is sitting quietly, this breathing pattern is called quiet respiration and the amount of air that enters and leaves is about one-half liter. When we measure this amount of air, we are measuring the tidal volume of air. An examination of Figure 2.10 depicts quiet respiration as well as a number of tasks that are discussed in the following section. Kent (1997) reported that 3-year-olds produce 20 to 30 breaths per minute, and as children get older (at age 10) they develop a more adultlike rate of 17 to 22 breaths per minute. When we get involved in activities that are strenuous and require greater volumes of air, we use forced respiration, or respiration that requires the active use of many more muscles to move larger volumes of air. As we require more air for various activities, we begin to use more than the tidal volumes required for quiet

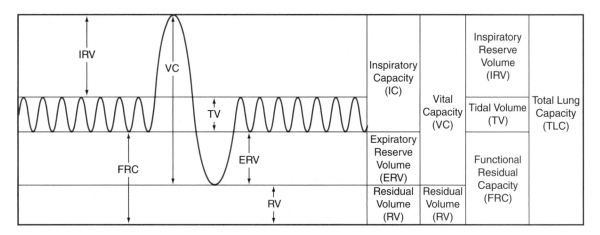

FIGURE 2.10
Lung volumes and capacities.

breathing. As we take larger breaths to get more air into our lungs, we use inspiratory reserve volume, and as we exhale this air, we use expiratory reserve volume. When we add up the inspiratory reserve volume + tidal volume + expiratory reserve volume, the total equals vital capacity, or the maximum amount of air the lungs can hold following a maximum inhalation and exhalation. It is interesting to note that after an individual exhales as much air as possible, there is still about one and one-half liters of air left in the lungs to help maintain their structure. This volume of air is referred to as *residual volume*. If we add the vital capacity + residual volume, we have total lung capacity. Total lung capacity is about 6 liters of air.

Although breathing for speech requires movement of air, the process is very different than the breathing we do to sustain life. Breathing for life requires unimpeded movement of air in and out of the lungs to maximize the body's ability to exchange oxygen and carbon dioxide. Breathing for speech requires a number of modifications to this process. For speech, it is necessary to impede the flow of air at the larynx in order to build up enough pressure to blow the vocal folds apart and cause vibration, or impede the air behind structures like the tongue or lips in order to create speech sounds. An extensive discussion of this topic will occur in sections to follow. In addition to increased pressure requirements, speech breathing requires greater volumes of air. For quiet respiration we require approximately 10% to 15% of vital capacity, but conversational speech requires 25% of vital capacity, and loud speech requires up to 40% of vital capacity. A third difference we find for speech breathing relates to the amount of time we spend during inhalations and exhalations. For normal breathing or exercise, we spend an equal amount of time inhaling and exhaling. However, during speech, a large change occurs in this process. During speech we shorten the inhalation process to about 10% of the total respiratory time, while 90% of the time is spent exhaling. As speech occurs during the exhalation process, it makes sense that we adjust the system to use the air more efficiently.

Recognizing that the respiratory system will provide the energy necessary to produce speech sounds, we will now explore the second component of the speech production system, the laryngeal, or phonatory, system. In the section to follow, we will examine the anatomy and physiology of sound production.

Laryngeal System

The laryngeal system, also known as the phonatory system, derives its name from the *larynx,* or voice box. The structures of the larynx are involved in two important processes related to speech. The first process involves the larynx as a valve or structure that controls the flow of air. The structure of the larynx enables us to open and close the vocal folds so that air can pass for the production of consonants that do not require the use of the vocal folds. These are called voiceless sounds. The second function of the larynx is to produce vocal-fold vibration that serves as the foundation for the production of vowels and the remaining sounds requiring vocal-fold vibration. This production of sound at the larynx is called *phonation*. In the sections that follow, we will examine the anatomical structures associated with the larynx and their associated functions.

Anatomy of Sound Production

The largest structure of the larynx is the *thyroid cartilage* (see Figure 2.11). The thyroid cartilage has a prominence in front that we know as the "Adam's apple." The thyroid cartilage serves to protect the vocal folds that attach behind its front wall. The thyroid cartilage attaches to the *cricoid cartilage*, often described as a signet or initial ring. Because of its location, the cricoid has also been described as the topmost tracheal ring. As air moves through the trachea, it passes through the cricoid cartilage on its way to the vocal folds. Sitting on top of the cricoid, opposite to the thyroid cartilage, we find two *arytenoid cartilages* (see Figure 2.12), shaped like pyramids. The vocal folds attach to the arytenoids and thyroid cartilage.

In addition to the cartilaginous structures of the larynx, we have a group of muscles that are involved in the production of sound. These muscles attach and insert into the cartilages of the larynx, and are involved in the opening (*abduction*) and closing (*adduction*) of the vocal folds.

Examination of the vocal folds in Figure 2.12 reveals that they are a paired muscle that attaches to the backside of the thyroid cartilage, crosses at the opening of the cricoid cartilage, and attaches to the paired arytenoid cartilages. The space between the vocal folds is called the *glottis*. When the vocal folds adduct, or close to produce a voiced sound, the edges of the muscle come together so that vibration can occur. When taking a breath, it is very important for our system to take in the necessary air without anything obstructing the passage of air. To breathe, we need to abduct, or open our vocal folds to allow an unobstructed pathway.

Physiology of Sound Production

Historically, the best explanation for our ability to produce sound was provided by the *myoelastic–aerodynamic theory of sound production*. While the name may look complicated, we can explain the theory by understanding the meaning of the title.

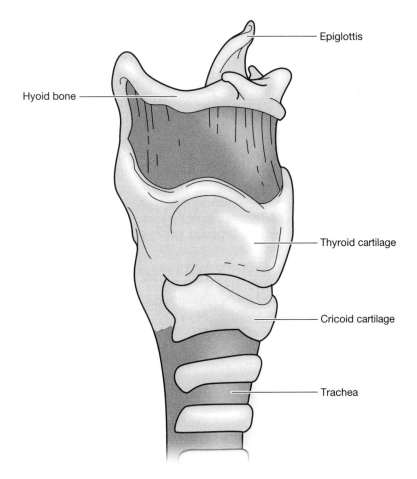

FIGURE 2.11
Cartilages of the larynx.

The prefix *myo-* refers to muscles, while *-elastic* refers to the stretchable properties of these muscles (the vocal folds). The term *aerodynamic* refers to moving air. Given these definitions, let's examine how a vowel or voiced consonant (e.g., /a/, /b/, or /z/) is produced. We would like you to know that it is customary to use "/ /" to indicate a phonetic symbol for a sound being represented.

The process begins when an individual closes, or adducts, the vocal folds. When the vocal folds are closed, the air in the lungs is trapped and the pressure below the vocal folds begins to increase. We previously described the space between the vocal folds as the glottis; therefore, the space below the vocal folds is the *subglottic space*. The subglottal air pressure builds up to a point where it can overcome the resistance of the closed vocal folds. When the subglottic air pressure is greater than the forces of resistance, the vocal folds are blown apart and the air rushes through the opening.

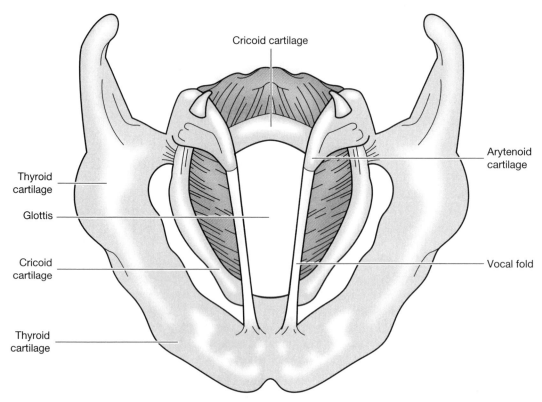

Cricoid cartilage

Thyroid
cartilage

Glottis

Cricoid
cartilage

Thyroid
cartilage

Arytenoid
cartilage

Vocal fold

FIGURE 2.12
Superior view of the larynx: the arytenoid cartilages.

At this point we need to examine the properties of the moving air as it rushes through the glottal space. According to the *Bernoulli principle*, as the speed of a moving fluid (air is a fluid) increases, the pressure associated with this movement will decrease. This principle helps to explain the lift of an airplane wing and the fact that your shower curtain is determined to stick to your body as you shower. The movement of the water in the shower causes a decrease in air pressure in the shower. As a result, the air pressure on the outside of the curtain pushes the curtain in, resulting in you being stuck to your shower curtain. Getting back to our explanation of sound production, we noted that the vocal folds were blown apart by the subglottic air pressure, and the moving air resulted in a decrease in air pressure. We also noted that the vocal folds are muscular tissue with elastic properties. When these folds are blown apart, they return to their original resting position because of their elastic properties and the Bernoulli principle. This entire process is known as one cycle of vocal-fold vibration. As soon as the vocal folds return to the closed position, the process begins again and again as the person produces a sound. Although the myoelastic–aerodynamic theory has been used to help explain vocal-fold vibration, more recent research has suggested that the process is more complicated. It has been reported that "the vocal folds move in a wave-like motion from bottom to top, with the bottom edge leading the way" (Titze, n.d.). This movement comes about because the vocal folds are a multilayered structure that enables independent movement of the top and bottom portion of the vocal folds. The description of the vocal folds as a multilayered structure has been referred to as the *body-cover model* and was first proposed by Hirano (1974). According to Titze, the ability of the vocal folds to close from bottom to top helps to account for pressure differences within the larynx and provides a more accurate explanation for the continuous vibration of the vocal folds. (See the Anatomy of Voice Production section on pp. 165–166 for a more detailed description of the vocal folds as a multilayered structure.)

It has been reported that, for males, this rapid opening and closing of the vocal folds occurs on average 125 times per second, and for females the average is 225 to 250 times per second. When looking at vocal-fold vibration in children, we note that their vocal folds can vibrate as fast as 400 times per second. These differences are due in part to the length and thickness of the individual vocal folds.

The rapid opening and closing of the vocal folds results in the collision of air molecules immediately above the vocal folds. If an individual had a microphone placed just above his or her vocal folds, the resulting sound would be a buzzing noise. If the product of phonation is a buzzing sound, the question arises as to how this buzzing noise is ultimately perceived as the sounds of our language. To understand this process, we have to examine the articulatory system to learn how the buzz is transformed into speech sounds.

Quiz on the Fly 2.2

1. Energy = Pressure × Volume is known as _____ law.
2. Opening of the vocal folds is called laryngeal _____.
3. The vocal folds attach to the _____ cartilage and the _____ cartilage.
4. The production of sound at the larynx is called _____.
5. Vocal-fold vibration is assisted by the _____ principle.

Articulatory System

Anatomy and Physiology of Shaping Sounds

The production of speech sounds occurs within a long tube that we call the vocal tract. The vocal tract begins just above the vocal folds and ends at the lips and the nose. The vocal tract is made up of three air-filled spaces known as *cavities;* these can be seen in Figure 2.13. The first cavity begins at the vocal folds and appears

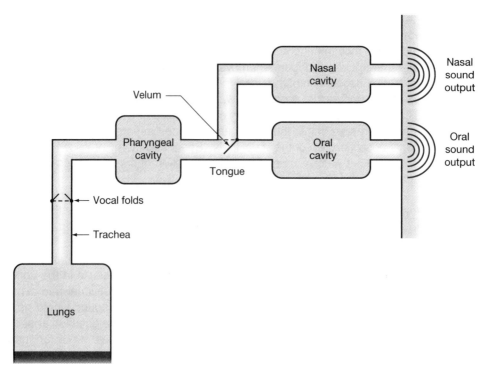

FIGURE 2.13
Schematic view of the vocal tract.

as a trumpet-shaped tube that ends behind the mouth and nose. This is the *pharyngeal cavity*. The second cavity is the *oral cavity*, which begins at the lips and ends at the back of the mouth, connecting to the pharyngeal cavity. In a similar manner the *nasal cavity* begins at the opening of the nose and ends in the back at the pharyngeal cavity. The sound generated at the larynx travels throughout the vocal tract and vibrates within these three cavities. Humans are able to change the shape and the length of the vocal tract; as a result, we are able to produce different speech sounds. For some sounds, we leave the vocal folds open or abducted (voiceless sounds), but for other sounds, the vocal folds are closed, or adducted (voiced sounds). In English, all vowel sounds and about half of the consonants are voiced sounds. The remaining consonants are classified as

---

Quiz on the Fly 2.2 Answers

1. Energy = Pressure × Volume is known as **Boyle's** law. **2.** Opening of the vocal folds is called laryngeal **abduction**. **3.** The vocal folds attach to the **thyroid** cartilage and the **arytenoid** cartilage. **4.** The production of sound at the larynx is called **phonation**. **5.** Vocal-fold vibration is assisted by the **Bernoulli** principle.

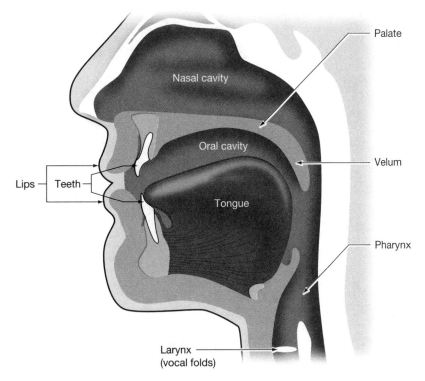

FIGURE 2.14
Lateral view of the speech articulators.

voiceless sounds. In order to understand how the buzzing produced at the larynx is converted into the speech sounds that we know, we need to examine our ability to change the shape and the length of the vocal tract. We make these changes using our *articulators* (see Figure 2.14).

The term *articulation* is often associated with movement. As a result, the articulators are movable structures that help to change the shape and length of the vocal tract. An examination of these structures will enable us to understand how speech sounds are produced.

The articulators include the tongue, hard palate, soft palate or velum, mandible or jaw, teeth, and lips (see Figure 2.15). Speech sounds are typically made by positioning the articulators in a specific location to produce a sound. We use these articulators to change the shape and length of the vocal tract. The lips are formed by a group of muscles that are active in the production of the /p/, /b/, /m/, and /w/ and a number of vowel sounds. To produce a /b/ sound, we close our vocal folds because /b/ requires phonation. At the same time, we close our lips to build up the necessary air pressure in the oral cavity to produce the sound. When we release the tension in our lip muscles and explode the air, a /b/ sound is produced. The lip movement associated with /b/ sound production is an example of changing the shape of

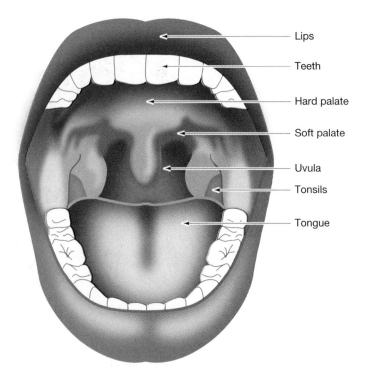

Lips

Teeth

Hard palate

Soft palate

Uvula

Tonsils

Tongue

FIGURE 2.15
The oral cavity and associated articulators.

the vocal tract. It is interesting to note that the production of the /p/ sound requires the same lip muscle activity, the same buildup of oral cavity air pressure, but does not require phonation in the larynx. The /b/ sound is considered a voiced sound, while the /p/ is a voiceless sound. The lips are also involved in sound production that requires lengthening the vocal tract. By protruding or extending our lips, we are able to make our vocal tracts longer, a task that is required for production of sounds like *oo* in the word *blue*. Because of the unique properties of our articulatory system, when we produce the word *blue* we note that our lips are beginning to lengthen well before the production of the actual *oo* sound. This process is known as *coarticulation* and enables humans to produce sounds in an efficient manner by anticipating upcoming sounds. Thus we can see that the lips are involved in the production of a number of sounds and work to change the shape and length of the vocal tract.

The *soft palate*, or *velum,* is another articulator. The soft palate acts as a movable bridge that helps to separate the nasal cavity from the oral cavity. As the velum rises, it makes contact with the back of the throat (the posterior pharyngeal wall) and enables air pressure to build up in the oral cavity. As we discussed for the /b/ and /p/ sounds, this oral air pressure is necessary for the production of these sounds. When the velum is unable to close off the nasal air cavity from the oral air cavity, as we often see in children and adults with cleft palate, air escapes into the nasal cavity and too much sound vibrates in the nasal cavity, resulting in nasal-sounding speech.

The tongue is a large bundle of muscles that help in the production of numerous speech sounds. The tongue makes contact with the hard palate (roof of the mouth) to make sounds like /t/ and /d/. For the production of many sounds, the tongue acts to block the flow of air so that noise occurs from this blockage. For example, the /s/ sound is a voiceless sound, yet there is perceptible noise associated with this sound. The sound does not come from the larynx but rather from the movement of air against the tongue. In contrast during vowel production, the tongue and the jaw are the primary articulators that determine which sound is produced. Our ability to position our tongue within the oral cavity, assisted by the movement of the mandible, determines the nature of the vowel produced. Additional discussion of vowel production will occur in the chapter on speech sound development (chapter 3).

SUMMARY AND REVIEW

The focus of this chapter has been an examination of the anatomical structures and their associated physiology required for the production of speech and language. The discussion began with an exploration of the nervous system as a foundation for communication and was followed with detailed information regarding the respiratory, laryngeal, and articulatory systems. The respiratory system was described as the energy component of the speech production system, and the laryngeal system was described as using that energy in order to produce sound. Finally, the articulatory system was described as the system that helps in the formation of speech sounds by transforming the sound produced at the larynx into meaningful speech and modifying the vocal tract in such a way that enables the production of both voiced and voiceless speech sounds.

Central Nervous System

What are the components of the central nervous system?

The central nervous system is made up of the brain and the spinal cord. The brain is divided into four lobes that have specific functions. Speech production, motor planning, and emotional control all originate in the frontal lobe. The parietal lobe contains the primary sensory area, and the temporal lobe is the location for the primary auditory cortex and the brain's language center. The occipital lobe is the part of the brain that deals with vision. The spinal cord is continuous with the brain stem and serves to transmit information from the central nervous system to the peripheral nervous system and vice versa.

Peripheral Nervous System

What is the role of the cranial nerves in the peripheral nervous system?

The peripheral nervous system is all of the nervous tissue outside of the brain and the spinal cord. The cranial nerves are a special component of the peripheral nervous system that transmit smell, vision, hearing, and taste information to the brain. These same nerves are also involved in transmitting information regarding voluntary movements of the eyes, mouth, lips, tongue, and larynx.

Anatomy and Physiology of Speech Production

What is the role of the respiratory system during speech production?

During speech production the respiratory system provides the energy that moves the vocal folds and results in vocal-fold vibration. In addition, the moving air helps us to create noisy speech sounds (e.g., /s/ and /f/). The resulting vibrating air is shaped into speech sounds.

What is the role of the laryngeal, or phonatory, system during speech production?

Voiced sounds require the vibration of the vocal folds to produce sound. As a result, the laryngeal system is actively involved in the rapid opening and closing of the vocal folds during voiced sound production, and during connected speech, the laryngeal system is abducting and adducting to enable the system to produce both voiced and voiceless sounds.

What is the role of the articulatory system during speech production?

As the vocal folds are vibrating and producing sounds associated with various speech sounds, these sounds must be shaped by the articulators into those sounds that we recognize as part of our language. It is the speech articulators found within the vocal tract that enables us to shape the sounds.

WEB SITES OF INTEREST

Brain Anatomy and Discussion of Traumatic Brain Injury
http://www.brainline.org/multimedia/interactive_brain/the_human_brain.html?gclid=COnV4Lex46ACFRMNDQod-jl7Lw

Cross-Sectional Anatomy
http://www.lumen.luc.edu/lumen/meded/grossanatomy/vhp/visible.htm

How Lungs Work
http://www.lungusa.org/your-lungs/how-lungs-work/?gclid=CM2g47mw46ACFQ0eDQodcDeBDw

Views of the Larynx
http://www.entusa.com/larynx_videos.htm

Vocal Tract Visualization Lab
http://speech.umaryland.edu/index.html

3

Speech Sounds, Articulation, and Phonological Disorders

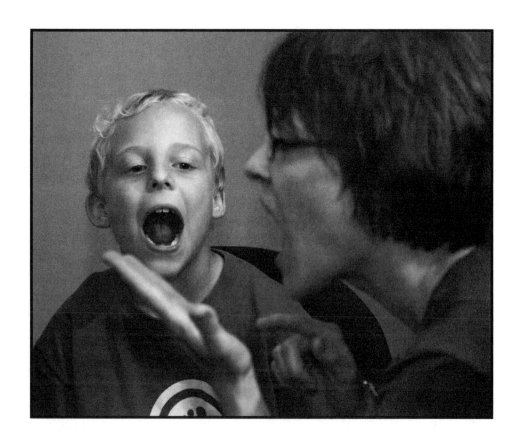

This chapter will focus on the normal development of speech sounds, followed by discussions on the evaluation and treatment of speech sound disorders. We will provide a number of definitions that will help you to differentiate language from speech and follow this with definitions that will help you to understand the speech sounds that we produce and the variations that we perceive regarding speech.

LANGUAGE AND SPEECH

According to the American Speech-Language-Hearing Association Committee on Language (1983), *language* has been defined as a system of symbols that can be spoken, written, or signed and used for communication and thought. Our ability to relate meaning to the human voice is defined as *speech* (Kent, 2004). As speech involves the production of various sounds, we need to examine the sounds in a more formal manner. *Phonemes* have been described as an abstract concept, an internal, idealized version of specific speech sounds. If you can imagine a central storage unit within your brain that houses the mental representation of a sound, then you can understand a phoneme. When we change a phoneme within a word, we change the word meaning. For example, when we change *cap* to *cab*, we have replaced the phoneme /p/ with the phoneme /b/ and completely changed the meaning of that word. Phonemes are often written with slashes, as in /kæp/. When we say the word *cap*, we recognize that every time we try to produce the word, there are going to be slight variations in how the sounds are produced. Sounds are influenced by adjacent sounds as well as our ability to move our articulators. As a result, if we repeat *cab* five times in succession, each production of /b/ will be slightly different. The individual production of the phoneme is called a *phone* and the variations that occur from production to production are *allophones*, also labeled as *allophonic variation*. To think about this process in another way, consider that if we change a phoneme in a word, we change the word meaning, but if we change the phone in a word, the word is the same but it sounds a little different. A more dramatic example can be seen in the experience of my friend Tricia, who moved from Long Island, New York, to Iowa City, Iowa. On a cold winter day, Tricia went to the store and ordered a "hot chawclate." The clerk looked at her and asked, "You want a hot chaclate?" In both cases the first vowel sounds were intended to be the same although it was obvious that these words sounded slightly different. Both listeners knew that the meaning of the word remained the same but the sounds that were produced were variations of the intended phoneme /a/ in the word *chocolate*. Given these definitions, we will now examine how these sounds are represented in English.

SOUNDS IN ENGLISH

When we look at the manner in which we write words using our traditional alphabet, we note that there are 21 consonant graphemes and 5 vowels that enable us to communicate by writing. Closer examination of the written word suggests that, in English, one, two, or three letters, or combinations of letters, may be used to represent the same sound. For example, if we consider the sound "f," we see that this sound appears in the word *tough* as *gh*, but in the word *flute* the sound is represented by an *f*, and in the word *photo* the "f" sound is represented by *ph*. The inability of our written alphabet to efficiently represent the sounds of English led to the development of the *International Phonetic Alphabet* (IPA).

The IPA has a symbol for every human speech sound. English only uses about 40 of the phonemes represented by the IPA. As each sound has its own unique symbol, the IPA helps us to avoid the confusions found in languages where multiple letter combinations are used to represent the sounds being produced. In the practical application of the IPA, a speech–language pathologist (SLP) can sit down with the recording of a child's speech and transcribe exactly what was being said by using the IPA to represent the sounds of English. For example, when a child said, "My mommy goed," the clinician would have transcribed /maɪ mami god/. While the symbols may look strange to the untrained reader, a transcript of this conversation would be understood by anyone familiar with the IPA.

Classifications of Speech Sounds

The characteristics of sounds in English help us to categorize these sounds into meaningful classes. At first glance we can divide sounds into vowels and consonants. Further examination of consonants can be completed by classifying the sounds according to their location of production, how the sounds are produced, and the presence or absence of vocal-fold vibration. Let's begin by examining vowels and consonants.

Vowels

In our previous discussions of anatomy in chapter 2, we indicated that all vowels are voiced sounds requiring vocal-fold vibration. In general, vowels are made with a relatively open vocal tract, and the differences that we note from vowel to vowel occur as a result of the different shapes of our vocal tract that we create through tongue and jaw movements. Vowels are classified according to tongue height (high, mid, low) and tongue position (front, central, back). Thus we can examine a vowel /i/ as in *beet* and classify it as a high front vowel but /a/ as in *pod* would be classified as a low back vowel. Figure 3.1 depicts a vowel chart where the vowels are plotted according to tongue height and position within the mouth.

Tongue Height	Tongue Position		
	Front	Central	Back
High	i beet		u boo
	ɪ bit		ʊ book
Mid	e bait		o boat
	bet ɛ	ə allow	
Low	æ bat		ɔ saw
	a bad		ɑ pod

FIGURE 3.1
Vowels as represented by the International Phonetic Alphabet.

Source: Reprinted with permission from The International Phonetic Association. Copyright 2005 by International Phonetic Association. (http://www.langsci.ucl.ac.uk/ipa/vowels.html)

In English we have a unique category of vowels called diphthongs. A diphthong is a combination of two vowels as in the word *buy* that is symbolized as /bai̅/. During production of a diphthong, a person actually moves from one vowel to another by changing the shape of the vocal tract. In the word *buy* the person moves from production of the /a/ vowel to a second vowel /ɪ/ to produce this complex combination. The line above the symbol lets the reader know that a diphthong was produced.

Consonants

Consonant sounds in English are classified in three different ways. These sounds can be classified according to where they are produced within the vocal tract (*place of production* or *place of articulation*), the type of constriction and how the breath stream is managed (*manner of production*), and, finally, whether the sound is made with or without the vocal folds (*voicing*) (see Figure 3.2).

Place of Production. The location where a sound is made within the vocal tract is known as the place of articulatory production or place of articulation. Consonant sounds are produced by the articulators and the place of production is identified by the articulators that are involved in the sound production. There are eight places of production and these are described in the following paragraphs.

　Bilabial sounds are made with two lips (*bi* = two, *labial* = lips). In English we have /p/, /b/, /w/, and /m/ as bilabial sounds.

　Labiodental sounds are made with the lips and teeth (*labio* = lips, *dental* = teeth). Put your lips over your lower teeth and try to make a sound. We see that /f/ and /v/ are the two labiodental sounds in English.

　Linguadental sounds, sometimes referred to as *dental* sounds, are made with the tongue and teeth (*lingua* = tongue, *dental* = teeth). Now place your tongue

Manner of Production	Place of Articulatory Production							
	Bilabial	Labiodental	Linguadental	Alveolar	Palatal	Velar	Labiovelar	Glottal
Stops or Plosives	p pit b bit			t tot d dot		k car g go		
Fricatives		f fat v vat	θ think ð bathe	s so z zoo	ʃ shoe ʒ measure			h how
Affricates					tʃ church dʒ judge			
Glides	w wall				j yellow		w wow	
Laterals or Liquids				l lip				
Rhotic or Liquids					r rice			
Nasals	m mother			n no		ŋ going		

Black type represents voiceless; colored type represents voiced.

FIGURE 3.2
Place, manner, and voicing.

between your teeth and produce the sound. The resulting sound is /θ/ as in tee**th** or /ð/ as in ba**th**e.

Lingua-alveolar sounds, sometimes referred to as *alveolar* sounds, are made with the tongue positioned at the alveolar ridge, the bumps behind your front teeth (*lingua* = tongue, *alveolar* = alveolar ridge). If you place your tongue behind your teeth, you will find that you make quite a few sounds in that position. Note that you can make /t/, /d/, /s/, /z/, /n/, and /l/ all in this same location.

Linguapalatal sounds, sometimes referred to as *palatal* sounds, are made with the tongue against the roof of your mouth (*lingua* = tongue, *palatal* = hard palate). If the wide portion of your tongue is positioned against your hard palate, you can produce /ʃ/ as in **sh**oe, /ʒ/ as in mea**s**ure, /dʒ/ as in **j**ewel, /tʃ/ as in **ch**ew, /r/ as in **r**ed, and /j/ as in **y**ellow.

Linguavelar sounds, sometimes referred to as *velar* sounds, are made with the back of the tongue and the soft palate (*lingua* = tongue, *velar* = soft palate). Place the back of your tongue against your soft palate and notice that you produce the /k/ sound, the /g/ sound, and /ŋ/ as in **k**i**ng**.

Labiovelar sounds are made by the lips and soft palate. Although we initially placed the /w/ in the bilabial category, some people consider the /w/ a labiovelar as there is a lip-rounding component to the sound, but at the same time the back of the tongue is rising toward the velum. Say ***wow*** and focus on both your lips and tongue.

Glottal sounds are made in the space between your vocal folds (*glottal* = glottis). Try to make a sound by keeping your vocal folds apart and forcing air through the space. Make a noisy breath and you produce the /h/ sound.

Manner of Production.   A second method of classifying sounds relates to how the breath stream is managed within the vocal tract and the method of constriction used to modify the stream of air. These constrictions are typically made using the lips and tongue. The seven categories of manner of production are as follows.

Stops (also called *plosives*) are sounds made by completely blocking off the vocal tract, building up air pressure behind a constriction, and exploding the sound. For example, to produce a /p/ sound, we put our lips together and build up pressure within our oral cavity. When sufficient air pressure has built up, we explode the sound by releasing the constriction of our lips to produce the sounds. Stop consonants include /p/, /b/, /t/, /d/, /k/, and /g/.

Fricative sounds are made by using our tongue to creating a constriction within the vocal tract and then forcing the breath stream through the constriction. The air moving through the constriction causes the production of noise and it is the noise that is associated with these sound productions. Fricatives include /s/, /z/, /θ/ as in tee**th**, /ð/ as in ba**th**e, /ʃ/ as in **sh**oe, /ʒ/ as in mea**s**ure, /f/, /v/, and /h/.

Affricate sounds are made by combining a stop consonant with a fricative. To make an affricate sound you first have to stop the air behind a constriction (e.g., tongue) and then release the sound to produce the noise associated with the fricative sound. In English we have two affricate sounds: /dʒ/ as in **j**ewel and /tʃ/ as in **ch**ew.

Glide sounds are also called semivowels and are made by gradually changing the shape of the vocal tract. For example, as we make the /w/ sound the lips are rounded and gradually change shape according to the following vowel. In English /w/ and /j/ as in **y**es are the two glide sounds.

Lateral sounds (also called *liquid* sounds) are made by having the air travel around the constriction within the vocal tract. The sound /l/ is produced in this manner, because the air flows out to the sides of the tongue while the tongue tip touches behind the teeth.

Rhotic sounds (also called *liquid* sounds) are produced with the tongue in a variety of different positions, resulting in a complex manner of production. The /r/ sound is the only rhotic sound in English.

Nasals are produced with an open velopharyngeal port. Unlike most sounds where constriction and management occur within the oral cavity, nasal sounds are produced within the nasal cavity. These sounds include /m/, /n/, and /ŋ/ as in goi**ng**.

Voicing.   A third method of classifying sounds in English is voicing. As described in chapter 2, voiced sounds are made by vibrating the vocal folds and shaping that sound with the articulators. In English, all vowel sounds are voiced. When we examine consonants, we note that consonants often form pairs of sounds for which the place and manner of production of that sound will be the same, and the only difference between those two sounds is the presence or absence of voicing. For example, the /p/ and /b/ sound are both bilabial stop consonants; the /p/ is the voiceless consonant and the /b/ is the voiced consonant. Sounds that differ by voicing alone are called cognates. Other pairs include /t/ and /d/, /k/ and /g/, /s/ and /z/, /f/ and /v/, /θ/ as in tee**th** and /ð/ as in ba**the**, /ʃ/ as in **sh**oe and /ʒ/ as in mea**s**ure.

Although we can hear the production of some voiceless consonants (e.g., /s/, /ʃ/), the resulting sound is noise created at the constriction within the vocal tract and not the vibration of the vocal folds. To test out this statement, place your hand on your larynx (Adam's apple) and make an /s/ sound. Note that you can hear the sound but do not feel any vibration in your larynx.

Quiz on the Fly 3.1

1. The category of speech sounds based on where the sounds are made is the _____ category.
2. Sounds that are made by totally blocking the moving air are _____.
3. The variations associated with sound production are _____.
4. Sounds made with two lips are _____.
5. The category of sounds determined by breath-stream management is the _____ category.

In the preceding section we have described three methods of classifying speech sounds. The three methods of classifying sounds have included place of production, manner of production, and voicing. Understanding where sounds are produced and how they are produced can help us to better understand the sound system when we observe that sounds are produced incorrectly. More specifically, an SLP can use this information to help to plan treatment. In the section to follow, we will describe the various stages of sound development from birth to the production of first words.

SPEECH SOUND DEVELOPMENT DURING THE FIRST YEAR OF LIFE

The development of speech sounds occurs in a systematic manner beginning at birth. In this section, we will explore sound production as it appears in association with various life processes and continues up to the production of a child's first word.

Newborns

The sounds produced by newborns are called *vegetative* sounds and occur as a result of activities for sustaining life. These include sucking sounds, crying sounds, breathing sounds, and swallowing sounds. These activities are called *reflexive,* which means that the child is responding to internal and external demands and is not voluntarily producing the sounds. It has been demonstrated through research that newborns are also capable of discriminating between two different sounds (Eimas, Siqueland, Jusczyk, & Vigorito, 1971). These studies have shown that newborns will change a behavior (e.g., increase or decrease sucking behavior) when two different sounds are perceived. At this stage, the infant is responding to the change without really understanding a difference between the two sounds.

2 to 3 Months

At this stage of development, children are starting to produce some velarlike consonants (/k/) and additional vowel-like sounds at the back of the mouth. The sound most often heard is an *oo*-like (/u/) sound; as a result, this stage has been referred to as the goo or cooing stage (Oller, 1980).

4 to 6 Months

During this stage, the sounds being produced begin to move from the back of the mouth toward the front of the mouth. Children are experimenting with sounds and the listener will hear a variety of sounds that range from growling and yelling to burp-like noises made with the lips. In reality the sounds being produced are not the adult like sounds of speech but rather close approximations to adult like forms. The child in this stage is putting consonant like sounds together with vowel-like sounds to produce longer strings of sounds (e.g., yayayayaya). The occurrence of these combinations varies on a daily basis as the child appears to be experimenting with sound usage. Because these strings of sounds are approximations of adult like sounds, the utterances are referred to as *marginal babbling* (Oller et al., 1999). Stark (1980) has referred to this stage as *vocal play*, and Oller (1980) has called it the *expansion stage*.

7 to 10 Months

For the first time, the sounds being produced actually resemble the sounds of the language and as a result are referred to as *canonical babbling*. In addition, the child begins to combine sounds and repeatedly produces the sounds in nonvarying repetitions often referred to as *reduplicated babbling* (e.g., bababababa). The stage is also characterized by single-consonant babbles such as "ba" or "ada" (Oller, 1980).

11 to 12 Months

During this stage of sound development, the child is experimenting with sound productions by combining vowels with consonants, combining consonants with vowels and consonants, and producing a variety of sound combinations. A child in this stage may produce combinations that sound like "hapa," "atopa," and "goba." Oller (1980) has referred to this stage as *variegated babbling*. While the child is combining sounds together, the child is also starting to use the stress and rhythmic patterns of the language so that the combinations that are produced sound like real words, although they are meaningless. These meaningless combinations that sound like words are called *jargon*.

During this same time period, the child is moving closer to the actual production of words. However, prior to real word productions, children produce sound combinations that appear consistently but are not related to any object or meaning associated with an adult language form. These sound combinations have been termed *protowords* and appear to be part of a transitional stage toward the production of real words.

It is important to recognize that the events that have just been described do not occur as discrete events where one stage is totally completed before the next stage begins. This process of speech development involves the mastery of one skill while the next skill is emerging. As a result, it would not be unusual for a child to be mastering vocal play or marginal babbling while at the same time starting to use variegated babbling. These stages overlap with a lot of variation noted from child to child. As the child continues to mature, words and word combinations are produced as language develops. These words are formed using the developing speech sounds and as a result it becomes important to understand the sequence of speech sound development.

SPEECH SOUND DEVELOPMENTAL MILESTONES

Historically the study of speech sound development has attempted to determine the age when a child will master a specific sound. We need to remember that most consonants occur in three positions within a word. For example, the /s/ sound appears in the initial position of the word *soup*, the medial position of the word *missing*, and the final position of the word *bus*. When we examine the development of speech sounds, it is important to identify the individual sound, its location within a word, and whether the child was able to say the sound correctly. Ultimately this information may be important for parents, teachers, physicians, SLPs, and test developers. Knowing the age when a speech sound is mastered can help a physician make an appropriate referral to an SLP, help the SLP determine the need for therapy, and help parents determine whether their child's speech is developing appropriately.

Most investigators interested in speech sound development typically use a *cross-sectional* method of investigating the development of speech sounds in children. In cross-sectional testing, the investigators sample a large population of subjects representing the ages of interest as they relate to speech sound development.

Quiz on the Fly 3.1 Answers

1. The category of speech sounds based on where the sounds are made is the **place of production** category. **2.** Sounds that are made by totally blocking the moving air are **stops** (also called **plosives**). **3.** The variations associated with sound production are **allophones**. **4.** Sounds made with two lips are **bilabials**. **5.** The category of sounds determined by breath-stream management is the **manner of production** category.

For example, a number of studies were interested in the development of speech sounds. Children from 2 years of age through 8 years of age were examined. The investigators tested a large group of children at each of these age levels and determined the sounds that were mastered for specific ages. However, it is somewhat difficult to compare across these studies as mastery may be defined as correct production of sounds in three word positions in 75% of the children (Templin, 1957) whereas other studies define mastery as correct sound production in two word positions by 75% of the children (Prather, Hedrick, & Kern, 1975; Smit, Hand, Frelinger, Bernthal, & Bird, 1990).

A second, more practical method of reporting this information was provided by Sander (1972) (see Figure 3.3). In this study, Sander summarized two early studies of speech sound development (Wellman, Case, Mengert, & Bradbury, 1931;

Years of age

Sound	2	3	4	5	6	7	8
p	▓	▓					
m	▓	▓					
h	▓	▓					
n	▓	▓					
w	▓	▓					
b	▓	▓					
k		▓	▓				
g		▓	▓				
d		▓	▓				
t		▓	▓				
ng		▓	▓				
f		▓	▓				
y		▓	▓				
r			▓	▓	▓	▓	
l			▓	▓	▓		
s			▓	▓	▓		
ch			▓	▓	▓	▓	
sh			▓	▓	▓	▓	
z			▓	▓	▓	▓	
j			▓	▓	▓	▓	
v			▓	▓	▓	▓	
th (the *th* in thumb)			▓	▓	▓	▓	
th (the *th* in this)			▓	▓	▓	▓	
zh (the sound heard in mea<u>s</u>ure)				▓	▓	▓	▓

FIGURE 3.3
Speech sound development.

Source: Reprinted with permission from the American Speech-Language-Hearing Association. Sander, E. (1972). When are speech sounds learned? *Journal of Speech and Hearing Disorders, 37,* 55–63.

Templin, 1957) and reported that "customary production" of a sound occurs when a child correctly produces the sound in two out of three word contexts 50% of the time. This result is indicated by the left portion of the horizontal bar. Mastery of the sound occurs when 90% of children correctly produce the sound in all three word positions. This is represented in the table by the right side of the horizontal bar.

When we explain to parents that speech sound development is variable and occurs over time, we can direct the parents to Figure 3.3 and show them their child's chronological age, the sound in question, and where along the continuum their child's speech development is. This explanation enables an SLP to help mollify parental concerns if necessary. In this manner, we can encourage the parent to help to create an environment that facilitates speech development rather than create an environment that demands the production of sounds that are still emerging.

In summary, the results of these studies reveal that the development of speech sounds is a predictable occurrence. Children develop speech sounds according to their chronological age. It appears that nasals, stops, and glides are acquired early but fricatives, affricates, and consonant clusters are acquired later (Vihman, 2004). While these group studies reveal a method of examining speech sound development, it is also important to examine methods of classifying these sounds when development is delayed.

IN THE CLINIC

Linda is a speech–language pathologist who works with preschoolers who have demonstrated speech and language problems or are at risk to develop them. During a kindergarten roundup in which all incoming kindergarten children are screened for speech and language problems, Linda talks with a 4-year-old named David and his mother. Linda observes that David's speech is developing normally although there are clearly errors in his productions of the /r/ sound. David tells Linda that he likes to sing "wow wow wow your boat" and he likes to eat "owanges." David's mom says, "See I told you, he makes mistakes like this all the time and it's just so embarrassing." He needs to attend therapy to correct his /r/ sounds. Following this initial screening, Linda sits down with David's mom and explains that the /r/ sound is mastered by 50% of children at 3 years of age and 90% of the children by age 6. In addition, David does not seem to be concerned about his speech; however, with continued discussion and corrections, the mom could be creating a problem for her son when no problem really exists. Linda encouraged David's mom to provide good models for her son, occasionally repeat a word that he mispronounces with a correct production, and then just observe the development of his speech. David's mom was advised that it may take 2 additional years for the sound to develop. She was also advised that should David become more concerned about his mispronunciation or if kids began teasing him, an evaluation could be scheduled and further discussion could take place.

DISORDERS OF ARTICULATION

A Traditional Method of Classifying Speech Sound Errors

In order to determine the nature of the client's speech sound errors or *misarticulations*, SLPs use a classification system to describe the nature of the sound errors being produced. This classification system focuses on substitutions, omissions, distortions, and additions. When children produce one or two misarticulations, SLPs use this traditional method of classification.

Substitutions

The most common type of misarticulation is the speech sound substitution. Most people recognize this type of speech problem when a child substitutes a "th" sound for an "s" as in *thoup* for *soup*. Many untrained observers will comment, "Isn't that cute the way she says thoup." However, as children continue to grow and develop, misarticulations call attention to a child's speech, often in a negative way. Depending upon the age of the child, speech sound errors need to be addressed as a problem rather than dismissed as a cute way of talking. Other common sound substitutions include *w* for *r*, as in *wabbit*, or *y* for *l*, as in *yamp*, the device that provides light in the house. The reader might quickly recognize that many Warner Brothers cartoon characters exhibit misarticulations, and in particular we can identify Elmer Fudd's speech when he says to Bugs Bunny, "You wascally wabbit."

Omissions

A second classification of misarticulation is the sound omission. Sound omissions often occur at the end of a word and often occur in multiple words. When the child omits sounds in multiple words, it becomes extremely difficult for an untrained or unfamiliar listener to determine what the child is saying. For example, the mom asks her child, "Where's the ball?" and the child responds, "I pu i i the bo." In the same room, the child's grandmother asks, "What did he say?" and the mom responds, "He said I put it in the box." This type of misarticulation makes it difficult to understand what the child was saying, making his speech sound *unintelligible*, or difficult to understand.

Distortions

In this classification of speech sound error, the child is typically producing a sound that does not normally occur within the English language. For example, a child will attempt to say the word *soup*. While he produces the entire word, the /s/ sound may be produced by having air move laterally over the tongue. In this case, the movement of the air and tongue results in a "mushy" sounding /s/. This type of distortion can be observed when Sylvester the Cat in cartoons says "Sufferin' succotash" with both initial /s/ sounds being distorted.

Additions

Additions appear to be the least common type of misarticulation and occur when a child adds an additional sound to the word being produced. The most common type of addition occurs when an extra sound is added to the middle of a word as in "balack" for *black* or "sunow" for *snow*.

DISORDERS OF PHONOLOGY

When children are producing multiple speech sound errors, the SLP will examine the error patterns of an individual's speech production so that hypotheses about the individual's internalized underlying phonemic representations can be made. By examining the nonrandom, predictable manner in which children simplify and modify adult words, SLPs are able to identify the rules or processes that children use as part of normal language development. It is important to note that these *phonological processes* enable a child to communicate while at the same time simplifying the words being produced.

Various explanations have been provided for a child's use of phonological processes. These include a child's misperception of the adult model; the child's motor system is immature and to accommodate this immaturity, the sound is modified to enable communication; or the child lacks the underlying representation of the adult sound model.

For most children, the majority of these rules are modified or mastered by age 4. When a child is using a large number of processes, speech intelligibility is reduced. In addition, when these processes persist and are not suppressed, the child will continue to have speech sound errors that continue to affect communication. Examination of these errors across all sounds is called error pattern analysis, in which the child's phonological error patterns are noted. Phonological patterns are often classified into categories based upon their effect upon words. Syllable processes modify the syllable structure of words while segment change or substitution processes result in a sound substitution involving the place or manner of articulation. In the section that follows, we will discuss some of the more common phonological processes.

Syllable Structure Processes

Final Consonant Deletion

When a child uses this rule, he or she omits the final consonant of the intended word. For example, a child wants to say "cup" but instead produces "cu." In many cases the deletion of the final consonant may occur across many of the words in a sentence. As previously noted in the section on traditional classification of articulation errors, a child might say "I pu i i a bo" for the intended "I put it in a box." In this case the child is using a rule to simplify the production of the sentence but the sentence will be unintelligible to most listeners. As will be noted later in this chapter, the identification of the rule that the child is using to simplify the production of words will be targeted during both the evaluation process (e.g., error pattern analysis) and during therapy (linguistic or phonological therapy) so that a therapy program can be directed toward teaching the rule, rather than teaching individual sounds.

Reduplication

This process is often seen in younger children and involves the repeating of a syllable or part of the syllable to produce the word. We often hear younger children say "wawa" for *water* or "dada" for *dad*.

Consonant Cluster Simplification

In this process, the child will simplify the production of a complex string of consonants to effectively communicate the meaning of the word. Younger children will say "mi" for *milk*, "bed" for *bread*, and "top" for *stop*. During the winter time, a young child may look out the window and note that "it nowing outside." In this case, the child has simplified the consonant cluster in *snowing* and communicated to us that the white stuff was falling outside. A listener will note that the child effectively communicated his thought while at the same time simplifying the complex structure of the consonants.

Segment Change or Substitution Processes

Stopping

For this phonological rule, the intended target sound is a fricative consonant and the child produces a stop consonant in its place. For example, a child might say "bacuum" for *vacuum* and "dis" for *this*.

Fronting

Children typically learn sounds in the front of their mouths first, and as sound development progresses, the sounds move farther back in the mouth. As a result, when a child's system has not fully developed and is unable to say the sound in the back of the mouth, he or she will say "otay" for *okay* and "dun" for *gun*.

Gliding of Liquids

In this example, children will substitute for the liquid sounds (e.g., /r/, /l/) when they appear before vowels. For example, a child will say "won" for *run* and "yewo" for *yellow*.

ARTICULATION AND PHONOLOGICAL DISORDERS ASSOCIATED WITH DEVELOPMENTAL AND PHYSICAL DIFFERENCES

While the majority of articulation and phonological problems in children occur with no known explanation for their onset, there is a smaller percentage of children who exhibit these problems because of developmental and physical differences. In this section we will examine a number of different groups of children and relate their physical differences to the articulation and phonological problems that they exhibit.

Cleft Lip and Palate

During embryological development, the lip and palate are formed during the first trimester of a woman's pregnancy (Peterson-Falzone, Hardin-Jones, & Karnell, 2001). This development occurs as the lips and palate grow from the sides of the embryo and join at the midline. When these structures fail to develop, a child might be born with an opening in his lip or palate and this is called a cleft lip or a cleft palate. Children may exhibit clefts of the lip, hard palate, or soft palate. Clefts can be on one side (unilateral) or both sides (bilateral) and all have the potential to affect the development of the child's speech.

For children born with cleft lips and palates, their treatment is often coordinated through a hospital cleft palate or craniofacial team. Team members can include a plastic surgeon, otolaryngologist (ear, nose, and throat specialist), SLP, audiologist, psychologist, social worker, and nurse. Treatments for these children often involve multiple surgeries to repair the cleft, insertion of tubes in the child's ears to help to equalize ear pressures and prevent middle-ear infections, counseling sessions for parents regarding the services the child will require, and ultimately discussions regarding methods for improving the child's speech.

As cleft lip and palate often affects the movement of the lips and the soft palate, it is not unusual for sounds associated with these structures to be affected. If a child has had lip surgery to repair a lip cleft, he or she might require speech therapy to improve the production of bilabial sounds (e.g., /p/, /b/). When children exhibit clefts of the soft palate, this problem often results in excessive air traveling through the nose (*nasal air emission*) and abnormal resonance because vowels are often produced in the nasal cavity (*hypernasality*). This is because the soft palate is not able to make contact with the back of the throat (*velopharyngeal insufficiency: velo* = velum, or soft palate, + *pharyngeal* = pharynx, or back of the throat). As a result of a child's inability to build up pressure within the oral cavity, the sounds requiring air pressure will be affected. These include most stop consonants, fricatives, and affricates. As children learn to make sounds, they will often attempt to compensate for their inability to build up sufficient air pressure within the nasal cavity and develop compensatory articulatory strategies in attempts to correctly produce sounds despite their physical limitations. These misarticulations are attempts to stop the flow of air into the nose and attempts to use the tongue to try to build up increased air pressure in the oral cavity. While these strategies make sense to the child, they often result in sound production that is unintelligible. The SLP will take an active role in helping these children to learn to produce sounds correctly and maximize their articulatory abilities given the physical limitations of their speech production system.

Dysarthria

When a child or adult exhibits weakness and discoordination in his or her speech muscles as a result of a neurological problem, the speech problems associated with this weakness are called *dysarthria*. Dysarthria is often associated with cerebral palsy in children. *Cerebral palsy* is defined as damage to the developing brain affecting the motor areas that are responsible for smooth coordinated movements. In addition to weaknesses observed in the muscles of speech, the muscles of respiration and phonation may also be affected. Problems with respiration, phonation, and articulation will have a direct impact on the child's ability to produce speech. Dysarthria can also be associated with children and adults who have had strokes, traumatic brain injury, brain tumors, or other types of neurological conditions.

When an individual's speech is dysarthric, the production of consonants is often imprecise and sometimes slurred. The soft palate works more slowly, often resulting in a nasal voice quality or, in some cases, hypernasal speech. The client's speech intelligibility may be affected as the sounds that are being produced may be more difficult to understand because of the slurring and nasal quality. Many college students create a similar situation when they overdo their partying on a weekend evening and notice the impact that alcohol has on the speech production system. For some dysarthric clients, there will also be weakness in the respiratory muscles and the energy needed to produce the sounds will be reduced, making it difficult for the client to continuously produce three or four words on a breath. Given that the individual has permanent damage to his or her neurological system that is affecting speech production, the SLP will work with these individuals to determine the sounds that are most affected by the disorder, the client's ability to make changes to his or her speech, and the client's ability to learn to compensate for the physical limitations.

Apraxia of Speech

Apraxia of speech (also called *verbal apraxia*) is defined as a speech programming problem that is often associated with brain damage to the frontal lobe. Apraxia of speech is seen in adults following a stroke and may occur in the absence of any motor weakness or other language problems. Adults with verbal apraxia exhibit articulation errors that are inconsistent in that they may appear on different sounds or different words from sentence to sentence. As word length increases, these clients will have greater difficulty programming their speech production systems and more errors will be noted. *Childhood apraxia of speech* (CAS) appears to be a condition similar to that described for adults, although there is no direct evidence of neurological damage. In addition these children often exhibit normal hearing, normal receptive language skills, and IQ scores within normal limits. As a result, this diagnosis of CAS has been misused and inappropriately assigned to children with severe phonological disorders. These children appear to be a smaller subset of children with severe phonological disorders. Bankson and Bernthal (2004a) provided a summary of characteristics that help to define this speech disorder. Among these characteristics are severe speech sound difficulties that persist, unintelligible speech, increased number of sound errors as word length increases, difficulties sequencing sounds in syllables and words, and inconsistent speech sound errors. It was also noted that these children make very slow progress in therapy.

I CAN'T DO THIS ALONE

Corey Emert is the occupational therapy (OT) evaluation specialist for the Broward County, Florida, Schools where it is his job to observe and assess students to determine if they have significant skeletal, muscular, or motor problems that limit their ability to participate in educational activities. In order for students to be observed by an occupational therapist, they must have a primary ESE (Exceptional Student Education) eligibility. Eligibilities include autism, physical impairment, other health impairment, or the most common eligibility, speech and language delay.

After a complete review of the student's ESE file, Corey meets with all of the staff that makes up the student's Individualized Education Plan (IEP) team and, most important, the person who provided the original referral. Many of the referrals are made by the school's speech–language pathologist (SLP). "My meeting with the SLP usually deals with the SLP's observations of the child and her suggestions for how OT can help this student maximize his or her learning potential."

Apraxia of speech and oral motor difficulties are the most common difficulties reported by the SLP. Most SLPs that work in the Broward County school system will not address oral motor issues such as feeding or oral defensiveness. The occupational therapist in the Broward County school system receives the referrals for these children. Many times the SLP reports that a student is having a lot of difficulty with tongue placement for sound production. "It is my observation that many students with oral dyspraxia have difficulties in other areas as well." Handwriting difficulties are very common problems with students with global dyspraxia and the number one reason for an OT referral in our schools.

A total team approach is critical for the educational planning for a student. "It is my opinion that an IEP that has been developed without input from all of the professionals working with this child is setting up the student for failure. We must all be on the same page and work on collaborative goals in order to ensure a student's success in the educational environment."

Contributed by Corey Emert, MS, OTR/L, Generations Therapy, Parkland, Florida.

Hearing Loss

Our ability to hear sound is a significant factor that influences our ability to learn to produce speech sounds. When a child experiences a hearing loss, his or her ability to hear and perceive sound is going to be affected by the early identification of the problem, the nature of the hearing loss, and early access to treatment that includes amplification. While these factors will be discussed at length in subsequent chapters, we need to address the impact of hearing loss on the development of speech sounds. Children with significant hearing loss often experience problems associated with voicing distinctions such as *bag* and *back* or *pit* and *bit*. In addition, individuals with hearing loss may also experience difficulties with vowel distinctions such as *beat* and *bit* as well as problems with sounds that look alike, such as *poor*, *more*, and *bore*. The speech of those exhibiting a hearing loss is quite variable and it is difficult to identify one specific pattern associated with hearing loss.

ASSESSMENT OF ARTICULATION AND PHONOLOGICAL DISORDERS

The evaluation of articulation and phonological disorders is completed in a systematic manner by first determining the presence or absence of the problem and then selecting measures to determine the nature of the problem being exhibited. Once the information is collected, the SLP will use this information to determine the need for therapy, the type of therapy to provide, and the point at which to begin therapy. In addition, the data collected at the evaluation will serve as a baseline of the child's abilities so that as the child progresses through therapy, progress can be measured as it relates to the evaluation data. This evaluation process will focus on screening measures, hearing testing, oral–facial examination, speech sound inventories, conversational speech sampling, error pattern analysis, and stimulability testing. Upon completion of the evaluation, decisions are made regarding the treatment and/or follow-up.

Articulation and Phonology Screening

We are going to focus our discussion on the process of screening for the presence of articulation and phonological disorders. However, it is important to understand this process of screening. To begin with, we want the reader to envision that we are running a quarry and we are concerned with collecting speckled rocks that are 1 inch or larger. To accomplish this process we use a wire mesh screen with holes that are slightly smaller than 1 inch across. As we dig from the quarry, we dump a lot of rocks on the screen, and everything that is larger than 1 inch will remain on the screen while everything that is smaller will pass through the screen. What we have accomplished is separating those rocks that we think we want from those rocks that don't meet our size criterion. As we indicated that we only want speckled rocks, we recognize that we will now have to examine each of the rocks that is 1 inch or greater and sort the speckled rocks from the other rocks that we've collected. At this point the reader is probably asking what this has to do with articulation and phonology. For many school districts around the country, large numbers of children will be screened for speech and language disorders. Screening is a process of evaluating a large number of children in a short period of time. Because of the number of children involved, complete, full-scale evaluations of every child would be impractical. As a result, each child will be evaluated during a short period of time, and like the rocks, those children who appear to meet the criteria of having a speech sound problem will be identified, but those children who do not appear to have the problem will not be selected for further evaluation. As noted with our speckled rocks, further evaluation will be necessary to determine how many of the children in the first group actually do meet the criteria for a speech sound problem.

We also recognize that some of the rocks might squeeze through the opening despite the fact that they meet our criteria, and occasionally a child will not be identified despite the fact that the child's parents "know" the child has a problem. In those cases, the parents often contact the school and ask that the child be retested. Some other children identified as having a problem may in fact, upon further testing, fall within normal limits for speech sound production. The screening process is not an absolute measure but just part of the process that is necessary for initially identifying those children who appear to exhibit speech sound errors.

When a child's speech is screened, the SLP may ask the child to identify pictures, repeat sentences, describe a picture, or tell a story. During this process the SLP is noting the number of sound errors produced by the child, the child's chronological age, and the expectations for correct sound production when the child in question is compared to other children of similar age. Upon completion of this relatively short task, the clinician will decide whether the child requires additional testing or whether the child's speech is developing normally. As previously noted, there are occasionally false positives when a child appears to have a problem but it is later determined to not have a problem, or false negatives when the child does not appear to have a problem but has a problem that is not identified. Although screening is the initial method of identifying speech problems for children entering school, classroom teachers and school administrators can be useful referral sources when a child's problem is not identified during the screening.

Hearing Screening

In a manner similar to speech screening, all young children entering kindergarten are required to undergo a hearing screening. In addition, whenever the presence of a speech problem is suspected, it is always recommended that the child's hearing be checked as various types of hearing loss have the potential to delay or impair the development of speech sounds. An SLP is trained to do hearing screenings but complete hearing evaluations fall within the role of the *audiologist.* An audiologist is a trained specialist in the nonmedical diagnosis and treatment of hearing disorders. During future chapters, we will discuss a complete hearing evaluation and the role of the audiologist. During a hearing screening, the SLP and in some cases the school nurse will use a portable audiometer, which is a device for testing hearing. The tester will ask the child to respond to various sound frequencies by raising his or her hand when a tone is presented. The frequencies or tones used during this screening process are the frequencies most associated with speech sound production. If a child fails a hearing screening, the testing can be repeated; however, the child will more likely be referred for a complete audiological evaluation to add information to the complete speech evaluation.

Oral–Facial Examination

As previously described, some speech sound disorders are associated with structural problems (e.g., cleft lip and palate) of the speech sound articulators. As a result, a routine part of the speech evaluation is a visual examination of the observable speech articulators during rest and during speech and nonspeech activities. By examining the articulators, the clinician will be able to make some determination regarding the structure and function of the child's articulatory system. In general, the examining clinician is going to look at the child's face, lips, teeth, tongue, hard palate, soft palate, and pharyngeal walls and take note of any structure that is grossly abnormal. As there is a large range of variation from child to child, most oral–facial evaluations are unremarkable. However, even during routine oral–facial examinations it would not be unusual for an SLP to note poor oral hygiene, enlarged tonsils, and structural deviations of the teeth, or drooling. While we live in a world of improved health care, including medical and dental services, at times an SLP might be one of the first professionals to look within the mouth of a child to note a lack of good hygiene, poor dentition, or a structural abnormality that might require a referral and further medical or dental attention.

In addition to visually inspecting the oral structures, it is advisable for the clinician to make some determination of the functioning of the child's speech articulators during speech and nonspeech activities. Although the relationship between speech and nonspeech activities continues to be debated within the speech literature, assessing the functioning of the articulators during both types of activities can provide important information regarding the state of the child's articulatory system. In general an SLP will examine children's ability to purse and retract their lips, produce a smile, blow up their cheeks, rapidly move their tongue from side to side, demonstrate range of motion of the tongue, and raise and lower their soft palate. These activities in isolation provide an initial level of information regarding the nature of the articulatory system. More important, when the SLP combines the information seen and heard during the speech evaluation with the observations obtained during the oral–facial examination, the clinician is able to provide a more comprehensive picture of the total child and the child's abilities to produce speech sounds.

Speech Sound Inventory

There will be many readers of this book who have at some point in their life worked in a job where they were required to take an inventory of the products within the department where they worked. In my case, I had to count every item in the toy department of a large department store following the Christmas season. It was our job to account for everything that was left within the department. When we want to account for, or evaluate, all of the sounds that a child produces and look at all of these sounds within their possible contexts within a word, we use a speech sound inventory. Many speech sound inventories will examine consonants, consonant blends, and less often include vowels. Vowels are typically mastered early and vowel distortions are a less common occurrence than consonant errors. As consonants appear in the initial, medial, and final positions of words, a speech sound inventory is designed to assess these sounds in the word positions where they occur in English. There are many commercially available speech sound inventories that might be used by an SLP. The test usually includes a set of pictures that targets a specific sound in a specific position of a word. For example, a clinician points to the first picture and asks the child to name the picture. The child identifies a cup and the clinician notes that the child correctly produced the /k/ sound in the initial position of the word. As subsequent pictures are presented, the clinician uses a score form that lists the targeted word and highlights the targeted sound. When a child incorrectly produces the sound, the clinician will indicate the nature of the misarticulation by noting any substitutions, omissions, distortions, or additions.

It is recognized by most clinicians who use speech sound inventories that the child's speech is being sampled within the limitations of single-word productions and is sometimes following a model provided by the examiner. Recognizing that speech sounds are influenced by the sounds and words that precede and follow their production and recognizing the limitations of sampling one word at a time, clinicians will then obtain a conversational sample of the child's speech, making sure to make an audio and/or video recording of the child so that the entire sample can be phonetically transcribed for future analysis.

Conversational Speech Sampling

An SLP is interested in obtaining a sample of the child's speech during activities that reflect similar activities to those that occur outside of the therapy room. For younger children, a number of toys may be provided and the child and clinician will interact during this play activity. For some older children, a child might be asked to read, discuss a specific topic ("Tell me about Cub Scouts"), or just converse with the clinician. The clinician recognizes that the more talking that the child does, the larger the sample of speech sounds that can be collected. The clinician will make statements like "Tell me about the car" rather than "What color is the car" so that the child has the opportunity to provide a natural response that goes beyond a one-word utterance. While the clinician can use this speech sample to assess speech sound development, it is likely that the same sample will be used to also assess the child's expressive language skills. It is important for the clinician to use an audio and video recorder so that the speech sample is permanently recorded and analysis can occur at a later time. It would be very difficult to analyze the child's speech while also playing with the child. However, as many younger children are often unintelligible, it will be important for the clinician to take notes during the interaction so that the context of the conversation will be recorded and specific events and words can be recalled at a later date. When trying to analyze a conversational sample of a child who is difficult to understand, the more information that the clinician has and the more detailed notes that were taken, the easier it will be to develop an analysis.

The conversational speech sample will be used in conjunction with the information obtained during the speech sound inventory. As noted by Bankson and Bernthal (2004b, p. 205) conversational samples "allow one to transcribe phoneme productions in a variety of phonetic contexts, to observe error patterns, and to judge the severity of the problem and the intelligibility of the speaker in continuous discourse." The clinician will play back the audiotape and/or videotape following the evaluation and use the IPA to transcribe exactly what the child has said.

The clinician will then examine the nature of the speech sound errors and compare these with the errors noted during the speech sound inventory. It is not uncommon to find that a child will be able to adequately produce sounds during

IN THE CLINIC

Javier, a speech–language pathologist who works with preschool children, has just completed transcribing his interaction with Jessica, a 3-year-old child attending the Early Learners Program at the Naperville Community Center. In the first sample below you can find the text of Jessica's utterances written out using the English alphabet. In the second sample you will note the transcribed set of utterances written in the International Phonetic Alphabet.

English Alphabet:

The baby is sweeping. She's tired. I not tired. I wanna pway. Where my mommy? I done now.

International Phonetic Alphabet:

ðʌ bebi ɪz swipɪŋ. ʃiz taɪ͡əˆd. aɪ nat swipi. aɪ wʌnə pwe. wɛr maɪ mami. aɪ dʌn naʊ.

---

the single-word task and yet have difficulty producing the sounds in context. To some clinicians, this might suggest that the sounds are in the process of developing and the child is still figuring out how to master the production of these sounds in context. For other children, specific sound errors are noted during the speech sound inventory and are also evident during the conversational sample. In both cases, a clinician will then be interested in determining whether a child can be prompted to produce the correct sounds. As we conclude this portion of the evaluation, we are determining the number of sound errors that the child is exhibiting and the child's speech intelligibility. When the child is exhibiting multiple misarticulations and his or her speech intelligibility is reduced, the SLP will then complete a more in-depth examination of the nature of the child's speech sound errors.

Error Pattern Analysis

As we described earlier in the Disorders of Articulation section (see p. 53), the multiple speech sound errors produced by some children can be examined and classified as substitutions, omissions, distortions, or additions. However, by using *error pattern analysis* the SLP can begin to examine the phonological processes that the child is using to simplify sound productions, modify sound productions, or modify the syllable structure of words (Bankson & Bernthal, 2004b). Using these processes enables a child to communicate but often affects the intelligibility of the words being produced. The error pattern analysis enables the SLP to compare the child's error patterns to the adult standard and use the results of this analysis to plan therapy and serve as a baseline when examining therapy progress.

In a manner similar to those described previously, an error pattern analysis can be completed by examining single-word productions or a conversational speech sample. A clinician might use a series of pictures with targeted sounds and also use a conversational speech sample that has been transcribed. There are a number of commercially available phonological tests that can help in the identification of phonological patterns (e.g., Hodson, 1989). When the clinician completes the error pattern analysis, decisions need to be made regarding the nature of the child's problem and the need for treatment. After we have examined the speech sound errors that the child is producing, we need to examine the child's ability to correctly produce these sounds following a model provided by the clinician.

Stimulability

Stimulability is a method of determining the child's ability to produce the correct form of the sound, sometimes referred to as the adult form (Bankson & Bernthal, 2004b), with some form of stimulation.

By examining stimulability in a variety of contexts, an SLP can make determinations regarding the likelihood that a sound will be acquired without therapy, a point where therapy might begin, and the child's ability to follow the clinician's model and apply the newly learned sound to another context. Children who demonstrate poor stimulability are likely to require immediate therapy and therapy may progress at a slow rate as a result of the poor stimulability skills.

Assessing Speech in Context

The consistency of speech sound errors is a factor in determining whether to enroll a child in therapy. If a child is enrolled, determining the contexts in which the child is able to correctly produce the sound can provide important information

IN THE CLINIC

Jennifer, a graduate student speech–language pathologist, is working with 4-year-old Ashley to determine Ashley's ability to produce a correct /s/ sound. Jenn says to Ashley, "I'm going to say some words and I want you to try your best and say the words just like I do. Let's try soup." Ashley replies "thoup." "Now let's try see." Ashley replies "thee." Jenn quickly determines that Ashley is having difficulty following her models. Jenn decides to now make the task less difficult by producing the sound in isolation. Jenn says to Ashley, "I want you to try and say sssssssssss." Ashley responds with "thththth," obviously having difficulty with isolated sound production as well. Jenn further simplifies the task by asking Ashley, "Put your tongue behind your teeth and say sssss." Ashley follows Jenn's suggestion and produces a correct /s/ sound. The clinician has identified a task in which the client can produce the sound correctly and decides to use this task as a starting point for therapy.

regarding a point to begin therapy and the type of activities that might be selected. As sound production is influenced by those sounds that precede and follow the target sound, examining sounds in specific sound contexts might enable a clinician to determine environments in which the sound can be correctly or incorrectly produced. McDonald (1964) developed a test that enables the examiner to vary the sounds that immediately precede and follow a sound so that the examiner can determine contexts in which the sound might consistently be produced and other contexts in which the child is unable to produce the sounds.

What Do I Do with All of This Information?

When the SLP completes the articulation and phonological evaluation of the child, a large amount of information needs to be examined so that a decision can be made regarding whether a problem exists and, if a problem exists, what form of treatment will be provided. Factors such as speech intelligibility, number of speech sound errors, number of phonological processes produced, types of phonological processes used, and age appropriateness of the phonological processes are all factors that must be taken into consideration when deciding if a problem exists. Bankson and Bernthal (2004c) suggested that a general guideline for starting therapy focuses on a child who exhibits errors that are more than one standard deviation below the age-expected norms on standardized tests. In addition, with children who are younger than 3, unintelligible speech is a strong indicator for enrollment in therapy. For children 3 to 8 years of age, speech intelligibility and the number and variety of phonological processes used by the child will help to determine the necessity of therapy.

TRADITIONAL ARTICULATION THERAPY

When a child is exhibiting one or two speech sound errors, traditional articulation is often provided. This approach to therapy typically focuses on the motor aspects of speech production and requires that the child learn to produce the sound in a new, correct way. One approach to traditional articulation therapy often uses a three-component model of treatment that focuses on *establishment*, *generalization*, and *maintenance*. The goal of therapy is to teach the child to correctly produce the sound (establishment), learn to use that sound in words and sentences both within the therapy room and outside of the therapy room (generalization), and then be able to correctly produce the sound during speech away from the therapy room without cues or prompts from parents or the SLP (maintenance).

During the establishment stage, specific skills are taught through repeated practice of a task. For example, when a child incorrectly produces a speech sound by substituting a /θ/ for an /s/ sound in the word *soup*, the SLP will try to determine the best place to begin therapy. As we discussed in the section on stimulability, the clinician needs to determine in which context the child is able to correctly produce the sound. The clinician recognizes that therapy progresses from simple tasks to more complex tasks. A task at the bottom of this list might involve the clinician sitting in front of a mirror with a child and stating, "Put your tongue behind your teeth to say the sound." When the child completes the task, the clinician rewards the child's behavior so that the child will be more likely to repeat the behavior when asked to produce the sound again. As the ultimate goal of treatment is to get the child to be able to produce the correct sound during conversational interaction, the clinician will begin to introduce tasks so that the child can learn to generalize the correct production of the sound to words, phrases, and sentences. In addition to the speech production skills described previously, some SLPs also include various listening tasks that address that child's ability to not only produce the correct sound but also understand the differences when a sound is substituted or a sound is omitted at the end of the word. These tasks are frequently used when a child has omitted final consonants. The description that follows helps to illustrate this type of activity.

The second component of this treatment model focuses on generalization. During this stage of the treatment, the child is taught to expand his or her ability to produce the sound from one context or one situation to a variety of words and sentences and then learn to consistently produce the correct sound in many different situations. For example, if a child can correctly produce an /s/ in words like *see* and *sit* (/s/ + high vowels), the clinician will work with the child to generalize the speech production skills to other /s/ + vowel combinations like *so*, *sue*, and *saw* (/s/ + low front vowels) (Bankson & Bernthal, 2004c). When the child can successfully produce the sounds in single words, the clinician develops activities to teach the child to correctly produce the sound during more linguistically complex speaking activities like describing pictures or telling a story. The ultimate goal of generalization is for the child to be able to converse with the clinician while producing the sound correctly. Ultimately, the clinician wants the child to learn to correctly produce these sounds and words outside of the therapy. As a result, the clinician will work closely with the child's parents so the child can participate in activities outside of the therapy room that reflect the same activities that are completed within the therapy room. In this manner the child will learn to correctly produce the sounds during different speaking activities both within and outside of the therapy room.

The final stage of this traditional articulation program will focus on the maintenance of the corrected sounds outside of the therapy room. While generalization and maintenance are discussed as discrete activities, the reality is that maintenance will begin before the generalization stage is completed because the clinician is interested in having the client assume a greater role in the correction of the targeted speech sounds. In order for the child to ultimately be successful, he or she has to learn to correctly produce the target sounds without prompting so that the newly learned sound becomes a routine part of the child's speech sound repertoire. To that end the clinician is going to gradually reduce the frequency of therapy sessions while encouraging the child to take a more active role in monitoring and correctly producing the sounds that were being addressed in therapy. The child will continue to do homework in gradually more complex situations (e.g., conversing with mom) and return to the therapy session to report on progress. Ultimately, the clinician will dismiss the client from therapy when the sound has been successfully integrated into the child's conversational speech outside of the therapy room.

LINGUISTIC OR PHONOLOGICAL-BASED THERAPY

When a child exhibits multiple speech sound errors, the child's speech is often difficult to understand and sometimes unintelligible. Traditional articulation therapy is often viewed to be inappropriate for addressing the complex nature of the child's speech sound problems. Teaching the child one sound at a time would probably have the child continuing in therapy until adulthood. As a result, linguistic or phonological-based therapies focus on teaching sound contrasts and the use of appropriate phonological patterns (Bankson & Bernthal, 2004c).

While teaching sound contrasts, the clinician will decide to work on pairs of words that are differentiated by one feature. These features might include voicing differences as in *pit*/*bit* (/p/ is voiceless and /b/ is voiced), final consonant differences as in *bow*/*boat*, or sound class differences like *sew*/*toe* (phonological process of stopping). Clinicians will develop activities that involve perceptual tasks such as identifying differences between two words that are presented by the clinician and production tasks in which the clinician might present a picture, ask the child to correctly name the two pictures, and note the sound contrasts.

In addition to working on contrasts, SLPs will use various therapy approaches that target the appropriate use of phonological patterns. One of the more popular approaches for dealing with children who exhibit multiple sound errors is the cycles approach (Hodson & Paden, 1991). The cycles approach to therapy focuses on the length of time in which the child practices sounds rather than the child reaching a specific performance level. Within this program, a phonological pattern or process will be targeted depending upon the type of process being used, the frequency with which the child uses this rule, and the child's stimulability for change. Treatment cycles can last from 5 to 16 weeks, depending upon the number of sounds being addressed and the child's ability to make changes. When the clinician selects a

IN THE CLINIC

Sarah, a speech–language pathologist, noted during the evaluation of Jeff, a preschool child, that he was consistently omitting final consonants in a number of words. Based on the errors noted during the evaluation, Sarah developed a list of word contrasts to help Jeff hear the differences between words such as *boo* and *boot* and *bye* and *bike*. As a result, Sarah finds pictures to depict each of the word contrasts and presents the pictures side by side while asking Jeff, "Show me boot." When Jeff correctly identifies a picture, he gets to put a block in a bucket as a reward for the correct identification of the word. At the end of the activity, Jeff can exchange the blocks for 5 minutes of playtime, a sticker, or save the reward for a larger reward during the next session. To make the task more complex or as Jeff continues to successfully identify the correct word that was presented, Sarah asks Jeff to correctly produce the word so that he starts to make the connection between the words that he is hearing and his ability to correctly produce final consonants.

phonological process that will be addressed, it is recommended that each sound within that class of sounds be addressed for 60 minutes before moving on to the next sound within that same class of sounds. During each session the clinician will use a variety of activities that include both production tasks and listening tasks. A unique component of this program involves *auditory bombardment*, when the client is required to listen to word lists containing the targeted sounds. It is recommended that each process be addressed for 2 to 6 hours depending upon the number of deficient sounds. At the conclusion of this cycle, a second pattern may be introduced if the child is having problems with other phonological processes. For children who are unintelligible, the clinician will work through a cycle of activities, move on to a second cycle of activities, and then continue to address these cycles of activities until the target sounds are evident during the child's spontaneous conversation. Hodson (1989) suggested that a child may require three to six cycles of therapy that last 30 to 40 hours before a child's speech becomes intelligible. For an examination of a typical sequence of activities that takes place during a therapy session using the cycles approach, see Figure 3.4.

---

1. Review—Client and clinician review the production words from the previous week's therapy session.

2. Listening Activity—Clinician requires the child to listen to a list of 12 words that contain the target sound (auditory bombardment). The clinician is also encouraged to use some type of amplification system (e.g., FM system) to increase the child's ability to focus on the words being produced and keep the child's attention.

3. Target Word Cards—The child will draw, copy, paste, or color pictures of three to five target words on cards. The name of the picture is also written on the card.

4. Production Practice—Five target words are selected for practice. The clinician will use a number of modalities to help stimulate the child and improve his or her chances for success. These modalities include auditory, tactile, and visual tasks that may assist the child's ability to correctly produce the targeted words. The clinician recognizes the need to modify activities every 5 to 7 minutes to retain the child's interest and vary the task from single-word productions to sentences to conversation.

5. Stimulability Probing—The clinician will assess a child's ability to produce another sound associated with the phonological error that is being targeted.

6. Listening Activity—The clinician conducts a second activity that uses auditory bombardment with amplification.

7. Home Program—The parents are instructed to read the list of 12 words to the child every day. In addition, the parents are encouraged to use the five picture cards that the child created and practice producing these words on a daily basis.

FIGURE 3.4

Instructional sequence of activities for cycles therapy.

Source: Based on "Treatment Approaches" by N. Bankson & J. E. Bernthal in J. E. Bernthal & N. W. Bankson (Eds.), *Articulation and Phonological Disorders* (5th ed.). Boston: Pearson/Allyn & Bacon, 2004.

SUMMARY AND REVIEW

The focus of this chapter was normal speech sound development, classification of speech sounds, and then an examination of the identification, evaluation, and management of speech sound problems. We first examined classification of speech sounds, the development of speech sounds from birth to 12 months, then speech sound developmental milestones for children older than 12 months. We then examined methods for classifying disorders of articulation and phonology and then discussed developmental and physical differences that can result in articulation and phonological problems. To complete the chapter we examined a comprehensive approach to evaluating articulation and phonological disorders and concluded with an examination of traditional articulation therapy and phonological therapy.

Language and Speech

What is the difference between language and speech?

Language is a set of symbols that conveys the meaning of words while our ability to relate meaning to sounds is speech. Speech involves our ability to use sounds to convey the meaning of words and language.

Sounds in English

How are sounds classified according to place and manner of production?

Place of production describes the location within the vocal tract where sounds are produced. For example, the /b/ sound is made with two lips and is classified as a bilabial sound. Manner of production has to do with where a constriction occurs within the vocal tract and how the stream of air is managed. For example, an /s/ sound is a fricative or noisy sound. The tongue forms a constriction in the mouth so that the moving breath stream collides with the tongue and the air passes around the constriction to create the noisy /s/ sound.

How are sounds classified in English?

The sounds in English can be represented by a set of symbols known as the International Phonetic Alphabet. We classify sounds as vowels and consonants, and recognize that the sounds can be classified according to where they are produced within the vocal tract, how the breath stream is managed to produce the sounds, and whether the sounds are made with or without the vocal folds.

Speech Sound Development During the First Year of Life

What are the precursors to speech sounds?

During the first year of life, children begin to produce sounds in a systematic manner that approximate adult sounds. Children experiment with sound productions and, as they get older, the sounds produced begin to sound more and more like the sounds of the language.

Speech Sound Developmental Milestones

Is speech sound development predictable?

As a result of a number of investigations, we have determined that speech sounds develop in a predictable manner. These investigations have identified the chronological ages when children typically master specific sounds. We noted that nasals, stops, and glides are often acquired early but fricative, affricates, and consonant clusters are acquired later.

Disorders of Articulation

How do we classify speech sound errors?

Traditional classification of speech sound errors focuses on individual sounds and classifies these errors as substitutions, omissions, distortions, and additions.

Disorders of Phonology

How are phonology disorders classified?

Phonological disorders are associated with the rules of speech sound development and language. These rules of development are often applied to groups of sounds rather than individual sounds, and enable SLPs to provide therapy programs for children with multiple misarticulations who are unintelligible. Phonological patterns are often classified into categories based upon their effect upon words. Syllable processes modify the syllable structure of words, and segment change or substitution processes result in a sound substitution involving the place or manner of articulation.

Articulation and Phonological Disorders Associated with Developmental and Physical Differences

What physical conditions might lead to articulation and phonological disorders?

Conditions that lead to structural differences may be associated with articulation and phonological disorders. With cleft lip and palate we see the failure of the lip and/or palate to form, resulting in the need for surgery and ultimately speech therapy to compensate for physical difficulties. Neurological impairment may cause weakness in speech muscles resulting in slurred and nasal sounding speech. Damage to the frontal lobe of the brain (speech motor programming areas) can result in speech apraxia. Finally, the nature of a child's hearing loss and the amount of amplification required will be factors in determining the nature of speech sound difficulties exhibited by children with hearing loss.

Assessment of Articulation and Phonological Development

What is involved in evaluating a child's articulation and phonological development?

The evaluation of a child's speech sound problem involves a number of important components that begin with speech and hearing screening to determine whether a problem exists. When it is determined that a child exhibits speech sound errors, his or her speech will be evaluated in single words and conversation to determine the nature of the speech sound errors. The clinician will also determine the child's ability to produce these sounds following models and instructions provided by the clinician. When the evaluation is completed, the clinician will determine the need for therapy and use the evaluation results to help to plan a therapy program.

Traditional Articulation Therapy

What is involved in traditional articulation therapy?

Traditional articulation therapy is often provided for the child who has one or two articulation errors. This therapy focuses on the motor aspects of speech production. One approach to therapy uses a three-component model that focuses on establishment, generalization, and maintenance of the sounds in question.

Linguistic or Phonological-Based Therapy

How is linguistic or phonological-based therapy different from traditional articulation therapy?

Linguistic or phonological-based therapy is often used for children with multiple speech sound errors whose speech is unintelligible. This therapy often includes a lot of auditory as well as speech production tasks, and requires that the child and parents complete daily assignments. As described in the Hodson program, parents also take an active role at home to help their child improve speech production.

WEB SITES OF INTEREST

The International Phonetic Association
http://www.langsci.ucl.ac.uk/ipa/

The National Institute on Deafness and Other Communication Disorders
http://www.nidcd.nih.gov/health/voice/speechandlanguage.asp

Phonology Project and Clinic
University of Wisconsin
http://www.waisman.wisc.edu/phonology/index.htm

4

Language Development in Children

Bernard Grela, PhD
University of Connecticut

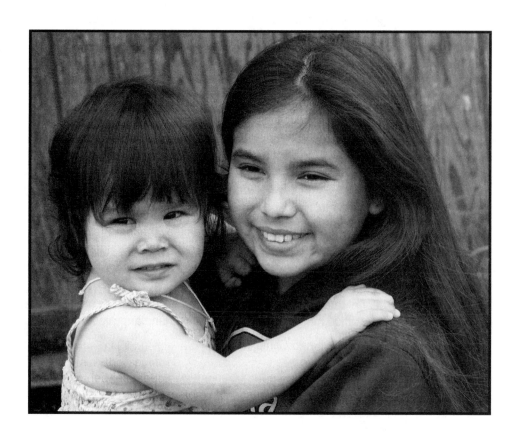

The purpose of this chapter is to familiarize the reader with terminology used in the study of language development and to introduce the stages of language development found in typically developing children. The chapter begins with a description of different modes of communication and the components of language, and continues with a discussion of theories of language acquisition. The remainder of the chapter will focus on language development illustrated by case examples examining five typically developing children. First, we will follow the development of a boy named Alex during his first year of life (birth to 12 months). We then study his older brother Aidan from 12 to 24 months (2 years of age). We will then be introduced to Kyela who was born a year before Aidan and is acquiring the language skills appropriate for a child between 25 and 36 months (3 years of age). Sara is a preschooler (3–5 years of age) who is well on her way to developing adultlike language and is mastering the skills that will be important for her to succeed in school. Finally, we will read about Brenden, who is learning to read fluently and is moving through his school years (beginning with kindergarten). Overall, we will follow these children as they move from limited communicative abilities to the process of reading. The children are following a typical developmental pattern and demonstrate language behaviors that are expected for children within the same age ranges.

MODES OF COMMUNICATION

Three modes of communication are critical for the understanding of child language: *gesture*, *oral language*, and *written language*. Gesture is the use of nonverbal communication (such as eye or hand movements) as a method of expressing, or assisting with the expression, of one's ideas or desires. It is often accompanied by oral language or vocalizations, but in very young children it may be the only means of communication. Oral language is the use of spoken language to communicate one's wants and needs. For typically developing children, oral language is learned effortlessly and does not need to be explicitly taught. Written language is a form of communication that utilizes an alphabetic system and is found in books, notes, text messages, e-mails, and other formats. Written language is thought to be the most complex mode of communication because it cannot be learned without formal instruction. Therefore, all children receive instruction in reading and writing when they enter school in order to acquire these skills. A strong foundation in oral language is considered to be essential for children to learn to read and write effectively (Catts & Kamhi, 2005).

In general, children first use gestures accompanied with vocalizations to communicate with others. For example, a child may squeal and laugh while pointing to her pet cat that has just jumped up onto a nearby chair. As the child learns words, oral language replaces gestures as the more efficient mode of communication. However, gestures often accompany oral language to enhance the intended message. In the same situation, a child will excitedly exclaim "Kitty!" while pointing to indicate that her cat has arrived. Finally, the development of oral language is seen as an essential prerequisite for the development of written language. For example, a child in the fourth grade may write a story about her trip to the pet store with her dad to buy a new kitten, as well as tell the story to her friends. In comparison, another fourth-grade child with a history of oral language impairments will have difficulty writing a similar story.

COMPONENTS OF LANGUAGE

The concept of language was introduced in chapter 3 where it was defined as a rule-based system using an arbitrary set of signs or symbols to convey a message to members of a particular community. In this section, we will view language as consisting of five subcomponents that children must acquire in order to communicate effectively: *phonology*, *pragmatics*, *semantics*, *syntax*, and *morphology*. We define phonology as the rules associated with sound combinations within a language. Pragmatics is the function or use of language in appropriate contexts. Semantics refers to children's understanding and production of words. The term *vocabulary* is often used to describe children's semantic development. Syntax refers to rules governing word order and word classes such as nouns and verbs. Finally, morphology includes words and inflections that attach to words. Morphology functions as the smallest unit of meaning within a language. Because phonological development was discussed in chapter 3, this chapter will focus on the development of pragmatics, semantics, syntax, and morphology. In addition, the foundations of written language will be described during different stages of oral language development. Prior to our discussion of the components of language, we first need to examine two different perspectives of language development: Is language developed by an internal process where children are born with the tools necessary for acquiring language effortlessly? Or is language acquired through an external process where children learn exclusively by interacting with people in their environment?

THEORIES OF LANGUAGE ACQUISITION: NATURE VERSUS NURTURE?

It is well known that for most children language develops easily, in a predictable sequence, and in a relatively short period of time. What accounts for this ease of acquisition? The answer is not so simple because there are two opposing views of language development in children. First, there is the *nurturist* perspective that suggests that children acquire language as a result of the direct interaction with caregivers (parents and siblings) in their environment. One of the most influential proponents of this perspective was B. F. Skinner (1957). Skinner believed that children are born with no knowledge of language and they learn language through the principles of *operant conditioning*, a form of learning in which behaviors are increased through the use of rewards (*reinforcement*). For example, a child may vocalize a string of syllables such as "mamama" when his mother is present. The mother immediately reacts to her child's vocalization by hugging her son and voicing her excitement that her child has produced something that sounds like her name. The child is thus rewarded for this vocalization with attention and affection from his mother. This pairing of the child's vocalization with a reward (hugging) increases the likelihood that the child will produce this string of syllables again. Eventually the child will associate his vocalization with the presence of his mother because she continues to reinforce the vocalization when it is produced. This association will eventually become a productive word for the child because it is only used to label the child's mother. Vygotsky (1978), another proponent of the nurturist perspective, emphasized that the social interaction between children and their caregivers is an important factor that contributes to the acquisition of language. Through everyday social interactions involved with caregiving (e.g., feeding, dressing, and playing) infants, with the assistance of their caregivers, are able to acquire language. For example, while changing her son's diaper, a mother may say, "You are wet. Let's change your diaper. You are such a good boy." The child will acquire words and learn about language by hearing his mother talk. Along these lines, Tomasello (2003) proposed that the social nature of language serves as a motivator for children to learn to talk. In other words, children learn language because they attend to their caregivers and realize that there is an intention associated with this interaction. They begin to imitate these intentions and eventually produce words and sentences spontaneously. Finally, Piaget (1970) hypothesized that language was a secondary behavior of cognitive development. According to this theory, language is learned because children perceive and organize their experiences into meaningful units of information. These organizational units allow the children to make sense of the unfamiliar words and sentences that they hear. Eventually the organizational units become language.

The second perspective, proposed by the *naturists*, focuses on the belief that language is an innate ability and children only need exposure to language for these inborn abilities to be set in motion. Noam Chomsky (1965) was one of the main proponents of the naturist perspective for language acquisition. He popularized the notion of a *language acquisition device*, an abstract mechanism located somewhere within the brain that allows children to acquire language at a rapid pace and to be creative in their sentence constructions. According to Chomsky, children are "prewired" with a basic set of *linguistic universals,* or grammatical rules, that all languages have in common. The child's task during language acquisition is to sort through these linguistic universals and determine which ones apply to the language he or she is learning. *Ambient language* is frequently used to refer to the native language that children are learning. Other researchers (Gleitman, 1990; Pinker, 1989) take a more conservative approach to language acquisition. Gleitman (1990) proposed that children are born with a basic understanding of word categories, such as nouns and verbs. When children are exposed to novel words in a sentence, they are able to use their innate understanding of grammar to decipher the meaning of the novel words. She referred to this ability as *syntactic bootstrapping*. For example, children have a general understanding of a verb as an action word; when they hear a novel verb in a sentence, they are able to determine the meaning of the action based on how it is used in a sentence. A typical Gleitman study involves children being exposed to an unfamiliar action (e.g., Cookie Monster pushing Big Bird so that he bends at the waist) while hearing a sentence such as "Cookie Monster is *tunking* Big Bird." Immediately following exposure to the novel action, children are shown two video clips while hearing the target word *tunking*. One of the video clips depicts the action they just heard (*tunking*) and the second shows an unfamiliar action. The experimenter notes which video the child attends to the most. The assumption is that if children look at the target action longer, they have bootstrapped, or learned the meaning of the target verb. From a slightly different perspective, Pinker (1989) believed that children use their inborn conceptual knowledge to create grammatical categories, and then use that knowledge to acquire words. This is known as *semantic bootstrapping*. For example, children have a general idea of what an object and an action are and use that knowledge to understand that a novel word functions as a corresponding noun or verb.

Both groups of theories have contributed to our understanding of language development in children and are summarized in Table 4.1. In addition, these theories are influential in selecting the styles of intervention that are used with children with language impairments. It is likely that the ultimate theory will be a combination of both perspectives although continued research will be required to answer this question.

TABLE 4.1
Summary of two language-learning perspectives

Nurturist Perspective

- Basic premise: Children are born knowing nothing of language.

    Skinner—Language is learned through operant conditioning.

    Vygotsky—Language is learned through social interactions with caregivers.

    Tomasello—Social interaction serves as a motivator for children to learn language.

    Piaget—Cognitive development influences language development.

Naturist Perspective

- Basic premise: Children are born with basic linguistic principles or capacities for learning language.

    Chomsky—Language acquisition device (LAD) aids development.

    Gleitman—Innate knowledge of syntax aids development (syntactic bootstrapping).

    Pinker—Innate conceptual knowledge aids development (semantic bootstrapping).

Quiz on the Fly 4.1

1. Gesture, oral language, and written language are all _____.
2. A proponent of linguistic universals is _____.
3. A component of language that describes the use of language in appropriate contexts is _____.
4. The native language that children are learning is known as _____.
5. The _____ theory suggests that children learn words because they have an innate understanding of grammar.

PERIODS OF LANGUAGE DEVELOPMENT

Prelinguistic Communication

Alex was born a healthy, full-term baby with a birth weight of 8 pounds and 9¼ ounces. His first vocalization consisted of a birth cry that indicated he was breathing and could exhale sufficiently to vibrate his vocal folds to produce a strong, loud cry. Alex responded to unexpected sounds in his environment by blinking and crying. He also looked at his mother's face and fed quietly as she held him. Therefore, Alex has the essential sensory tools (vision, hearing, touch, smell, and taste) to help him learn language. During this period of development, Alex will be building the foundation of language. He is ready to learn any language of the world, but because his parents speak English, this will be the language he acquires. Alex's primary development will be deciphering the English phonological system, understanding a small number of words, and learning that he can relay basic desires to his parents through nonverbal communication. He is not expected to produce words during his first year of life.

Semantics

In this section, we will follow Alex during the *prelinguistic period*, which ranges from birth to approximately 12 months of age. The prelinguistic period is the stage of communicative development prior to the production of the first word. During this period, Alex is using vocalizations and gestures to interact with his parents and is beginning to build a *receptive vocabulary*, which consists of words that he understands but does not produce yet. He will understand 3 to 50 different words by his first birthday and will demonstrate this by pointing to common objects as his parents name them. However, at this time Alex will be unable to say the names of the objects. Additionally, Alex has no *expressive vocabulary*, which is defined as words that are produced by children. Even though he is not producing real words at this point, he is cooing and beginning to babble when he interacts with his family.

Perception

At birth, Alex, like all other children, had the ability to perceive the difference be-tween all sounds used in the English language as well as all sounds used in other languages of the world. By about 9 months of age, he has lost this ability and can distinguish between English sounds only. How do we know this and what do we think accounts for this perceptual change in children? Before we dis-cuss the changes that occur in a child's perception, we first need to explain how perception can be assessed in infants. We know that during most speech perception studies with older participants, they are often asked to respond by pushing a button or raising a hand to indicate that they have heard a differ-ence between two sounds. Infants during the prelinguistic period are unable to respond in this manner. There are at least two types of procedures that have been designed to assess speech perception in infants. *High-amplitude sucking* (Jusczyk, 2003; Jusczyk, Friederici, Wessels, Svenkerud, & Jusczyk, 1993) is one procedure used to assess speech perception in children from birth to 6 months of age. During this procedure, infants are given a pressure-sensitive pacifier that measures their rate of sucking. During the initial phase of this study, baseline data is recorded by measuring the infant's sucking rate per minute. The child is then exposed to a novel syllable string (e.g., ba ba ba ba) that is repeated for a specified period of time. Initially, infants will suck at a faster rate when they are first exposed to the syllable string and then their sucking rate decreases to a baseline measure as they become more accustomed to the syllable string. The experimenters will then introduce a different string of syllables (e.g., da da da da) in an effort to determine whether the child responds to the new, different sound. If the infant perceives a difference in the newly introduced string of syllables, the sucking rate will increase again.

A second perception procedure can be introduced with children around 6 months of age when they have developed the ability to sit upright with little or no support. For these infants, an experimental technique called the *head-turn paradigm* (Conboy, Sommerville, & Kuhl, 2008) can be used to assess their per-ception. In the head-turn paradigm, operant conditioning is used to train or teach children to look in the direction of a toy that lights up when a new or novel stim-ulus is introduced. Once a child has been conditioned to respond to the toy, the experimenter plays a continuous string of syllables for the child to hear. When the syllables are first introduced, the infant looks in the direction of the toy. As the infant becomes more accustomed to the syllable string, the toy no longer maintains his attention. Shortly thereafter, the experimenter introduces a new string of syllables. If the infant perceives a difference between the new and the old syllable string, he will look in the direction of the toy in anticipation of it being activated.

Having explained how we can go about assessing perception in prelinguistic children, we will discuss those factors that contribute to infants' change from perceiving all sounds to only sounds in their ambient language. One factor that may contribute to this change is that children have become accustomed to their ambi-ent language. Through repeated exposure to their ambient language, children suppress the ability to perceive differences in other languages because these sounds are not important for the acquisition of words in the language they hear every day (Jusczyk, 1997). Another important phenomenon is the parents' use of *child-directed speech* that may assist infants in learning their ambient language (Fernald, 1994). Child-directed speech occurs when caregivers use a reduced rate of speech, increased pitch variation, long pauses between utterances, and frequent repetition of utterances when interacting with infants. Infants also attend for longer periods of time when caregivers use child-directed speech in comparison to adult-directed speech. It is thought that child-directed speech assists infants in learning about speech sounds, word boundaries, and clausal boundaries in their ambient language. Parents also use *joint reference* to help children learn new words (Franco, Perucchini, & March, 2009). Joint reference occurs when a caregiver labels an object or action when both the caregiver and the child are attending to that object or action. These factors may help children attend to sounds and words that are important in their ambient language.

Pragmatics

As Alex's control of his arms and facial muscles improves, he responds to his parents' speech by smiling and laughing. He is beginning to understand that language serves a social function and is beginning to show *intentionality*. Intentionality refers to Alex's use of verbal and nonverbal behaviors to indicate his wants and desires. These are also called *illocutionary acts.* Alex is likely to squeal and point to an object of interest to get his parents' attention. His parents respond by verbalizing what they think that Alex is trying to say. For example, as Alex looks at their cat and vocalizes, his parents will respond by saying, "That's the kitty. The kitty is walking." The parents' interpretation of his utterances is known as *perlocutionary acts.*

As defined earlier, the awareness of the social use of language is known as pragmatics. Dore (1974) described early prelinguistic behaviors organized according to social function. These prelinguistic behaviors are known as *Dore's primitive speech acts.* The primitive speech acts describe vocalizations and gestures that are used to label, request objects or actions, refuse an object or action, call attention to something, and repeat vocalizations (see Table 4.2). The speech acts are considered to be primitive because infants at this stage are not using words or sentences to accomplish a communicative attempt, but are using vocalizations, gestures, or both.

Quiz on the Fly 4.1 Answers

1. Gesture, oral language, and written language are all **modes of communication**. **2.** A proponent of linguistic universals is **Noam Chomsky**. **3.** A component of language that describes the use of language in appropriate contexts is **pragmatics**. **4.** The native language that children are learning is known as **ambient language**. **5.** The **syntactic bootstrapping** theory suggests that children learn words because they have an innate understanding of grammar.

TABLE 4.2
Examples of Dore's primitive speech acts

Speech Act	Example Behavior
Labeling	Alex picks up a toy car, shows it to his parents, and vocalizes. The assumption is that he is attempting to name the car.
Requesting an object	Alex wants a drink of juice. He reaches toward his bottle, vocalizes to gain his parents' attention, and indicates that he wants his bottle of juice.
Refusing an object	Alex closes his mouth and turns his head away when his parents attempt to give him a spoonful of baby food.
Calling attention	Alex notices his mother walking by while he is in his playpen. He makes a loud sound to get his mother's attention.
Repeating	Alex imitates the pitch variation his father uses during child-directed speech.

Summary of Alex's Development (Birth to 12 Months)

Two subcomponents of language have shown development during the first year of Alex's life: semantics and pragmatics. Alex understands 3 to 50 words by his first birthday. His receptive vocabulary is emerging because he has the ability to perceive differences between sounds produced in the English language. This provides evidence that he is beginning to make sense of his ambient language. Alex's expressive vocabulary has not emerged yet; therefore, we say that he is still within the prelinguistic period. He has developed an understanding of the purpose of language and is using vocalizations and gestures to get the things that he wants.

First Words

Shortly after his first birthday, Aidan produced his first word, which was "no." This word was typically used when he did not want to eat any more food during meal-time. He continues to use "no" consistently when he does not want something that his parents try to give to him or when he does not want to do something. Aidan is now in the process of acquiring his first 50 words that he will use and will be producing some two-word combinations by his second birthday. The important changes during this period are that his receptive and expressive vocabularies are growing. However, he is still using a combination of jargon along with real words. These communicative behaviors are typically seen in children between the ages of 12 to 24 months.

Semantics

A significant area of growth for children aged 12 to 24 months is the development of both receptive and expressive vocabulary. Aidan's receptive vocabulary will consist of approximately 500 words and his expressive vocabulary will grow from one word to approximately 250 words by his second birthday. He demonstrates recognition of words by pointing to objects as his parents name them. An examination of his first 50 words reveals that approximately 60% consist of nouns and proper names for people and animals (*momma*, *daddy*, and *kitty*). Another 15% are early action words such as *up*, *go*, and *kiss*. A smaller percentage of words consist of social interaction words such as *hi* and *please*, and descriptive words such as *pretty* and *mine* (Nelson, 1973; Rescorla, 1989). Aidan may begin to combine two words to form simple sentences such as "Hi mommy" or "bye daddy." However, the number of two-word utterances is relatively small.

Even though Aidan is using a small number of real words, the majority of his utterances consist of unintelligible strings of syllables with *protowords* and real words embedded within the jargon. Protowords, also known as *phonetically consistent forms*, describe wordlike productions that Aidan uses consistently to label a particular object or action. A protoword bears no resemblance to the adult form of a word, but caregivers learn what object or action it refers to when the child produces it. For example, he calls his favorite toy car "pooty" and only uses this word to refer to his car. This is an important milestone because it indicates that he understands that words can refer to objects. Eventually, Aidan will learn the actual name for the objects or actions and the protoword will be replaced by the real word.

Pragmatics

Aidan continues to use a combination of vocalizations and gestures to indicate his wants and needs. Therefore, Dore's primitive speech acts continue to be utilized. However, Aidan is also beginning to use real words to request and label objects. He is using social words to interact with others (e.g., *hi* and *bye*). The use of real words, or language, to communicate is known as *locutionary acts*. Aidan is beginning to demonstrate his knowledge of language by using mostly single-word utterances.

Preliteracy

Aidan has shown an interest in books. Even though he is not able to read, he selects his favorite books for his parents to read to him. Aidan holds books in their upright position and turns pages from front to back. These are two important *preliteracy skills*. The term *preliteracy* refers to behaviors relating to books that children demonstrate before they begin to read. These behaviors include showing an interest in books, holding books in the correct orientation, starting to look at a book from the beginning, and turning pages from left to right. This shows that Aidan understands the conventions of reading. These preliteracy skills are important developmental milestones that will function as the foundations of reading. In addition, he is learning about vocabulary and language when his parents describe pictures in books as they read to him.

Summary of Aidan's Language Development (12 to 24 Months)

Aidan continues to build his language skills in the areas of semantics and pragmatics. His receptive vocabulary has increased to around 500 words and he is producing approximately 250 words at 24 months. We can see that he understands more words than he produces. Aidan is also beginning to combine words in his expressive vocabulary to form a few two-word combinations. His use of language is emerging from vocalizations and gestures to the use of real words to obtain what he wants. However, he continues to use features described under Dore's primitive speech acts. Aidan is beginning to show an interest in books and this will lay the foundation for reading later in life.

Early Language Development

Kyela is a typical 2-year-old girl. She began this age with an expressive vocabulary of 250 words, but will understand approximately 900 words and produce 500 different words by her third birthday. She is using less jargon in her utterances and we are starting to observe the development of sentences. Kyela will begin to use her utterances for a variety of purposes and her sentence length will increase as she combines more words in sentences. Her understanding of language is slightly advanced in comparison to her production. Therefore, Kyela can comprehend sentences of five to seven words in length that her parents use with her.

Semantics

Kyela's receptive and expressive vocabularies are growing so rapidly that her parents are unable to keep track of the new words she is producing. She is going through a phase known as the *vocabulary spurt*, when she can learn up to five new words a day (Bloom & Markson, 1998). A concept known as *fast mapping* (Carey & Bartlett, 1978) is thought to account for this rapid growth in vocabulary. Fast mapping refers to children's ability to hypothesize the meaning of a new word after hearing it used only one or two times.

In addition to this rapid increase in vocabulary, Kyela is combining words to form two- and three-word sentences. *Semantic relations* refer to the relationship that words within a sentence have with each other. For example, Kyela produces the sentence "more cookie" to indicate that she would like to have another cookie. This semantic relation is known as *recurrence*. She also uses sentences such as "no cookie" either to *reject* (she does not want another cookie), to indicate *disappearance* (her cookie is gone because she ate it), or to *deny* (someone gave her a chip instead of a cookie). Kyela is also using action words in combination with nouns to indicate *agent + action* (e.g., doggy barking) and *action + object* (e.g., hide cookie).

In addition, Kyela is *overextending* and *underextending* words in her expressive vocabulary. Overextending occurs when she uses one word for many different objects. For example, Kyela uses the word *daddy* to refer to every adult male she encounters. She is also underextending some of her words. Underextending occurs when Kyela uses one word to only label an object that is specific to her. For example, she uses the word *doggie* to refer to her dog, but not the neighbor's dog or other dogs that she sees walking down her street.

Syntax and Morphology

With the increase in Kyela's expressive vocabulary and the appearance of word combinations to form sentences, we see the emergence of *syntax* and *morphology*. As indicated in the beginning of the chapter, syntax refers to the rules dictating the combination and order of words in sentences. Morphology refers to the smallest unit of meaning. Morphemes can be either *freestanding* or *bound.* Freestanding morphemes consist of words (nouns, verbs, adjectives, articles, prepositions) and bound morphemes are *grammatical inflections* that attach to words to change their meaning. For example, the plural morpheme -s attaches to a noun to change it from singular (e.g., dog) to a plural (e.g., dogs), and the third-person-singular morpheme -s attaches to verbs to indicate that an action has duration and can take place at any time (e.g., She play*s* soccer). During this year of her life, we will see Kyela's sentences increase from two morphemes per sentence to three to four morphemes per sentence. The number of morphemes in a sentence, rather than words, is used as a measure of language development in preschool children (Brown, 1973; de Villiers & de Villiers, 1973). When we average the number of morphemes per sentence, we get a measure of syntactic and morphology development called *mean length of utterance* (MLU).

Fourteen grammatical morphemes have been found to develop between 3 and 5 years of age. The 14 morphemes were identified by Roger Brown (1973) in his study of three young children. These morphemes are used to measure language development in typically developing children and children with language problems. Brown's 14 grammatical morphemes can be found in Table 4.3. These

TABLE 4.3

Brown's 14 grammatical morphemes

Morpheme	Example
1. Present progressive -ing	Mommy cook*ing*.
2. Plural -s	Two car*s*.
3. Preposition *in*	Daddy *in* car.
4. Preposition *on*	Daddy *on* chair.
5. Possessive -s	Mommy*'s* car.
6. Regular past tense -ed	Kitty jump*ed* over chair.
7. Irregular past tense	Doggy *ate* food.
8. Regular third person -*s*	Horse run*s*.
9. Articles *a* and *the*	*The* boy is funny. *A* girl is going home.
10. Contractible copula *be*	She*'s* a big girl.
11. Contractible auxiliary *be*	He*'s* playing ball.
12. Uncontractible copula *be*	*Is* she a big girl?
13. Uncontractible auxiliary *be*	*Is* he playing ball?
14. Irregular third person	He *does* dishes.

Source: Information from *A First Language: The Early Stages,* by R. Brown, 1973, Cambridge, MA: Harvard University Press.

morphemes develop in a progressive sequence, with the present progressive appearing earliest and the irregular third-person singular appearing later in the preschool years. The grammatical morphemes that are developing in Kyela's age group are the bound morphemes, including the present progressive -ing, the plural -s, and the possessive -s, and the freestanding morphemes including the prepositions *in* and *on*. The other grammatical morphemes will emerge during the next stage of development.

Pragmatics

Single words, short sentences, and gestures are Kyela's primary mode of communication with the people around her. She is progressing from Dore's primitive speech acts and we can begin to describe the purpose of her interactions using *Dore's conversational acts*. Dore's (1978) conversational acts describe the purpose of Kyela's communicative intent when she uses words and sentences to request information, respond to her parents' questions, and make comments (see Table 4.4). Therefore, Kyela is using a larger repertoire of communicative functions in comparison to Alex and Aidan because she can use words and sentences to verbalize her wants and needs. As her language development continues, the sophistication of her conversational acts will improve.

Preliteracy

Kyela is interested in having her parents read books to her. She helps hold the book and turns the pages. She points to pictures in the books and asks her parents, "What's that?" Kyela labels familiar objects, animals, and characters in the books. However, she is not yet aware that it is the text of the book that tells the story and not the pictures.

TABLE 4.4
Examples of Dore's conversational acts

Speech Act	Definition	Example
Request	Utterance used to request information or action.	Kyela: "Where mommy?"
Response to a request	A response to a request, including answering questions, repeating information, or compliance with a command to do something.	Mother: "Kyela, what are you doing?" Kyela: "Drinking juice."
Description	Utterance used to describe an event or object.	Kyela: "Kitty playing with ball."
Statement	Utterance used to state facts, rules, feelings, or beliefs.	Kyela: "Mommy, my tummy hurt."
Acknowledgment	Utterance used to indicate recognition of another's utterance.	Father: "I am going to work now." Kyela: "Okay, daddy."
Organizational device	Utterance used to begin or close an interaction or topic of conversation.	Kyela: "Daddy, know what?" or "I done."
Performative	Utterances used to register a complaint, a joke, teasing, or a warning.	Kyela (when her mother tries to give her water instead of juice): "I not want water."

> ## Summary of Kyela's Language Development
> ## (25 to 36 months)
>
> Kyela's vocabulary is growing rapidly. She is going through a vocabulary spurt where she can learn up to five new words a day. At the end of this period, her receptive vocabulary consists of approximately 900 words and her expressive vocabulary is around 500 words. Kyela is combining words to produce two- and three-word sentences on average. These early word combinations can be described by the way the words relate to each other, but a basic syntactic structure to her sentences is also emerging. Kyela is beginning to use the early grammatical morphemes identified by Brown (1973). She is using more words and sentences in comparison to vocalizations and gestures to indicate her communicative intentions. Kyela is interested in books and is labeling common objects she sees in books. She does not understand that the text of the story is important, but pays more attention to the pictures.

Preschool Language Development

Sara is a 4-year-old girl. We will describe her development from her third to fifth birthday, which is often referred to as the preschool years. At about 3 years 4 months, Sara's receptive vocabulary consisted of approximately 2,000 words and her expressive vocabulary was close to 1,500 words. At around her fifth birthday, her receptive vocabulary will have close to 3,000 words and her expressive vocabulary will grow to around 2,000 words. Sara's MLU at the beginning of this stage was around three morphemes and will be over five morphemes by her fifth birthday. She is consistently using all of Brown's 14 grammatical morphemes but she is still making some errors with irregular past tense. Sara understands long sentences with multiple commands within the sentences. For example, her mother tells her to "Go put on your pajamas, brush your teeth, and get ready for bed." Her use of language continues to be varied as she is using a variety of sentences to make her desires known.

Semantics

As was seen with the younger children, Sara understands more words than she produces. Therefore, we can say that her receptive vocabulary continues to grow at a faster rate than her expressive vocabulary. The majority of these words are nouns, but she is also acquiring words in all the major word categories including verbs (e.g., *play, kick, fall*), adjectives (e.g., *pretty, good, heavy*), adverbs (e.g., *down, fast, up*), prepositions (e.g., *to, behind, under*), pronouns (e.g., *he, she, I, me*), articles (e.g., *a, the, an*), negatives (e.g., *not, won't, don't*), and wh-words (e.g., *who, what, where, why*).

Syntax and Morphology

With the increase in her expressive vocabulary, Sara is combining these words to form longer sentences. Her MLU increases significantly as she combines these newly acquired words to form adultlike sentences. This is accomplished by adding adjectives, adverbs, articles, and verb inflections to sentences (e.g., "The little dog's eating his dog food." "I was running really fast yesterday."). In addition, Sara is using conjunctions (e.g., *and, but, if*) to form *compound sentences* such as "The boy is playing *and* the girl is jumping." She is also beginning to form *complex sentences* by imbedding phrases within sentences, as in, "The girl *who had blond hair* was jumping." During this period of development, children's sentence structure appears to be adultlike in grammatical form. The sentences are relatively error free and children are capable of talking about a variety of topics that include events that are currently taking place, events that occurred in the past, and events that will occur in the future. By her fifth birthday, Sara will be using all 14 of Brown's grammatical morphemes, but may continue to have difficulty with the use of irregular past tense verbs (e.g., "The girl falled down.").

Pragmatics

With the increase in her vocabulary and sentence length, Sara is using language for a variety of purposes. We can compare Sara's conversational acts with those of Kyela from the Early Language Development section (see Table 4.4). First, Sarah is using language to request information ("Why can't we find mommy?"), request actions ("Can you open this?"), ask for clarification if she does not understand ("What did you say?"), and request attention ("Hey, you know what?"). Second, she is sharing information by making comments ("Mommy took me to the playground."), making statements about feelings ("I don't like that."), disagreeing with others ("That's not mine!"), announcing challenges ("Bet you can't catch me."), and issuing warnings ("Watch out."). Third, she is responding to others during a conversation by answering questions, answering others when they ask for clarification, and acknowledging or agreeing with others ("Okay. I know.").

Sara is capable of carrying on an extended conversation with adults or peers. She is using devices to initiate a topic of conversation ("Hey, know what?"), maintain a topic ("And then he . . ."), and end a topic of conversation ("I am done now."). She is using these conversational devices to build friendships with other children in her neighborhood or preschool.

Narratives

Sara's language has developed to the point where she is capable of telling stories about things she has experienced, seen on television, and heard in storybooks. These stories are known as *narratives*. Sara has learned that stories have a beginning, a setting, an interaction between characters, and a conclusion. Initially, her narratives consisted of a description of characters and objects present in the stories, but by the end of this developmental period, she is including information about the relationship between characters, events that have created problems within the story, and a resolution to the problems. The narratives are told in correct sequence and may include an interpretation of beliefs. Sara's understanding and use of narratives is highly predictive of her potential to learn to read and write. Children with good narrative abilities do well academically because they become good at reading and writing (Liles, 1993).

Preliteracy Skills

Another skill that develops during this period is *phonological awareness*. Phonological awareness is described as a complex linguistic skill by which children become aware that sentences are composed of words, that words are composed of syllables, and that syllables are composed of individual phonemes (Torgeson, Al Otaiba, & Grek, 2005). Sara shows an awareness of this skill by identifying words that rhyme (e.g., *hair* and *bear*), identifying words that begin with the same sound (e.g., *sun, soap, sock*), and by changing the first sound in a word to create a different word (e.g., *hello* and *Jell-O*™). Like narrative structure, the ability to identify and manipulate sounds is highly predictive of children's ability to learn to read. Children who have good phonological awareness abilities typically become good at reading.

Sara has become aware that the story is not carried by the pictures but is carried by the words and text in a book. Her parents will assist her by pointing to words as they read to her. Sara is beginning to recognize some of the words by their shape but not yet by the letters. She likes to have her favorite stories read to her and she will correct her parents if they deviate from the story's plot. Sara likes to pretend that she can read. She demonstrates this by pointing to the words in a book and making up her own story or retelling a story that she has heard many times. Sara is also able to identify her favorite restaurants (McDonald's and Burger King) by the signs they have displayed outside their buildings.

Summary of Sara's Language Development (3 to 5 Years of Age)

Sara has grown significantly in the areas of semantics, syntax, and morphology. With an increase in her vocabulary and acquisition of Brown's grammatical morphemes, she is producing longer sentences, including both compound and complex sentences. This has seen her MLU grow from three to over five morphemes per sentence. Her growth in these areas of language has also increased the variety of pragmatic skills she is using. Sara is capable of requesting, commenting, and providing information on request. This allows her to recall events and tell stories. This ability to sequence events is one of the foundation skills viewed as an important language skill that will help her to learn to read and write. In addition, she is developing an awareness of phonemes, which is also thought to be an important skill for learning to read.

The School Years

Brenden is a 9-year-old boy and is entering the fourth grade. There are several important changes that occur during the school years. His vocabulary grows exponentially because he is learning new words from his teachers and also through reading. He understands and produces complex sentences, and tells narratives frequently in his interactions with others. His oral language development has

IN THE CLINIC

Jenny S., a student in speech–language pathology, often sat in her undergraduate classes and wondered why it was important to understand stages of language development, calculating MLU, and understanding grammatical morphemes. During Jenny's first week of graduate school she was asked to participate on a diagnostic team at the university speech–language hearing clinic. After examining the case history information provided by the client's mom, Jenny noted that the last comment from the parent was, "Is my child's language developing normally? All of my friends tell me not to worry but Jimmy's speech and language just doesn't seem right." As part of the diagnostic evaluation, Jenny was required to bring some toys into the therapy room and interact with the client. At the same time, this interaction was being audio- and video-recorded. While interacting with Jimmy, age 3 years 2 months, Jenny was trying to get Jimmy to talk about the toys. Jenny knew that she was going to have to transcribe everything that Jimmy was saying, so she tried to get him to verbally communicate. After 10 minutes, Jenny's supervisor asked her to return to the observation room while another team member tried to do some formal testing. While reflecting on her interaction with Jimmy, Jenny noted that most of Jimmy's answers were one or two words in length and they often appeared to be missing some morphemes that should have been present. When Jenny had an opportunity to transcribe the conversational interaction, she was surprised to note that Jimmy actually produced a couple of sentences that were four words in length, but the majority of his verbal interactions were one- or two-word responses that were consistent with his mom's reports. When writing up her test results, Jenny was able to examine a chart with the stages of language development and list of grammatical morphemes, and share her results with the other diagnostic team members. As it turned out, both Jenny's results and the other test results confirmed the mother's suspicions that Jimmy's language skills were slower to develop and required that Jimmy attend therapy to help him catch up. Furthermore, Jenny's understanding of the stages of typical language development will help her develop appropriate intervention goals for Jimmy. This way she will avoid working on skills that may be too far advanced for Jimmy's current level of functioning.

formed a strong foundation for his reading and writing skills. As Brenden becomes more proficient with his literacy, or reading, skills, he is going to use reading as a tool for enhancing his oral language. Through reading Brenden is going to increase his vocabulary, syntactic, and morphological skills and learn about the world.

Literacy

Literacy is known as the ability to read and write. As part of his kindergarten instruction, Brenden was introduced to the *alphabetic principle*, which is the understanding that phonemes have an associated *grapheme* (or letter of the alphabet). Brenden demonstrates his understanding of the alphabetic principle by recognizing the letters of the alphabet, naming each letter, and telling his teacher what sound each letter makes. The phonological awareness skills he developed as a preschooler were an asset to his acquisition of the alphabetic principle. Now, he is able to use his knowledge of the alphabetic principle to sound out unfamiliar words. The ability to sound out words is known as *decoding*. In addition to learning to decode, Brenden is building a *sight vocabulary*, which consists of words that he can recognize instantly without decoding. These consist of small words that occur frequently in books that children are exposed to at an early age. For example, a sight vocabulary may include words like *it*, *and*, *is*, *a*, and *the*. Children are able to recognize the combination of letters and immediately identify the words. This is a more efficient way of reading than decoding each word encountered in written text. During Brenden's first 3 years of school, he was learning to read. However, now that he has entered the fourth grade, the assumption is that he has learned to read fluently and now he is going to use material in school textbooks to "*read to learn*." This means that Brenden is going to gain knowledge about the world by reading. Brenden will now be taking classes such as literature, social studies, science, and math where he will be using textbooks to enhance his learning.

I CAN'T DO THIS ALONE

Gillian Smith, a speech–language pathologist at the Jackie Robinson Elementary School, works in collaboration with Julia White, the classroom teacher, to plan a lesson for her class. As both the teacher and speech–language pathologist are interested in improving the phonological awareness of the kids in the class, they have developed a number of different activities to help the children in class to become more aware of sound and syllables in words. During the first activity, Ms. Smith says to her class, "I'm going to say a sentence and I want you to tell me the beginning sound that is the same for three words in the sentence. Ready? The dog chased the big blue ball." José raises his hand and reports that the sound was "b." Ms. Smith continues with this activity for a while and then gives the following instructions, "Now I'm going to say sounds with big spaces between them and I want you to put these sounds together to make the word. Let's try one." Gillian proceeds to say, "B A T." Jenny in the front row raises her hand and says, "Bat." Ms. Smith tells Jenny that she's correct and moves on to the next activity. Finally, Ms. Smith decides to play a rhyming game with the class and tells them that she will say a word and when someone has a word that rhymes, that is, a word that sounds the same, they should raise their hand. Gillian is using a poster board to write down each of the responses so that the children will be able to hear the words and also see what each word looks like. Gillian recognizes that when these phonological activities can be completed on a consistent basis, the students in her class will have a solid foundation for future reading requirements.

Semantics

As Brenden's literacy skills develop, his enjoyment of reading continues and through reading he learns more about language. At the beginning of kindergarten, Brenden's expressive vocabulary consisted of approximately 5,000 words; however, that number will grow to over 10,000 words by the time he graduates from high school. Through reading, Brenden will encounter a larger variety of words than he would through day-to-day conversation. Therefore, his parents encourage him to read as much as possible so that he builds a strong receptive and expressive vocabulary. Another change that occurs during the school years is that Brenden will learn that words that sound the same (*homonyms*) can mean completely different things. This knowledge is assisted by Brenden's ability to recognize that words are spelled differently. For example, even though the words *sun* and *son* sound the same, they mean different things. He also begins to understand *figurative language*. Figurative language carries a meaning that is different from its literal sense and includes *idioms*, *metaphors*, *similes,* and *humor*. Idioms are considered to be expressions that carry an underlying meaning different from its literal form. For example, we say "he kicked the bucket" to indicate that someone has died. The literal form of this sentence has no relationship to the act of dying. Metaphors are comparisons of two things. For example, "He was a happy camper" means that someone was happy about something, but probably not camping. Similes are a direct comparison between two entities using the words *like* or *as* (e.g., She was as strong as an ox). Brenden will understand that an ox is a very strong animal and that the person mentioned in this sentence is strong as well. Finally, Brenden understands that telling jokes often requires knowledge of both figurative language and world knowledge. For example, he thinks the following joke is funny: "When is a car not a car? When it turns into a garage."

Syntax and Morphology

Literacy will assist children in learning about *derivational morphology.* Derivational morphology consists of prefixes and suffixes that we add to words that change the meaning of the words or the category of the word. An example of a derivational morpheme is the use of the prefix un-. We add this prefix to a word to make it the opposite of the root form of a word (e.g., **undecided** versus *decided*). Derivational morphemes can also change the class of a word. For example, by adding the suffix -er we can change the verb *compute* to the noun *computer*.

In his conversations with others, Brenden uses and understands multiple complex and compound sentences. When we compare his written language with his oral language, we find that the length and complexity of his sentences are greater for his written language than for his oral language. Therefore, Brenden understands that writing is a more formal form of communication than conversation in most instances.

Pragmatics

Brenden's level of sophistication with pragmatics continues to grow during the school years. His ability to use language is going to have a large impact on his ability to develop social networks and maintain friendships. Therefore, Brenden

---

Quiz on the Fly 4.2

1. The head-turn paradigm is used to assess _____.
2. Wordlike productions that are used by young children to represent objects or actions are _____, or _____.
3. During the vocabulary spurt, children can learn up to how many new words per day? _____
4. A linguistic skill by which children become aware that words are composed of phonemes is known as _____.
5. Something that attaches to words to change word class or word meaning is a _____.

---

has moved beyond using language to request and provide information, and has realized that he can modify his style of language depending on his communicative partner. For example, he knows that the language he uses with his teachers is different from the language he uses with his friends. The language he uses with his friends is the least formal, whereas the language he uses in the classroom is more formal.

Narratives

In comparison to Sara, Brenden's construction of narratives is much more detailed and complex. He is able to retell the events of a movie he has seen, including motivations of characters, reactions of characters, and multiple events within the story. Brenden can organize his thoughts to provide detailed instructions for the rules of a game. The development of complex narratives allows Brenden to understand stories that he has read and helps him organize essays that he writes for class assignments.

Summary of Brenden's Language Development (5 Years Plus)

Brenden's oral language continues to progress and expand in all areas. Since he has entered school, the emphasis of development has been on his reading and writing skills. As he becomes a proficient reader and writer, literacy becomes a major influence on his development of oral language. The more he reads, the larger his vocabulary becomes, the better he is able to understand complex sentences, and his knowledge of the world grows. Therefore, we can say that his oral language abilities have a significant impact on his ability to learn to read, and in return his reading ability has a significant influence on his further development of oral language.

SUMMARY AND REVIEW

Language is an efficient and effective means of communication. Children are born with a limited ability to communicate, but by about their fifth year of life they are using language that is similar to that of an adult. As children enter school and learn to read, their language abilities are further enhanced through literacy. Language develops at a phenomenal rate from birth to the school years. Two theories have attempted to account for this rapid development: the nurturist and the naturist perspectives. In the nurturist perspective, children enter the world with no knowledge of language, but learn to be proficient communicators by interacting with people in their environment. In other words, external factors such as reinforcements, social interactions, and experience influence the development of language. From the naturist perspective, children are born with the essential tools for learning language. The external world provides the input, but the children's internal abilities allow for language development to occur. Both sets of theories have contributed a wealth of knowledge to our understanding of language. Therefore, it is likely that language development is the result of a combination of both innate abilities and learned skills.

For most children, language develops with relative ease and in a predictable, stagelike progression. However, this is not the case for children with language impairments who struggle to acquire both an oral and written language system. Our understanding of the sequence of language skills and the process of language development is of interest to speech–language pathologists. We are interested in the developmental sequence of language because it helps us determine whether children are following a typical developmental pattern and are achieving important developmental milestones at appropriate ages. A speech–language pathologist is able to use his or her knowledge of typical language development to diagnose a child with a language impairment. Furthermore, the speech–language pathologist can use this knowledge to determine appropriate goals for intervention. Finally, by understanding the different theoretical perspectives of language development (nature versus nurture), the speech–language pathologist can utilize an appropriate intervention style that best suits the child.

Modes of Communication

What are three modes of communication?

Young, typically developing children utilize three modes of communication. These are gestures, oral language, and written language. Initially, gesture is the only

---

Quiz on the Fly 4.2 Answers

1. The head-turn paradigm is used to assess **speech perception**. **2.** Wordlike productions that are used by young children to represent objects or actions are **protowords**, or **phonetically consistent forms**. **3.** During the vocabulary spurt, children can learn up to how many new words per day? **5. 4.** A linguistic skill by which children become aware that words are composed of phonemes is known as **phonological awareness**. **5.** Something that attaches to words to change word class or word meaning is a **derivational morpheme**.

mode of communication. As children develop oral language, this is used in combination with gesture to communicate with others. Finally, written communication is learned through formal instruction in school. Unlike oral language and gesture, children must be formally taught to read and write. Therefore, it is viewed as one of the most complex forms of communication.

Components of Language

What are the five components of language?

Language can be thought of as consisting of five different but interconnected components. These are phonology, pragmatics, semantics, syntax, and morphology. Phonology is the set of rules associated with sound combinations within a language. Pragmatics is the function or use of language in appropriate contexts. Semantics is the understanding and production of words. Syntax is the rules governing word order and word classes such as nouns and verbs. Morphology is words and inflections that attach to words. It functions as the smallest unit of meaning within a language.

Theories of Language Acquisition

What is "nature versus nurture"?

There continues to be a debate among researchers about whether children are born with the essential tools for acquiring language (naturists) or whether language is learned exclusively through interaction with caregivers (nurturists). There has been no resolution to this debate, but speech–language pathologists use both theoretical perspectives to assess and provide intervention for children with language impairments.

Periods of Language Development

What is the general developmental sequence?

Prelinguistic Communication: From birth to about 12 months of age, infants are unable to communicate their wants and needs using words. This is known as the prelinguistic period because children do not have the motor skills or the language skills to use words. They are building the foundations for language by learning their phonological system, developing a receptive vocabulary (anywhere from 3 to 50 words), and learning to communicate through vocalizations and gestures.

First Words: From approximately 12 months to 24 months, children begin to move toward the linguistic stage. Their receptive vocabulary continues to grow and their expressive vocabulary should consist of at least 50 to 250 words by 24 months. Some two-word combinations appear. By this time, children are using a combination of words and gestures to obtain their wants and needs. They also show an interest in books and have a general idea of the orientation of books.

Early Language Development: This stage takes us from about 25 to 36 months of age. Children in this stage are showing a rapid increase in both receptive and expressive vocabulary. We are beginning to see the emergence of a syntactic structure in their sentence combinations with a sentence of approximately three or more morphemes by 36 months of age. Early developing grammatical morphemes appear. Children are beginning to use rudimentary conversational acts for social purposes. They are interested in looking at pictures in books and labeling the things they see in books. Children do not yet know that the words in a book convey the story. Rather they believe that pictures carry the story.

Preschool Language Development: The preschool period spans from 3 to 5 years of age. Vocabulary is continuing to grow rapidly. By the end of this period, children understand about 3,000 words and produce around 2,000. Their sentence structure and morphological use appear to be adultlike, but they still produce some grammatical errors. Children are using conversational acts for a wide variety of communicative purposes. These components of language are combined to produce stories, or narratives, that describe past events. Finally, children are showing phonological awareness abilities, which are highly correlated with reading and writing skills.

The School Years: This period spans from age 5 years to high school. The significant change during this period of time is that children are learning to read and write. During grades 1 through 3, children are learning to read. They are mastering the alphabetic principle and learning to decode words. They become fluent readers by the third grade. From the fourth grade on, children have mastered reading and reading is used as a learning tool. Reading significantly increases all aspects of oral language. By reading, children are increasing their vocabulary and understanding that there can be a figurative meaning to words and sentences. In addition, their sentence length and structure increases. This is assisted by writing assignments where they learn to put their thoughts down in words to write stories. They use reading and writing as a social tool, and send notes and e-mails to their friends.

WEB SITES OF INTEREST

American Speech-Language-Hearing Association (ASHA)
http://www.asha.org/public/speech/development/
http://www.asha.org/public/speech/development/communicationdevelopment.htm

Child Language Data Exchange System (CHILDES)
http://childes.psy.cmu.edu/

Education.com
http://www.education.com/reference/article/normal-language-development/

National Institute on Deafness and Other Communication Disorders (NIDCD)
http://www.nidcd.nih.gov/health/voice/speechandlanguage.asp

5

Language Disorders in Children

Nina C. Capone, PhD
Seton Hall University

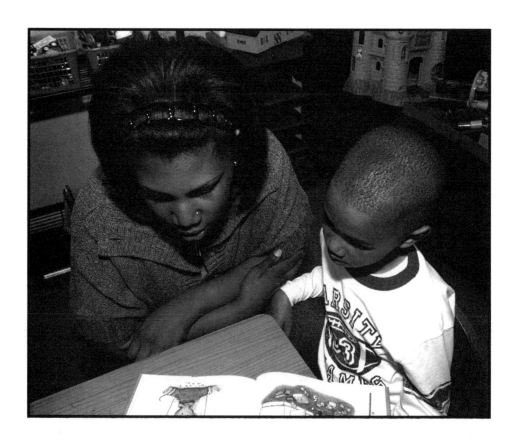

This chapter introduces the topic of language disorders in children. The term *language disorder* refers to the difficulty a child has in learning and communicating with language. Terms such as *language delay*, *language impairment*, *specific language impairment*, *early language delay*, *specific expressive language delay*, and *language learning disability* are also used to refer to children with difficulty learning and communicating with language. These terms may be considered synonyms although there are subtle differences between them. In this chapter, we will refer to children who have difficulty learning and communicating with language as having language impairment. In the section to follow, language is defined by its five rule systems and three functions.

THE DOMAINS OF LANGUAGE

Language is composed of five rule systems: phonology, morphology, syntax, semantics, and pragmatics. Each of these domains is governed by rules that can be grouped into three language functions. These functions are form (phonology, morphology, syntax), content (semantics), and use (pragmatics; Bloom & Lahey, 1978). The form of language is defined by two structural components: the sound system (phonology) and the grammar system (morphology, syntax).

Form

Phonology is the study of phonemes, syllables, and prosodic aspects of speech. A phoneme is a speech sound recognized as different from other sounds in the language (Nicolosi, Harryman, & Kresheck, 2004). It is the smallest unit of language that signals a change in meaning. For example, the sound change of /g/ to /d/ in the words *go* and *dough* is what signals a change in the meaning between the words. However, the sounds /g/ and /d/ on their own do not have meaning. Each consonant and vowel is a distinct phoneme. An important phonological skill is *phonological awareness*. Phonological awareness refers to the child's ability to think about and manipulate sounds and syllables in words. It also reflects the child's ability to separate a word's structure from its meaning (Gillon, 2004). Two examples of phonological awareness skills are *syllable segmentation* and *word manipulation*. Syllable segmentation refers to the ability to identify the number of syllables in a word. Word manipulation refers to the ability to decompose or compose words by deleting and adding words, respectively (e.g., substitute *bath* for *class* in classroom and you get bathroom). Good phonological awareness skills are positively linked to reading and writing development (Gillon, 2004). Conversely, children who have phonological difficulty early in development may have later difficulty learning these literacy skills.

Morphology and syntax are the grammar of language. The morpheme is the smallest unit of language that expresses meaning. As described in chapter 4, morphology is the rule system governing the use of morphemes. Syntax is the sentence-level structure of language that marks relationships between words and ideas. The syntactic domain is the rule system for constructing different types of sentences, such as declaratives, interrogatives, negatives, and passives, as well as for creating complex sentences. Complex sentences include those that are *noncanonical, conjoined*, or contain *embedded clauses. Noncanonical* sentences are sentences in which the subject–verb–object word order is reversed. We use non-canonical sentences to draw attention to important aspects of the message such that the important information occurs in the beginning of the sentence. For example, the sentence "The girl pushed the boy" is a canonical sentence because the person performing the action occurs first and the recipient of the action occurs last. However, it may be important to emphasize the boy is the one being pushed. Language processes that are beyond the scope of this text allow us to unconsciously move phrases around in systematic ways and add the relevant grammar to create "The boy was pushed by the girl." This noncanonical sentence is a passive voice sentence. It is just one type of noncanonical sentence.

The sentence "The boy climbed the tree and the girl read a book" is a *conjoined sentence* in which the conjunction *and* combines two ideas. Other conjunctions function to relate two ideas in specific ways. The word *because* is also a conjunction and it indicates a direct consequence, as in the sentence "The boy ran away because the girl pushed him."

In the sentence "The girl who pushed the boy is running," the phrase "who pushed the boy" is an *embedded clause* within the sentence "The girl is running." The embedded clause functions to modify the phrase "The girl." The conjoining and embedding of clauses makes communication more efficient because fewer utterances are needed to convey ideas and relationships between ideas.

Content

Semantics is the content, or meaning, system of language. Meaning can be expressed by single vocabulary items (e.g., *dog*) or the proposition expressed by vocabulary items in combination (e.g., mommy shoe = the shoe belongs to mommy; shoe mommy = a request for the child's shoe). Vocabulary development encompasses the number of words in a child's vocabulary as well as the richness of the child's knowledge of that vocabulary.

Later in development children must understand that words can have multiple meanings (Nippold, 2007). For example, the word *cold* can refer to temperature or to a person's personality. Multiple-meaning words are intrinsically linked to understanding important academic and social language such as metaphors, idioms, humor, and advertising. A *metaphor* draws comparisons between entities that are normally viewed as distinct (e.g., "The giraffe was a flagpole living at the zoo"; Nippold, 2007, p. 159). *Idioms* are expressions that have literal and figurative meanings (e.g., "It's raining cats and dogs"; Nippold, 2007, p. 183). They function like a single word because their meaning is stored in the entire phrase and does not come from analysis of the individual words.

Use

Pragmatics is the rule system for using the form and content of language. Pragmatic behaviors may include the intention of an infant's message (e.g., to request an object, to greet, or to comment on an object; Westby, 2009), using and understanding nonverbal behavior (e.g., eye contact, physical contact, and proximity), adjusting the social appropriateness of a message for a listener (e.g., professor, friend, stranger), and ensuring the appropriate amount of information is provided to a listener (i.e., avoiding too little or too much). Skill in the pragmatic domain is associated with social competence.

The domain of pragmatics encompasses a wide range of behaviors. The first communication behaviors to emerge in infancy fall under the domain of pragmatics and include eye contact, joint attention, and turn taking. They are the foundation behaviors of communication. *Eye contact* occurs when a child's eye gaze reaches the caregiver's eye gaze for communication. It serves to get or maintain attention. *Joint attention* refers to the sharing, following, and directing of a partner's attention to the same topic or activity (e.g., play, conversation; Tomasello, 1995). *Turn-taking* behavior can be verbal or nonverbal, such as speaking in a conversation, an exchange of vocalizations between caregiver and infant, or handing a block to and fro between caregiver and child. These three pragmatic behaviors are essential for the toggle between communication partners. Later in development, another pragmatic skill, *discourse,* is important for communicating social, academic, and vocational success. Conversation and narration are two types of discourse genre used to share information (Nippold, 2007). Discourse requires the integration of all language domains. In a manner of speaking, pragmatic development can be thought of as "book-ending" language development overall. We start developing language with three nonverbal pragmatic skills and culminate language development with the integration of all domains in discourse, which is also a pragmatic skill.

RECEPTIVE LANGUAGE
VERSUS EXPRESSIVE LANGUAGE

For communication to be successful, language must be understood as well as produced. The ability to understand or comprehend the domains of language is referred to as *receptive language.* The ability to produce or speak (sign, write, etc.) language is referred to as *expressive language.* Some examples of receptive language include the child's ability to follow a direction from his or her mother, follow the instructions given on an academic worksheet, and understand a conversation. Expressive language is what the child says (or signs, or writes). Some examples of expressive language include retrieving words from memory to name an object, writing an essay, asking a question, and taking a turn to respond in a conversation. Individuals must comprehend as well as produce language for communication to be successful.

The child's ability to comprehend a certain level of language often precedes the child's ability to produce the same language. For example, a child may follow a direction but may not produce the same length and complexity of sentence until many months later. In addition, receptive vocabulary size is generally larger than expressive vocabulary size. This relationship between receptive and expressive language is observed in both typically developing children and children with language impairments. There are those few children with language impairments, however, who present with more expressive language than understanding of language. This is considered atypical development.

LANGUAGE DIFFERENCES ARE NOT LANGUAGE DISORDERS

To add complexity to the clinical picture of language impairment, children may have co-occurring *language differences* that are not defined as a disorder. A difference is a variation of a symbol system used by a group. It reflects and is determined by shared regional, social, or cultural/ethnic factors (American Speech-Language-Hearing Association, 1993; 1998). Differences are observed in speakers who are learning *English as a second language* (ESL), speakers who are *multilingual*, and speakers of a *dialect*. Speakers who are ESL learners are defined as those born in another country who learned their first language before English. An accent would most likely be evident. An accent is a characteristic of one language that is carried over to a second language. For example, Chinese speakers say /w/ for /r/ because the distinction of /r/ is not learned in their first language. Multilingual speakers are defined as those people born in the United States who acquire English after another language that is spoken in the home (e.g., Spanish). Dialects are typically spoken by individuals born within the United States (English only). A dialect is a mutually intelligible form of a language used with a particular group. Groups can vary by region, style, ethnicity, age, gender, life experiences, and so forth. All differences are rule governed and can affect all language domains. Some dialects spoken in the United States are African American English, Appalachian American English, and Southern American English. It should be emphasized for the reader here that these language differences are neither language disorders nor incorrect English. They are systematic, abide by rules, and are shared by a group of individuals, the same characteristics that also define language. Language differences occur in all domains of language (for further discussion, see chapter 6, *Communication in a Multicultural Society*).

DEFINING LANGUAGE DISORDERS IN CHILDREN

A language disorder is an impairment of comprehension and/or expression of language form, content, and/or use in any combination (American Speech-Language-Hearing Association, 1993). Language impairment can be reflected in spoken, written, and gestured forms.

Children with language impairments are a heterogeneous group. Consider the following variations. Language impairment can occur for children with intact cognitive and intellectual functioning or it can co-occur with other disabling conditions (e.g., mental retardation/intellectual disability, hearing impairment, visual impairment). Language impairment can be developmental or acquired (e.g., traumatic brain injury, excised brain tumor). Some children are identified at birth with conditions associated with language impairment (e.g., Down syndrome [DS]) while other children are at risk for language impairment (e.g., higher order multiple birth). Language impairments can have a biological root (e.g., premature birth), an environmental cause (e.g., severe neglect), or both (e.g., prenatal alcohol and drug exposure). Children with language impairments can have difficulty in a single language domain or multiple language domains. For children with impairments in multiple language domains, there can be more impairment in one domain relative to another. Children can have a delay in expressive language with intact receptive language, or they can be impaired in both receptive and expressive language.

The assessment and intervention of language must also take into account nonlinguistic cognitive functions such as attention, perception, and memory because they are the support systems for language learning. If a child has difficulty with nonlinguistic cognitive functions, the speech–language pathologist will intervene on these domains as well as on language. Language differences add yet another level of complexity to the picture. A child can present with a language difference with no language disorder or the co-occurrence of a language disorder and a language difference. As you can plainly see, the business of language disorders is complex.

CHARACTERIZING LANGUAGE IMPAIRMENTS

Language impairment can be present in any or all domains of language. It is helpful for you to remember that for any or all domains it is possible to have a delay in any milestone. Therefore, if you have a solid knowledge base in the timeline and sequence of development of language, then any milestone delay will be evident to you. This section reviews some common delays in each domain. However, although we are highlighting a few of the more common delays, it is possible to have a delay for any expected milestone.

Form

Impairments in language form are characterized by difficulty learning the rules of sounds, syllables, and prosodic aspects of words (phonological impairment); grammatical endings (morphological impairment); and/or sentence types (syntactic impairment). During typical development, children make systematic phonological errors as they are first learning language but these resolve within predictable age ranges. Children with language impairments may present with language errors that persist longer than would be expected during typical development. We might take as an example the phonological process of velar fronting. Early in language development, children may produce an anterior sound instead of a sound produced more posterior in the mouth (e.g., saying "doe" for *go* or "tup" for *cup*). While part of normal development, the process of velar fronting is largely resolved by 36 to 42 months of age (Porter & Hodson, 2001). Children will gradually begin to produce more /k/ and /g/ consonants in words. Children who continue to front the posterior consonants beyond the 36- to 42-month milestone are considered delayed. There are also atypical phonological errors such as initial consonant deletion. In this case, the beginning sounds are deleted from words (e.g., saying "at" for *cat*). Initial consonant deletion is considered atypical because as part of typical development, children do not often omit initial consonants.

In addition to phonological processes, each phoneme in the language (consonant, vowel) has an expected age range of acquisition during which the sound will be accurately produced. For example, /m/ is an early developing sound and one of the first to be acquired before 18 months of age. On the other hand, /s/ is one of the later developing sounds to be acquired and is sometimes not acquired until 8 years of age. Children with language impairments can exhibit speech sound delays and the persistence of phonological processes that will require intervention. Intervention in this domain will also include improvements in saying all syllables of words, using prosodic features such as emphasis on certain words to clarify meaning, and developing phonological awareness skills.

Children with language impairments can have delays in acquiring morphemes (e.g., Rice, Wexler, & Hershberger, 1998). As previously discussed, there is a typical developmental sequence for morpheme acquisition. Children with language impairments tend to have delays in morpheme acquisition, and the morphology associated with verbs (tense and agreement) presents a particular difficulty for them. For example, Rice et al. (1998) documented the acquisition of early developing morphemes (e.g., plural -s, regular past tense -ed, "to be," etc.) in children with language impairments and two groups of typically developing children. Rice et al. showed that, while the typically developing 5-year-old children were consistently using verb tenses, the children with language impairments used them significantly less often and took up to 3 more years (i.e., to 8 years of age) to use verb tenses more consistently. Older children with language impairments can also have difficulty acquiring more advanced prefixes and suffixes that are necessary for academic success.

Children with language impairments also have delays in syntactic development (e.g., Ebbels, van der Lely, & Dockrell, 2007). Specifically, children with language impairments tend to produce less complex sentences and sentences with few conjoined or embedded phrases. These children are also delayed in using passive sentences and wh- questions, resulting in shorter mean length of utterances (MLUs). Delays are also exhibited for syntax comprehension.

Content

Children with language impairments often have delays in semantic development (e.g., McGregor, 2008; McGregor, Newman, Reilly, & Capone, 2002). The children take longer to learn new words and show weak word knowledge even for words they have learned. Children with language impairments tend to have smaller vocabularies and often use fewer verbs than a typically developing child. Many children with language impairments have difficulty retrieving words that they already know. Instead they will produce the wrong word (e.g., saying "pig" for *cow*) or produce nonspecific vocabulary terms (e.g., *thing*, *that*). Word retrieval errors are often semantically related to the intended target word. Other types of errors include phonological errors (e.g., saying "kitchen" for *chicken*) and visual misperceptions (e.g., saying "lollipop" for *balloon*). Typically developing children and children with language impairments make the same patterns of errors (i.e., more semantic errors than other types). However, children with language impairments make more errors overall when retrieving words from memory than their unimpaired peers. Children with language impairments also tend to have difficulty using sentences and surrounding discourse to glean the meanings of unknown words.

Use

Children with language impairments can also have delays in pragmatic development (e.g., Newman & McGregor, 2006). These delays include failing to make eye contact while communicating and less engagement in turn-taking and joint-attention activities. During conversation these children initiate talking and initiate new topics of conversation less often than a typically developing child. Children with language impairments can also have difficulty maintaining the topic of a conversation with their own contribution. Further, they are less likely to request or provide clarification when communication fails. The difficulties exhibited by language-impaired children with storytelling and conversation are discernable to both their parents and professionals.

Quiz on the Fly 5.1

1. Receptive language is the ability to _____ what is said, whereas expressive language is the ability to _____ language.

2. A language disorder is an impairment of comprehension and/or expression of language _____, _____, and/or _____ in any combination.

3. Three types of language differences are _____, _____, and _____.

4. Language impairment can be reflected in _____, _____, and _____ forms.

5. An evaluation will identify _____ and _____ of a child's ability to communicate.

EVALUATION OF CHILDREN WITH LANGUAGE IMPAIRMENTS

A well-planned and comprehensive evaluation of the child's language skills and abilities will be necessary to determine his or her strengths and weaknesses when using language to communicate. The results of the evaluation help the clinician to determine the need for intervention and how to proceed with management and treatment. The process is much like a physician who conducts a physical exam and medical tests before prescribing the right medication as treatment. An evaluation should assess the demands of communication activities and the child's ability to perform communication activities for social, academic, and vocational success.

The components of a language evaluation include a hearing evaluation; an interview with the caregiver to collect information about the child's medical history, timeline of milestones, and a family history of language impairment; a formal analysis of language during play, conversation, and narration; a battery of formal language tests; and trial treatment. An assessment of intraoral and facial structures, function, and sensory development is also completed to determine the relationship between the child's speech system and his or her ability to communicate. The speech–language pathologist (SLP) will generally complete all of these tasks but may modify the evaluation to focus more specifically on the parents' concerns about their child's language development. While concern is most often expressed by the child's parents, teachers, and other professionals who work with a child, the speech–language pathologist may be the first to identify and have additional concerns about a child who is having difficulty.

The child's hearing must be tested because hearing impairment is known to adversely affect language development. In addition, the results of a language test would be invalid if it turned out that the child could not hear the test directions. Even an intermittent hearing loss due to recurrent ear infections can influence language learning (Petinou, Schwartz, Gravel, & Raphael, 2001).

The interview with the parent or caregiver provides the speech–language pathologist with sufficient background information to make hypotheses about significant issues that might be contributing to a child's communication problems. Parents are also given the opportunity to share their specific concerns with the speech–language pathologist so that the clinician can make informed decisions at the conclusion of the evaluation.

The formal analysis of language occurs in a functional communication context. Specifically, a sample of the child's language is collected by the speech–language

---

Quiz on the Fly 5.1 Answers

1. Receptive language is the ability to **comprehend** what is said, whereas expressive language is the ability to **produce** language. **2.** A language disorder is an impairment of comprehension and/or expression of language **form, content,** and/or **use** in any combination. **3.** Three types of language differences are **English as a second language, multilingualism,** and **dialect. 4.** Language impairment can be reflected in **spoken, written,** and **gestured** forms. **5.** An evaluation will identify **strengths** and **weaknesses** of a child's ability to communicate.

IN THE CLINIC

After sharing some findings at the conclusion of an evaluation, the speech–language pathologist will reexamine the results of the interview, analyze the test results, and prepare an evaluation report that summarizes the results of all testing. The following descriptions will provide the reader with examples of statements provided in this report.

Evaluation Summary: Michael is a delightful 7-year, 2-month-old who demonstrates a mild receptive language delay and a mild–moderate expressive language delay. Michael also presents with language differences characteristic of the African American English (AAE) dialect. Nonlinguistic cognitive skills such as attention are age appropriate; however Michael has some difficulty with memory of verbal material.

Michael's mild receptive language delay is characterized by difficulty understanding directions and longer linguistic units. Michael's mild–moderate expressive language delay is characterized by a small vocabulary and difficulty retrieving words during conversation. Michael's strengths in communication are his motivation to interact with others and his ability to use gestures to facilitate communication. Michael is fully intelligible, with complete phonological development and intact structures, functions, and sensory aspects of the oral mechanism.

In addition to providing the results of the evaluation, the clinician will also provide recommendations for the parents and other professionals working with the child.

Recommendations: The following recommendations were discussed with and agreeable to Michael's parents.

I. Enroll Michael in speech–language therapy (60–120 minutes/week). Goals of therapy should include:
   Long-Term Goal: Michael will demonstrate age-appropriate receptive language skills to support functional communication for academic and social success.
   Short-Term Goal: Michael will expand his vocabulary around age-appropriate concepts (e.g., temporal and spatial concepts).

II. To aid Michael in comprehending auditory information in the classroom and at home, please consider the following strategies:
   1. Introduce new curricular vocabulary prior to lessons.
   2. Prior to giving directions, provide Michael with visual cues whenever auditory information is presented.
   3. Be sure Michael is seated in the front of the classroom.

pathologist during an interaction with the child or an interaction between the parent and the child. The communicative interaction between the child and adult is audio- and/or video-recorded so that an accurate transcript of the interaction can be completed. The speech–language pathologist will transcribe the interaction and then conduct several formal analyses that can include at least one analysis of each domain of language. For example, the child's phonological development can be assessed by making note of all phonological errors that are then categorized by type of error and frequency of occurrence. MLU is a common analysis of syntax and is a measure of the average length of an utterance in morphemes. A common analysis of semantics is the *number of different words* (NDW) analysis. This analysis requires that the speech–language pathologist tally each different word to get a measure of word diversity, or richness of word use. There are also formal analyses of narratives and Brown's (1973) 14 grammatical morphemes. For very young children Dore's (1978) analysis of conversational acts is used to analyze pragmatic skill.

There are numerous formal tests that tap all aspects of language development. Some formal tests survey a variety of language domains. For example, the Test of Language Development-Primary (TOLD-P; Newcomer & Hammil, 1997) has several subtests that include: Picture Vocabulary, Relational Vocabulary, Oral Vocabulary, Grammatic Understanding, Sentence Imitation, and Grammatic Completion. The scores from the subtests are combined in different combinations to yield composite scores for spoken language (all subtests), listening (Picture Vocabulary and Grammatic Understanding), organizing (Relational Vocabulary and Sentence Imitation), syntax (Grammatic Understanding, Sentence Imitation, and Grammatic Completion).

Other formal tests assess one domain in depth. For example, the Expressive Vocabulary Test (EVT; Williams, 1997) is a test that requires a child to name a series of individual pictures. The result is a measure of the size of the child's expressive vocabulary. The Test of Pragmatic Language (TOPL; Phelps-Terasaki & Phelps-Gunn, 1992) assesses the pragmatic skills of children ages 5 years to 13 years, 11 months.

The scores on these tests are compared to the scores of same-age peers to determine a child's relative performance. The speech–language pathologist will select specific tests so that a well-rounded picture of the child's language development can be obtained. Using formal tests enables the speech–language pathologist to focus on a wide range of language skills so that when the results of formal testing are examined in conjunction with the results of the functional communication assessment, the speech–language pathologist can feel confident that the results obtained during the evaluation accurately represent the child's language skills.

At the conclusion of the evaluation, the speech–language pathologist integrates the information obtained during the parental interview with the results of the language testing. As the speech–language pathologist has collected a lot of information during the evaluation and a lot of the data needs to be analyzed and interpreted, the clinician may provide the parents with some limited findings and inform the parents that all of the results will be documented in an evaluation report.

TYPES OF LANGUAGE-IMPAIRED POPULATIONS

It is important for you to remember that language impairment may be the child's only problem, or it can co-occur with language differences, intellectual impairment, articulation problems, or even cleft palate. In this section we will provide an overview of some populations of children who demonstrate language impairment. These are late talkers, children with specific language impairment (SLI), those with pervasive developmental disorder (PDD), and children with Down syndrome (DS). We will also discuss a population of children who deserve consideration, children who are at risk for language impairment. Although we tend to think of language or behavioral characteristics as being associated with a specific problem (e.g., children with autism having difficulty maintaining eye contact), it is important to recognize that not every child in a special population will exhibit all of the same language behaviors. As a result, although it is important to understand how a child's diagnosis (e.g., SLI) relates to language delay and overall development, it is most important to view each child as an individual with strengths and weaknesses that are revealed during the diagnostic evaluation.

Late Talkers

Children are referred to as *late talkers* when they demonstrate an early delay in language in the absence of cognitive (e.g., mental retardation or intellectual disability), motor (e.g., cerebral palsy), sensory (e.g., hearing) impairment, social or emotional disorders, and environmental deprivation (e.g., neglect). Their language delay is primarily manifested as an expressive language delay although there can be a delay in receptive language as well (Tsybina & Eriks-Brophy, 2007). There are other terms that refer to this group of children, including early language delay (ELD) and specific early language delay (SELD), but here we will use the term *late talker*. Late talkers are generally identified around their second birthday because parents notice that their child is not as talkative or doesn't have as many words as their peers (Whitehurst et al., 1991). Approximately 10% to 15% of 2-year-olds fall into this category.

Late talkers typically have small expressive vocabularies (Paul, 1996) and they fail to combine words such as "mommy shoe" to communicate (Rescorla, Roberts, & Dahlsgaard, 1997) at a time in development when these milestones should be met. Even though the language delay of late talkers is generally associated with semantics, late talkers are also found to have a small phoneme inventory and a delay when acquiring morphemes (Mirak & Rescorla, 1998; Rescorla & Schwartz, 1990). Rice and Bode (1993) found late talkers to also have small verb vocabularies. A verb vocabulary is important for learning the early tense and agreement morphemes, and it is these morphemes that are often delayed. For some late talkers, gesturing to communicate may be a strength (Thal & Tobias, 1992). Gesturing and good receptive language skills and play skills are good predictors of whether a late talker will outgrow his or her early language delay. Therefore, even though all late talkers will exhibit an expressive language delay, those late talkers with good gestural communication, play skills, and receptive language development will most likely be reclassified as *late bloomers* when their language eventually catches up (Thal, Tobias, & Morrison, 1991). It should be noted that late bloomers tend to be children who, despite having caught up, fall into the low average range of language skills. You should remember that low average is average nonetheless. Because many late talkers are actually late bloomers, Paul (1996) recommends a wait-and-see approach to intervention that incorporates monitoring language development over time (e.g., quarterly, yearly). Others argue that early intervention may improve language and other skills in a time-lier manner, and will provide a better foundation for subsequent skill learning (Tsybina & Eriks-Brophy, 2007). The late talkers who are not late bloomers but per-sist with language impairments into the preschool and school-age years will likely be diagnosed with specific language impairment (SLI).

Specific Language Impairment

Specific language impairment (SLI) is defined as a language impairment despite in-tact hearing and nonverbal cognitive function. It excludes diagnoses of autism spec-trum disorder (ASD) (to be discussed in the following section), mental retardation or intellectual disability, sensory impairment, social–emotional disorders, and environ-mental deprivation. Approximately 7% of preschool and kindergarten-aged children meet the criteria for SLI (e.g., Tomblin, Smith, & Zhang, 1997). A diagnosis of SLI is not made until after a child is 4 years of age because a large proportion of late talk-ers will outgrow their early language delay.

There appears to be a genetic component to SLI (e.g., Paul, 2007; Tomblin, et al., 1997) as it tends to run in families. Work from the Human Genome Project has found an associated gene although the details have not yet been borne out. Additionally, the brain morphology of children with SLI has been found to be differ-ent than that in typically developing children, and these structural differences are related to depressed language functioning (Gauger, Lombardino, & Leonard, 1997). Finally, recent work suggests that SLI may not be so specific to language after all. Rather there may be an overall delay in the maturation of the brain that affects other skills as well. For example, Webster et al. (2006) found children with SLI also tend to have delays in motor skills. Also, children with SLI demonstrate other neurologi-cal weakness such as clumsiness (Rescorla & Lee, 2001).

Children with SLI have language development that follows the typical course of development but is slower to develop. Their language development tends to look like that of younger children with the same MLU. Children with SLI can have delays in any or all domains of language, but the domains of morphology and syntax present relatively greater difficulty for children with SLI. In particular these children will have difficulty with the grammar of verbs, such as using tense and agreement morphemes and more complex argument structure. Argument structure refers to how many "players" are needed for a sentence to be grammatical. The verb deter-mines argument structure. Children with SLI also have difficulty producing more complex syntax such as conjoined and embedded sentences.

Children with SLI can also have difficulty with semantics. They tend to need more exposures to learn a word, and tend to have weaker word knowledge and smaller vocabularies. With these vulnerabilities in word learning and storage, children with SLI also tend to have difficulty retrieving words from memory. Therefore, they produce more word errors than their typically developing peers. This is a group that also has difficulty gleaning the meaning of new words from surrounding discourse (e.g., text preceding the new word; McGregor, 2008). Although pragmatics are considered a relative strength, children with SLI are less socially interactive and do show some pragmatic issues that were discussed earlier in the chapter. Phonological impairment may or may not be present.

Autism Spectrum Disorders

Autism spectrum disorders (ASDs) are a complex set of pervasive developmental disorders that include autism, Rett syndrome, childhood disintegrative disorder, Asperger syndrome, and pervasive developmental disorder–not otherwise specified (PDD-NOS). The diagnosis of an ASD is made using the criteria found in the *Diagnostic and Statistical Manual of Mental Disorders* (4th ed.; *DSM-IV-TR*; American Psychiatric Association, 2000). The ASDs are characterized by impairments in verbal and nonverbal communication and social interaction, and restricted, repetitive, and stereotyped patterns of behavior and interests. Some of these impairments include poor eye contact, lack of play skills, delay to gesture and speak words, language regression, and repetitively engaging in meaningless activity (e.g., spinning the wheel of a toy car) to the exclusion of other types of play and interaction. Children with ASDs are a heterogeneous group because the variety of symptoms exhibited by these children in each of these diagnostic categories can greatly vary between language and social skills categories and between children. Like children with SLI, children with ASD show neuroanatomical differences from the general population, and there also appears to be a genetic link to the disorder (Minshew, Sweeney, Bauman, & Webb, 2005; Rutter, 2005).

Rett syndrome and childhood disintegrative disorder are rare ASDs that are marked by a regression in development after a period of normal development of up to 2 years. Rett syndrome only occurs in females and is accompanied by repetitive hand-washing movements. Children with autism and Asperger syndrome have poor social and emotional responses to others, and do not spontaneously engage in shared enjoyment; they fail to develop peer relationships. The prognosis for individuals with Asperger syndrome is better than for individuals with autism. Individuals with Asperger syndrome can live and work independently, although their social impairments are part of their personality and considered to be lifelong issues. These individuals are sometimes characterized as eccentric. With the exception of Asperger syndrome, mental retardation or intellectual disability of varying severities co-occurs with the ASDs. PDD-NOS is a diagnostic category used for children who demonstrate impairments in the areas of social interaction, communication, and other behavior, but they do not meet all of the criteria of the other four diagnoses.

For children with ASD, some aspects of their language development follow a typical sequence of development with some delay whereas other aspects of language development are atypical. There are also children with ASD who do not verbally communicate. In fact, it is now recognized that children on the autism spectrum who achieve functional verbal communication by 5 to 6 years of age have a better prognosis for continued learning and communicating than those who do not verbally communicate (Paul, 2007). The primary impairment for ASD is pragmatics. Children with ASD often do not show early nonverbal behaviors such as eye contact, joint attention, and pointing for shared communicative purpose. They also do not interpret nonverbal social cues like eye gaze to associate the referent for learning a new word when they hear it (Baron-Cohen, Baldwin, & Crowson, 1997). It is also reported that children with ASD have difficulty with understanding the mental and emotional states of another person (i.e., theory of mind; Baron-Cohen, Tager-Flusberg, & Cohen, 1993).

One unique quality of persons with ASD is their loss of language, particularly expressive vocabulary, when they are young (McGregor, 2008). They start out saying a few words but then stop saying those words without adding new words. Smith, Mirenda, and Zaidman-Zait (2007) found that for children with autism, there were four predictors of vocabulary growth over time. These predictors are expressive vocabulary size in toddlerhood, verbal imitation skills, ability to use objects to pretend, and gesturing to initiate joint attention. Like children with SLI, children with ASD appear to have a typical mental organization of vocabulary but produce more word errors than typically developing peers, and they also tend to have difficulty using surrounding discourse to glean the meanings of new words (McGregor, 2008).

The form aspects of language (phonology, morphology, syntax) are relatively intact for children with ASD. Specifically, the development of language form appears to be in line with their cognitive level (Tager-Flusberg, Paul, & Lord, 2005). Children with ASD tend to be literal in their use and understanding of language overall (Tager-Flusberg et al., 2005). There are two characteristics of communication that seem to be more prevalent in the ASD population when compared with other populations of children with language impairments. These are *echolalia* and prosody that lacks the normal intonation and other qualities heard in normal speaking (Paul, 2007). Echolalia is the immediate or delayed repetition of language just spoken by another person. It is a repetition of language that does not reverse pronouns and so appears to be unanalyzed in terms of meaning. For example, a speech–language pathologist might say, "What do you call this one?" and the child replies, "What do you call this one?" The repetition has been described as parrot-like. Children with ASD appear to use echolalia when they do not understand the language spoken to them. Paul (2007) suggested that monitoring echolalia may be a good index of comprehension for children with ASD. That is, one indication of improved comprehension is that children produce echolalia less often.

Down Syndrome

Down syndrome (DS) is a genetic disorder associated with mental retardation or intellectual disability (Roizen, 2002). There are three types of DS: Trisomy 21, Translocation, and Mosaicism. Each type of DS has a different chromosomal mutation. Over 95% of children born with DS have Trisomy 21, in which the mutation is an extra copy of the 21st chromosome. Not all cells are affected in the child with Mosaicism, and they typically score higher on IQ testing and have fewer medical complications than the other DS types. Some of the clinical features of DS are flaccid muscle tone, flat facial profile, some facial differences, short stature, mental retardation or intellectual disability, and congenital heart disease. In addition to mental retardation or intellectual disability, children with DS can have multiple medical complications that can include congenital heart defects, as well as eye, hearing, and dental problems.

Language development for children with DS follows the typical sequence of development but is largely in line with their cognitive abilities. However, there is evidence that expressive syntax is relatively more impaired than would be expected for their cognitive level and more impaired than semantics for this population (e.g., Rice, Warren, & Betz, 2005). Mundy, Kasari, Sigman, and Ruskin (1995) also found an early difficulty in nonverbal communication with the intent to request. This delay was associated with poorer language development later. Children with DS have strengths relative to their morphosyntax delays. The strengths for children with DS are the number of words they understand, gesturing to communicate (Capone & McGregor, 2004), and the richness of information they express when telling stories (Miles & Chapman, 2002).

Children at Risk for Language Impairments

There are biological and environmental conditions that can place a child at risk for a language impairment. Biological risk refers to characteristics of the individual that make the child vulnerable, whereas environmental risk comes from circumstances outside of the child that have the potential to impact his or her development. One reason biological conditions are associated with risk is that concomitant medical conditions known to be associated with language impairments can occur. For example, intraventricular hemorrhage (IVH) or stroke can occur in children who are born prematurely because their neural systems are not robust enough to be outside the protection of the womb. Environmental conditions can place a child at risk because of fewer language learning interactions with a caregiver as well as nutritional deficiencies and limited access to medical care (e.g., Savic, 1980; Klerman, 1991). Nutritional and medical health contributes to brain growth and development, as well as intact hearing status (e.g., fewer middle-ear infections). Biological risk is a concern for those children who are prenatally exposed to alcohol and drugs, children born prematurely, and children with low birth weight. Environmental risks that can affect a child's language development include neglect, abuse, poverty, and multiple births. Children who are severely neglected and children who are abused perform more poorly on language comprehension testing than well-cared-for children (Fox, Long, & Langlois, 1988). However, Fox et al. (1988) reported that children who were severely neglected performed most poorly on testing when compared to abused children, who performed more poorly than generally neglected children.

The more risk factors a child bears, the more likely the child will evidence difficulty in learning language (Stanton-Chapman, Chapman, Kaiser, & Hancock, 2004). For example, Stanton-Chapman et al. (2004) found that low-income children were exposed to a greater number of risk factors than the general population. The risk factors studied included maternal and paternal education, marital status of parents, tobacco use, and traumatic birth history. The condition of multiple risk factors was also more strongly associated with language development in the girls that were studied. Therefore, there may be a biological influence of gender that also interacts with environmental factors.

Another group of children who present with biological and environmental risk factors are those children of multiple births. Twins and higher order multiples are more likely to be born prematurely and of low birth weight, and it is these conditions that are associated with a high incidence of language delays. Multiples also encounter shared adult interaction with less talk that is directed to each child less often. As a result, these interaction characteristics can also be associated with language delay. McMahon and Dodd (1997) found that twins and triplets were delayed in syntactic and phonological development when compared to singletons, with triplets more delayed than twins. Triplets also showed a delay in pragmatic development, with fewer conversational acts than twins or singletons. It should be noted, however, that in the face of biological risk, a socially enriched environment may provide a protective effect for the child's development (McGregor & Capone, 2004). The converse is probably also true that a particularly robust or resilient biological system can overcome environmental adversity.

INTERVENTION

Intervention can aim to capitalize on strengths, minimize weaknesses, modify environmental factors, and promote the learning of new language skills. Sometimes a speech–language pathologist helps the child compensate for weaknesses in communication through the use of *strategies*. A strategy is a plan of action with specific steps to achieve an outcome. Consider the child who has difficulty learning the meaning of new words from surrounding text in a textbook. The speech–language pathologist can teach the child a strategy of highlighting unknown or unfamiliar words and using a dictionary to determine the meaning. In other instances, the speech–language pathologist teaches the child a new language structure through the use of *scaffolds*. Scaffolding is a support that makes an aspect of a task more explicit so that the child can complete it successfully (e.g., Bransford, Brown, & Cocking, 2000). During the evaluation the speech–language pathologist administers some trials of treatment to assess the child's response to different types of scaffolds. Trial treatment can help to determine what types of scaffolds can result in the most progress for a child.

During the intervention process, the speech–language pathologist initially provides a lot of scaffolding to help the child learn a skill and then subsequently removes parts of the scaffolding over time as the child learns to be more independent, relying less on the speech–language pathologist. Consider the child who has difficulty creating complex sentences. One method of increasing the child's complex-sentence production is to take simple sentences that the child produces, introduce conjunctions, and illustrate the process of conjoining sentences. The scaffolds include visual cues from note cards and verbal prompts and models of how to combine sentences. Words, phrases, and conjunctions are written on note cards, and the clinician and child create conjoined sentences by manipulating the note cards and saying them aloud. A scaffold like this would be appropriate for a school-age child who has basic word-reading skills. As therapy progresses the speech–language pathologist might ask the child to manipulate the cards without any assistance. Therefore, the visual cues remain as a scaffold, but the child is gaining independence because he or she is less reliant on the speech–language pathologist's verbal prompt and model.

SUMMARY AND REVIEW

A language disorder is an impairment in the form, content, or use of language. A language difference is not a disorder. Therefore, a careful evaluation guides the speech–language pathologist (SLP) to an accurate diagnosis of a language disorder that is qualified and characterized by the skills that reflect the delay in each domain. The evaluation also guides the speech–language pathologist to recommend and plan intervention. The impact of a language impairment on functional communication is at the forefront of importance. Children with language impairments are a heterogeneous group. Even though there are general tendencies regarding the language development of individual populations of children with language impairments, each child will demonstrate different strengths and weaknesses. The goal of language intervention is to capitalize on strengths, minimize weaknesses, modify environmental factors, and promote the learning of new language skills. Speech–language pathologists embark on this journey with children to help them ultimately attain a functional level of communication to support lifelong academic, social, and vocational success.

The Domains of Language

What are the domains of language?

There are five domains or rule systems of language. These are pragmatics, semantics, phonology, morphology, and syntax. Pragmatics refers to how language is used. Semantics refers to the meaning system of language. Phonology is the sound system of language. Morphology and syntax are the grammar of language.

Receptive Language versus Expressive Language

What are receptive language and expressive language?

Receptive language refers to the language one understands. Expressive language refers to the language one produces.

Language Differences Are Not Language Disorders

What are language differences?

A language difference is a variation of a symbol system used by a group. It reflects and is determined by shared regional, social, or cultural/ethnic factors. Differences are observed in speakers who are learning English as a second language (ESL), speakers who are multilingual, and speakers of a dialect. A language difference is neither a language disorder nor incorrect English.

Defining Language Disorders in Children

How is a language disorder defined?

A language disorder is an impairment of comprehension and/or expression of language form, content, and/or use in any combination. A language disorder can be reflected in spoken, written, or gestured modalities.

Characterizing Language Impairments

How are language impairments characterized?

A child's language impairment can be characterized by difficulty learning and communicating using any of the five domains of language. Children with language impairments can have difficulty with the sound system (phonology), the grammar system (morphology, syntax), the meaning system (semantics), and/or the social-use system of language (pragmatics).

Evaluation of Children with Language Impairments

Why are children with language impairments evaluated?

A well-planned and comprehensive evaluation of the child's language skills and abilities is necessary to determine his or her strengths and weaknesses when using language to communicate. The results of the evaluation help the clinician to determine the need for intervention and how to proceed with management and treatment.

Types of Language-Impaired Populations

What are some examples of language-impaired populations?

Some examples of language-impaired populations include children diagnosed as late talkers, specific language impairment, autism spectrum disorders, Down syndrome, and those children who are at risk for language impairments. Late talkers and children with specific language impairment are children who have difficulty learning and communicating with language in the absence of cognitive, motor, sensory, social, emotional, or environment deficits, or other emotional/behavioral disorders. There are five autism spectrum disorders: autism, Rett syndrome, childhood disintegrative disorder, Asperger syndrome, and pervasive developmental disorder–not otherwise specified (PDD-NOS). Children with autism spectrum disorders have impairments in verbal and nonverbal communication and social interaction, and restricted, repetitive, and stereotyped patterns of behavior and interests. Down syndrome is a genetic disorder that is characterized by a language impairment associated with mental retardation and other sensory-motor difficulties. A group of children that we identify as at risk for language impairment are those that are exposed to biological and/or environmental conditions. Some at-risk children include those born prematurely, those who are abused or neglected, or twins and higher order multiples.

Intervention

What is the goal of intervention?

Treatment (or intervention) is provided to children with language impairments to capitalize on strengths, minimize weaknesses, modify environmental factors, and promote the learning of new language skills.

WEB SITES OF INTEREST

The American Speech-Language-Hearing Association
http://www.asha.org/

Language Intervention
http://www.mnsu.edu/comdis/kuster2/sptherapy.htm

National Institutes of Health: Autism
http://www.nidcd.nih.gov/health/voice/autism.asp

6

Communication in a Multicultural Society

Amy Weiss, PhD
University of Rhode Island

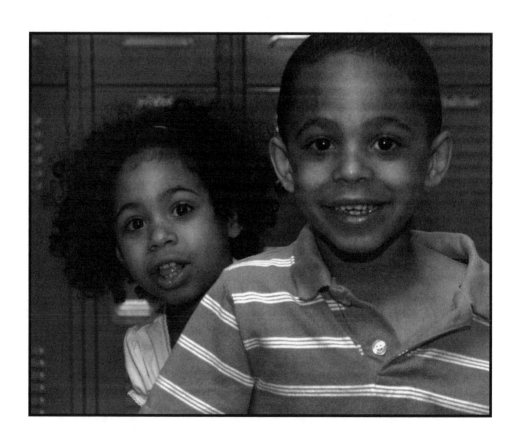

WHAT IS A CULTURE?

This chapter will focus on why it is important for professionals to recognize that the people with whom they will interact probably represent a variety of different cultures. We will discuss why ignoring cultural differences can lead to problems in providing best practices as we serve individuals with communication disorders.

To begin with, a *culture* relates to a person's values and beliefs about their place in the world (Hanson, 2004). For example, your cultural identification may influence the way you view your role in your family, even how you define *family*, your beliefs about a supreme being, and how you celebrate births and deal with death. Further, a person's cultural identification may be shaped by a number of factors including, but not limited to, religion, the language(s) spoken, the geographic region lived in (e.g., country of origin; region of the country; density of population such as rural, urban, or suburban), age, level of education, relative wealth, race or ethnicity, gender, and sexual orientation. Most people identify with more than one culture. For example, an individual might view herself as being a member of five cultures: female, American, white, middle aged, and Buddhist, each of them exerting particular influences on her worldview. That is, people interpret the world around them through their personal *cultural identification*. They will also use cultural identification to interpret what the concepts of ability and disability as well as illness and wellness mean to them.

These last considerations are particularly relevant for professionals to understand when they are developing working relationships with their students, clients, or patients because they will affect a clinician's ability to be effective (Hanson, 2004). That is, a person's cultural identity may influence the priority placed on seeking out speech–language therapy services or making a decision to wear a hearing aid. Several examples of how cultural identification may affect service delivery will be found later in this chapter.

There is still another way for preprofessionals and professionals to consider use of the term *culture*. We can say that different professional work settings have their own cultures. That is, certain terminology may be used in school settings (e.g., least restrictive environment, Individualized Education Plan, pull-out) that are not used in hospital settings (e.g., utilization review, bedside assessment). In addition to using different vocabulary, a hospital's culture may be expressed by administrative decisions regarding the provision of services. For example, despite the fact that a speech–language pathologist does not require a medical referral to work with patients, a hospital administrator may make the decision that, within his or her facility, all therapy services must be initiated by a physician. Because these beliefs or operating procedures may differ from hospital to hospital, we could say that an individual hospital has its own culture when it comes to determining how services will be provided. It is a critical piece of information for professionals providing services within a particular work setting to quickly learn: What is the culture of one's workplace?

WHY IS CULTURAL COMPETENCE IMPORTANT?

It is important for speech–language pathologists, audiologists, classroom teachers, and physicians to strive to become *culturally competent* in their professional practice (Lynch, 2004; Langdon, 2008). That means that in addition to learning about the nature of communication disorders and teaching reading, math, or the course of a specific disease process, professionals need to understand how cultural differences may impact the services they provide.

One of the major barriers to professionals providing the best, culturally appropriate clinical practices is the danger of overgeneralizing, or making assumptions about a client's cultural identity. Unfortunately, when clinicians make incorrect assumptions about the belief systems of a patient or client, it is often because they assume that there is a shared set of beliefs or culture between clinician and client. When this is an incorrect assumption, miscommunication can result. Miscommunication can lead to misdiagnosis and, in turn, to poor or inappropriate treatment of clients (Goldstein & Iglesias, 2002). Note that it is usually the case that members of the majority population (as defined by language, age, geographic region, etc.) are the ones who assume that members of nonmajority (or minority) populations are following the belief system of the majority. This may occur because persons in the majority culture are not typically forced to confront their majority status as often as persons in a minority culture are confronted by their minority status.

Here is another word of caution. When we consider differences between cultures, it can be tempting to generalize and decide that all people who identify themselves as members of a particular culture or set of cultures will behave in exactly the same, predictable way. This perspective is reflected in comments like, "I wasn't surprised he acted that way because he is from New York City." We must remember that there is as much variability within cultures as there is between cultures (Hanson, 2004; Langdon, 2008). For example, if we look at a group of people who are Jewish or Muslim, we would probably recognize a lot of variability in how their religions are practiced within their own groups; as a result, these individuals exhibit different cultural identities. For example, you cannot assume that all persons who are Jewish or Muslim follow all of the strict dietary laws that some persons of their faith would follow. We would also caution the reader to not assume that all families with Latino surnames speak Spanish as their first language. It would also be wrong to assume that a person who is African American is necessarily a Christian or that their church plays a central role in their lives, although for many families in the African American community these assumptions would be accurate (Willis, 2004).

Instead, the key to understanding the potential impact that one or more cultures may have on a family's values and beliefs, and thus how we use this information to treat the clients or patients we serve, is to treat each family in an individual manner. Clinicians who are culturally competent try very hard to not stereotype their clients (Lynch, 2004). This means that they take the time to learn about how each client or patient represents his or her culture. Said another way, culturally competent clinicians spend time finding out where each of their clients is truly "coming from" rather than making assumptions based on superficial categories. The term *stereotype* refers to the human cognitive tendency to categorize people on the basis of superficial characteristics (e.g., tall, skinny, brown-skinned, sophomores in college). Although stereotyping can be an unfair and dangerous practice, when it is done in a nonjudgmental way it probably happens because all clinicians by virtue of being human are working with brains that have limited capacities for holding information. For example, if I am a university instructor and I assume that all sophomores have the same skill set, it will save me a lot of time when planning classroom activities. In the same way, the use of stereotypes allows clinicians to take shortcuts in decision making, but when they do so, clinicians run the risk of making poor decisions, just as my assumption about college sophomores might leave me unprepared for dealing with the individual differences presented by my students.

Quiz on the Fly 6.1

1. A culture can be described as a person's _____ and _____.

2. Stereotyping is a poor strategy for decision making. Some clinicians may be tempted to use it because it serves as a _____.

3. Name three factors that can influence a person's cultural identification: _____, _____, and _____.

4. Professionals should strive to become _____ so that they understand the potential influence that their clients' cultures can have on the delivery of professional services.

5. If you are not a member of the majority culture, then you can be said to belong to a _____, or _____, culture.

CULTURE AND THE CHANGING FACE OF THE POPULATION

Unfortunately, the opportunity for miscommunication may be on the increase because the *demographics*, or description of the population according to age, race, ethnicity, gender, and languages spoken, of the population of the United States has been significantly changing during the last 30 years and continues to do so. Therefore, the description of the majority population is also changing. For example, consider the changes in the racial makeup of the United States for the last several census reports. In 1980, for example, the white population of the United States was estimated at 83.1%; in 2000 that percentage had decreased to 75.1%. At the same time, the percentage of persons identifying themselves as black increased from 11.7% to 12.3%. More striking is the increase in percentages of persons identifying themselves with racial groups that are neither black nor white: 5.2% to 12.5%. During the same period of time, the percentage of the population identifying themselves as Hispanic grew from 6.4% to 12.5% (Hobbs & Stoops, 2002). Another indication of the magnitude of the change in racial distribution is that, in 1900, 12.5% of the population of the United States was nonwhite. By 2000, that percentage had increased to 25%. The results of the 2010 census will provide additional information about the trajectory of U.S. population changes.

When an individual tries to fit into a group by adopting the social or cultural characteristics of that group, the process is called *acculturation*. Battle (2002) discussed three models of acculturation that require further examination. Throughout the history of our country we have traditionally adopted the *Anglo-conformity model*. This model requires individuals to give up their old-world ideas, language, and traditions and adopt the American way of doing things. While many of the readers might like to think that this model is part of our historical past, it can often be found in present-day debates about a national language and our neighbor's views about immigration. During the 19th century and early 20th century when we experienced one of the largest surges of immigration, new immigrants routinely tried to hide their foreign roots by aspiring to dress and speak as other Americans. Their goal was to assimilate or blend in rather than stand out and appear different. Given the attitudes of many in power at that time regarding recent immigrants, this assimilation process proved to be very useful when applying for jobs or attending school in the mainstream. This is not to say that immigrants did not preserve something of their native cultures in their homes, but they spent a lot of time trying to lose those characteristics that they thought made them look different and less "American."

With the increasing immigration during early 20th century, America was often described as a "melting pot" of people from different parts of the world although it was still assumed that typical Americans were white and spoke English. This *melting pot model* attempts to incorporate the characteristics of the minority culture and blend this with the existing American culture to form a new culture with both new and old traditions. It is not hard for you to understand that at one time in our country pizza, sushi, and salsa were nonexistent or characteristics of some

---

Quiz on the Fly 6.1 Answers

1. A culture can be described as a person's **beliefs** and **values**. **2.** Stereotyping is a poor strategy for decision making. Some clinicians may be tempted to use it because it serves as a **shortcut**. **3.** Name three factors that can influence a person's cultural identification: **geographic region, gender, race,** or **ethnicity. 4.** Professionals should strive to become **culturally competent** so that they understand the potential influence that their clients' cultures can have on the delivery of professional services. **5.** If you are not a member of the majority culture, then you can be said to belong to a **minority**, or **nonmajority**, culture.

international foreign culture. As a result of this melting pot model, these foods are readily available and have become part of the fabric of American culinary culture.

In recent years trends in population change in the United States clearly show that the perception of an American as a white, English-speaking individual is changing as a result of immigration patterns and differences in birth rates across racial and ethnic groups. Some estimates have suggested that within the next 50 years, there will be no clear racial majority in the United States. In addition, more and more Americans are speaking Spanish as their home language (34 million individuals 5 years of age and older out of 279 million total, according to the U.S. Census Bureau [2006]), and many non-Spanish-speaking Americans are recognizing that they will be better able to communicate with their neighbors and fellow citizens if they learn Spanish as a second language.

At the present time, we would like to think that the Anglo-conformity model and the melting pot model do not adequately describe the way that Americans view their cultural identification. That is, these models refer to no change or to gradual change from difference to sameness. As noted by Cole (1989), the melting pot represents the *e pluribus unum* perspective, suggesting "out of many, one." This perspective expects a population that is homogenous, or all blended, that will appear to be all the same. More recently, immigrants to the United States have demonstrated resistance to giving up their native culture, and promoted celebrating and maintaining the cultural differences within their communities, places of worship, and even in the workplace. This model has been called the *cultural pluralism model*, in which individuals are strong believers in an American way of life, are loyal to the laws of the country, but at the same time are able to maintain characteristics of their native culture, including foods, holiday celebrations, dress, and language. According to Cole (1989), this perspective could be referred to as the *e pluribus pluribus* point of view, suggesting "out of many, many." Cole's observation of 20 years ago is meaningful to clinical practitioners today because it further suggests that we cannot afford to ignore cultural differences. In fact, it may be even more important today that we recognize the impact of cultural differences on our methods of professional service delivery.

Although the current and future trends for the demographics of the United States population suggest dynamic growth, the membership of the American Speech-Language-Hearing Association (ASHA) has not reflected those same changes over the last few decades. According to data collected in 2008, more than 93% of the ASHA membership identifies itself as non-Hispanic white, compared with approximately 75% in the U.S. population, and the vast majority of the membership speaks only English. As current U.S. census figures tell us, the demographics of the United States are becoming increasingly nonwhite and Americans are increasingly using languages other than English as a first language. These changes would suggest that those individuals who will be providing services need to be aware of the culture of the clients with whom they will be interacting, as well as be aware of the languages spoken within the community so that appropriate resources can be utilized to provide the best diagnostic and treatment services that are appropriate for the community. ASHA has recognized the importance of cultural differences and has established clear guidelines for practitioners to determine who has the necessary competencies to provide therapy services to non-English-speaking clients (American Speech-Language-Hearing Association,

1985). Further, resources developed by ASHA specifically to assist its members in the enhancement of their knowledge of best practices for service delivery are frequently updated (American Speech-Language-Hearing Association, 2010c).

THE CHARACTERISTICS OF CULTURE

As previously discussed, cultural identity shapes the way we view the world and our role in it. One aspect of culture has to do with beliefs about children's development. This set of beliefs can be very important to speech–language pathologists who are working with children with communication disorders related to delays in language learning. Cultural differences may be reflected in the ways that caregivers and young children interact, when and who speaks to young children, and caregivers' beliefs about how language development occurs and whether they play a part in that development (Hammer & Weiss, 1999, 2000; Langdon, 2008; van Kleeck, 1994).

When we observe a wide range of young children growing up in different cultures and learning language, we may notice evidence of different interaction patterns between caregivers and their children. Most of the research that has shaped traditional ideas about language development has been collected from families that are white, from western countries, and considered to have at least middle-class socioeconomic status (SES, a measure of education and income). Because of this, many of the descriptions of normal language development have only considered how children in the majority population appear to learn language. Perhaps unintentionally, investigators have given the impression that there is only one way for language to be learned.

For example, when observing caregivers and their young children in typical white, western, middle-class households, it is common to find that caregivers attempt to include their linguistically immature children in conversations. Many of these caregivers structure their own conversation turns to allow even *infants* to take a turn, waiting much longer for the language-immature infant to signify a turn (e.g., by shaking its fist or turning to face the caregiver or smiling) than would ever be the case in conversation with another adult! On the other hand, in nonmajority cultures, caregivers typically do not treat language-immature infants as appropriate conversation partners. So in these families you will not see the same opportunities for practicing conversational turn-taking behaviors as you will in majority caregiver–child pairings. However, it is more likely that in nonmajority cultures you will observe young children being physically included in the conversations that go on between adults. Although they are not viewed as conversation partners and do not participate in the same way, these children are closely observing the back and forth and emotion of communication. See van Kleeck (1994) for a comprehensive discussion of this topic.

Here is an important question: If the caregiver's perspective on when a child is ready to be a conversation partner differs from culture to culture, does that mean that one perspective must be better than another for language-learning purposes? Taking into account studies of rates of typical language learning across cultures and languages, we believe that the answer to that question is no. There is no evidence to suggest that one perspective or culture is more correct or better at equipping their children for language learning than another. They are just different and reflect different cultural points of view. If children from nonmajority cultures consistently fell behind in their rate of language learning, then we could say that the majority point of view is likely to be the correct one. Because this has not been shown to be true, there is no reason to believe that the differences in language-learning environments that have been observed across cultures have greater or lesser value. They are just different. Of course, this is important for clinicians to know before making recommendations about how caregivers *should* talk with their children. In the absence of data showing that one or another interaction pattern is better, clinicians need to adopt the attitude of identifying differences, without adding negative judgments to that identification.

However, there is an important caveat to our explanation about language learning when we consider SES rather than cross-cultural differences. During a 2-year longitudinal study, investigators examined word learning in children from the time they began speaking to about 3 years of age and also looked at interactions among family members as a function of the child's SES (Hart & Risley, 1995). These investigators concluded that children who were growing up in households representing lower SES typically learned fewer words at a slower rate than those children growing up in households representing middle-class SES. Additionally, the children from the economically disadvantaged households had encountered significantly fewer experiences of word exposure than the other children. It appeared that several caregiver strategies predicted language-learning success and these included: caregiver responsiveness, provision of feedback, and the amount of language diversity provided to their children. As a result, it would be important for a speech–language pathologist to be familiar with these findings so that recommendations to families could focus on changes in the manner in which parents interact with their children. Equally important is the fact that we would be asking parents to learn new methods for interacting with their child and these changes will take some time and patience to implement.

Roles

We know that cultures may differ in terms of who is viewed as most knowledgeable about a child's development. In the majority culture that person is typically a parent. It is assumed that parents spend the most time with their children and therefore know them the best. A family consisting of the parents and children living together are referred to as a *nuclear family*. In minority cultures, it is not uncommon to view a family where a number of related family members and related generations (grandparents, great aunts and uncles) live together. This would be described as an *extended family*, and it may be an aunt or grandparent who spends the most time with the child and is the most knowledgeable informant.

Families also differ in terms of who makes the primary decisions for issues that involve family members, such as deciding whether a child should begin therapy in a local clinic. In some families this is a decision that one or another parent will make. For other families, a respected elder in the family makes that decision. In some cultures the parents maintain an equal share of the responsibility for their children's care. In other families, it is far more likely for the mother to be designated as the person who runs the day-to-day operation of the household, and it is the father's role to care for the family in terms of finances and protection (Lynch, 2004). It will be important to understand how the family you are working with operates when a decision needs to be made about seeking treatment, enrolling a family member in therapy, or purchasing a hearing aid.

Caregivers

It is a very good idea for clinicians to recognize how the roles of the family are distributed across family members. As previously noted, in the nuclear family, the parents are typically viewed as the primary caregivers. In an extended family or in the case where there are either many children or children separated by many years, older children may serve in the role of primary caregiver to younger siblings. Is it necessarily more or less beneficial to language learning to have different primary caregivers? So far, we do not have any reason to believe that there are inherent differences. If language learning involves receiving sufficient input and language modeling as well as opportunities to practice what you are learning, there does not appear to be any reason why one member of the family cannot be as good in this role as another. However, cultures differ in terms of who is most likely to be interacting with children and how this interaction might be accomplished (Goldstein & Iglesias, 2002). As previously noted, it will be important for clinicians to know who the primary caregiver for a particular client is, as this will help the clinician to obtain the most accurate case history information and provide therapy recommendations to the most appropriate individual.

In the majority culture, it is not unusual for caregivers to provide their child with a number of activities to help promote language development. However, this point of view regarding a parent's role in assisting language development is not universal. Clinicians working with families of children with language problems frequently make requests for parents to provide models for appropriate language and opportunities for their children to talk. However, for parents in nonmajority cultures, the parents may not understand the rationale for these suggestions and this type of request may not be understood (Hammer & Weiss, 2000; van Kleeck, 1994). The clinician has to be aware that cultural differences may account for a child's slow-to-develop first- or second-language learning, and not only explain to the caregivers why a suggestion for an activity has been made, but also provide some ideas of how the caregivers can be more engaged in their child's language development.

Professionals

The role of the professional within a culture may vary from group to group. As a professional speech–language pathologist, it is tempting for me to assume that because I have a doctoral degree and I'm certified as having clinical competence in speech–language pathology by ASHA, I possess state licensure in my home state of Rhode Island, and I'm a board-recognized specialist in child language, families that I work with will believe that I am an expert in communication disorders and have the knowledge needed to diagnose and treat their children. Letters following my name may be understood by some individuals who are knowledgeable about advanced degrees and, because of these letters, trust the decisions I make. However, not all families view a formal education as a reason to trust a professional (Lynch, 2004). Speech–language pathologists and audiologists may find that they are viewed as

I CAN'T DO THIS ALONE

A number of years ago I worked in a Midwestern state, known for its agriculture, that has a largely white population. During the years I lived there, the population of Mexican-born farm workers grew. Some were seasonal workers and others became year-round residents. In one community in particular located about 25 miles from where I lived, the population growth of this nonmajority group had exponentially increased. Several children from this community were brought for evaluations to the facility where I worked and were found to have true language disorders in their native Spanish (the reason for the term *true language disorder* will be explained later in the chapter). For all of these families, a bilingual, bicultural minister from a local church served as their *cultural ambassador*. His value to the family and to me was related to much more than his linguistic competencies. The minister was a trusted friend to the nonmajority community members, and he knew the families' strengths, needs, and concerns. The minister's ability to negotiate the cultural distance between the families and service providers was invaluable to them and to me. Through this cultural ambassador I was able to explain what I believed to be the best choices for the provision of speech therapy services and negotiate a therapy schedule. Once therapy began, the minister arranged transportation for the family to get to the clinic twice weekly and continued to provide support for the importance of consistent therapy attendance and other prescribed follow-up. I also received education from the cultural ambassador about the most appropriate way to address family members and convey respect for the family's method of decision making.

credible professionals only if they have demonstrated to the client or client's family their trustworthiness, sincerity, integrity, and so forth. This is another reason why cultivating a positive reputation in the community where you practice is always beneficial. If you provide speech–language pathology or audiology services in a community with a prominent culture other than your own, you may want to seek out someone who is bicultural, familiar, and accepted by both cultures (yours and theirs). This person could serve as your *cultural ambassador*, teaching you about the differences that exist between the two cultures and introduce you into the new community in a positive light.

THE ROLE OF COMMUNICATION WITHIN THE CULTURE

One of the most powerful factors that can connect people to a particular culture is a common form of communication. Although not all cultures have a distinctive language, they often use distinctive vocabulary (e.g., baby boomers may say "far out") or rituals of language (e.g., prayers in the Catholic mass) to set themselves apart or indicate membership in that specific group.

I am well aware that there are many terms that my students use in their daily communications that are a mystery to me. These are unique vocabulary words common to the group and may now also include text-messaging lingo. That is another major mystery. Because I do not understand, I am left out of their youthful culture—by their design. So languages and language types (e.g., *registers*) can be used to create outsiders and forge a more cohesive group of insider members.

A register is a set of language features that characterize the way a speaker talks in a specific context. For example, we use the expression "baby talk" to characterize the manner in which adults talk with young children. We can observe the adult using exaggerated and high-pitched intonation contours, facial expressions, body movements, and many more word repetitions than would be observed in typical adult-to-adult conversation. Another register example can be found when examining the speech and language of actors during the 1940s who were trying to portray characters from "high society." These actors used more formal language structures like *shall* ("Shall I get you a drink?") and too-precise articulation to characterize Hollywood's idea of persons from high society. When a speaker can easily slip back and forth between registers depending on the conversation context, we note that this person is skilled at code switching.

Verbal and Nonverbal Communication

The exchange of information can be accomplished verbally, with gestures, prosodic features of speech (e.g., intonation), and the context in which the communication takes place. Often communication is made up of a combination of verbal and nonverbal language. All languages appear to take advantage of both verbal and nonverbal communication tools. However, to someone unfamiliar with a particular culture, the nonverbal features of communication in that culture may be more difficult to learn than the verbal features. For example, in the majority culture it is common for young children to make eye contact with their conversation partner, even if that partner is someone who has a higher status (e.g., a teacher, a parent). In some nonmajority cultures, however, it is viewed as rude and inappropriate for an individual of a lower status to make eye contact with someone who has a higher status (Lynch, 2004). The teacher of children who follow a nonmajority culture's eye contact rule may believe that students are not paying attention or showing proper respect. Instead, the students are probably following the rules of their culture and not disrespecting the teacher by making eye contact. If anything, the children are demonstrating respect for the teacher. However, when the teacher is unfamiliar with these cultural differences, the child might be viewed as less intelligent or a behavior problem.

In another example, hand gestures that are commonly used in one culture may signify a completely different meaning in another. Pointing at someone may be considered impolite in many cultures. Hand holding between members of the same sex may be related to assumptions about sexual orientation in one culture but have nothing to do with sexual orientation in another.

These examples have been provided as evidence that clinicians who are working toward cross-cultural competence should not forget to consider the presence of meaningful nonverbal as well as verbal routines. Failure to do so could result in unintended miscommunication, another barrier to successful service delivery.

The emphasis placed on achieving successful communication may vary from culture to culture. For example, in American mainstream culture, there are unspoken beliefs about the connection between being an early language learner (precociousness) and intellect. Many parents have sets of expectations about their child's ability to communicate and anxiously await their child's first words. It is not unusual for these parents to remember their child's first words and share amusing anecdotes related to their child's early attempts at speaking. As a result, if the child of a mainstream family is demonstrating difficulty with language learning and appears to be falling behind the language abilities of his or her peers, family members will often notice. In other cultures, a parent's focus may not be as centered on closely monitoring language development, when compared to American culture (Hammer & Weiss, 2000). This is not a judgmental statement but rather an observation. On the other hand, other areas of development may be more closely watched in another culture. For example, motor development (e.g., walking and running) may be an area that is viewed with closer scrutiny. In this culture, a parent may pay closer attention to the time when their child is walking unassisted or running or has the balancing skills to walk across a teeter-totter (do not try this at home!). The point is that professionals should not expect that all caregivers value their children's language development in the same way as typical American parents (Lynch, 2004). When these parents are questioned regarding the onset of their child's speech and language or when their child first started to combine words, they might find it difficult to remember the exact time. These parents might question why this information is important and ask you to explain the significance as it relates to what the child is doing at the present time. It is also important to remember that just because parents are unable to provide this information does not mean that they are bad parents.

SPEECH AND LANGUAGE DIFFERENCES VERSUS DISORDERS

Definitions

In order to make appropriate decisions about who is eligible for therapy and who is not, we need to be sure that we are able to make the critical distinction between speech and language differences and speech and language disorders. To understand these differences, we need to review some of our previous discussion regarding speech, language, and communication. Languages are rule-governed, socially shared codes that are composed of groups of arbitrary symbols that enhance communication and the exchange of information between senders and receivers. The rules of language determine its form, its content, and how it is used. A *dialect* is a rule-governed variant of the language and *everyone* who speaks the language actually speaks a dialect of that language. The set of rules used by the majority of individuals who speak a language (i.e., people with the most education and influence) constitutes the standard dialect of that language. Those individuals who speak a nonstandard dialect of the language use a minimally different set of language features from the standard dialect, and these may include sound differences (phonology), vocabulary differences (semantics), grammatical differences (morphology and/or syntax), and/or pragmatic differences, or differences in how language is used in context.

There are two additional critical facts to remember about dialects. First, standard dialects are much more like nonstandard dialects than they are different. With very few exceptions, persons who speak a language's nonstandard dialect can understand the standard dialect of that language and vice versa. Second, there is nothing inherently better or more correct about a standard dialect when compared with a non-standard dialect. As linguists who study languages will tell you, all dialects are of equal value. It is society that inappropriately places value on one dialect over another.

We often encounter individuals who can speak more than one language. In fact, outside of the United States that is more the norm than an exception to the rule (Goldstein & Iglesias, 2002). Some of these people learned two or more languages at the same time from birth. We refer to these people as being *simultaneously bilingual*. Others learn one language first and then, sometime later, learn another language. We refer to these people as being *sequentially bilingual*. When we discuss the language of a sequentially bilingual individual, we refer to the first language as L_1 and the second language as L_2. So, if English was the first language you learned and Spanish was learned while attending middle school through college, English is your L_1 and Spanish is your L_2. Distinguishing between L_1 and L_2 is going to be an important issue when attempting to distinguish between the presence of a language difference and a language disorder.

Learning a second language takes time and there are many factors that contribute to the relative ease or difficulty of learning the second language. These include motivation, opportunities for exposure and practice, and the learner's willingness to take a risk. Risk taking means the willingness of an individual to accept a challenge like communicating even when unsure of the vocabulary or syntax. Cummins (1984) suggested that there are two levels of language proficiency; these are basic interpersonal communication skills (BICS) and cognitive academic language proficiency (CALP). It is important to note that a child may easily learn enough language to interact with his or her peers and teachers, but becoming proficient enough in a language to be successful on standardized tests often takes a much greater time. As a result, teachers and administrators need to resist the urge to withdraw learning accommodations just because a student appears to have mastered basic social language (Goldstein & Iglesias, 2002; Langdon, 2008). There may be several years between the achievement of BICS and CALP.

Examples of American Speech Dialects

Wolfram (1991) has spent most of his career studying the many dialects of American English. Probably the nonstandard dialects of American English that are spoken by most people are African American English and Southern American English. These dialects have more in common with Standard American English than they have differences. In fact, Southern American English and African American English have a number of similarities not shared by Standard American English. Dialects have all of the same properties that any language has: socially shared, rule-governed, and so forth. For some reason, however, people who speak Standard American English may make assumptions about speakers of African American English and Southern American English in terms of their race (not all speakers of African American English are African American and not all African Americans are speakers of African American English), intellect, or suitability for employment. Terrell and Terrell (1983) reported the results of a study that demonstrated that women applying for secretarial jobs with the same credentials were more likely to be offered the job if they spoke Standard American English rather than African American English during their interviews. When interviewed afterwards, the professionals interviewing the applicants stated that the persons offered the jobs, meaning the persons speaking Standard American English, were consistently viewed as more qualified. It is important to note that the interviewees in this study were the same applicants using both Standard American English and African American English in different interviews with different interviewers.

When a speech–language pathologist is asked to evaluate a speaker who uses a nonstandard dialect, one of the difficulties encountered involves the manner in which the individual might use the nonstandard dialect. A speaker of a nonstandard dialect might not use all of the features of the dialect or might not use the features in all contexts. For example, use of the plural morpheme is not obligatory, or required, in African American English but it is in Southern English. However, that does not always mean that a person who speaks African American English will never use a plural morpheme, just that the plural morpheme is optional.

Examples of Dialect Differences

In Table 6.1, we find some examples of differences in phonology, morphology, semantics, syntax, and pragmatics that could distinguish between speakers of Standard American English and African American English. Because they are predictable and

TABLE 6.1

Dialect differences between Standard American English and African American English

Five Components of Language	Speaker of Standard American English	Speaker of African American English
Phonology	bathtub, ask	baftub, aks
Morphology	I have three dollars.	I have three dollar(s).
	She works at Target.	She work(s) at Target.
	That's Mary's car.	That('s) Mary('s) car.
	[_ = *obligatory*]	[( ) = *optional*]
Semantics	home, car	crib, ride
Syntax	I take that bus to work every day.	I be taking that bus to work.
Pragmatics	Young children are considered to be appropriate conversation partners.	Young children speak only when spoken to.

rule governed, they represent language differences rather than language disorders. One of the primary differences between standard and nonstandard dialects of the same language is in their designation of what represents an obligatory (must be present to be considered grammatical) and what represents an optional (can be used inconsistently without a loss of grammaticality) grammatical element or structure. For example, in Standard American English (SAE), the plural morpheme is obligatory as in "I have three dollars." In African American English (AAE), the use of the plural morpheme is not obligatory, but optional, and is especially likely to be absent when the meaning of the morpheme can be conveyed in alternate ways. For example, in the sentence "I have three dollars" the descriptor "three" lets the listener know that more than one dollar is being considered. The use of the plural morpheme, although obligatory (the speaker is obliged to use it), is redundant in SAE.

Although only one example of a nonstandard dialect has been used here to make the point of "difference not disorder," you should be aware that there are many nonstandard dialects of American English. For further information, and with special attention paid to speech or phonological features of these dialects, you are encouraged to use McLeod (2007) as a very useful and current resource for information about Appalachian English, Spanish-influenced English, and Cajun English, in addition to African American English.

Once again, you should understand that when an individual uses a rule-governed variety of a language, a clinician should identify a *language difference* rather than a *language disorder*. However, that does not mean that disorders cannot occur in speakers of nonstandard dialects! It only means that the presence of a nonstandard dialect does not signal the presence of a disorder. To determine if a true disorder is present requires careful analysis of the speaker's communication patterns.

ASSESSMENT OF SPEECH AND LANGUAGE WITH CULTURAL AWARENESS

When planning an evaluation of speakers of nonstandard dialects, speakers who are learning English as a second language (ESL), or speakers considered to be English Language Learners (ELLs) who demonstrate proficiency in a language other than English, it is critical that the speech–language pathologist or audiologist is aware of and tries to minimize the effects of *test bias* as much as possible. Test bias has been described as external variables that may unduly influence the results of the test. These external variables can be membership in a specific group or race, with the results of the test showing statistically different results than the population in general.

There are a number of ways that unintentional bias can become a part of the assessment process. When test instruments and procedures are biased against a certain cultural group or language-based group, they do not yield accurate results and both the client's time and the clinician's time are wasted. The best advice to be given for test administration and interpretation is to try to limit all biasing features. Excellent reviews and descriptions of this topic can be found in Goldstein and Iglesias (2002) and Wyatt (1998).

One of the easiest ways to determine potential bias in testing is to carefully consider whom the test designers had in mind when they created the test. This information should be readily available in the manual that accompanies the test. For example, if the authors of a test stated in the manual that the test was developed to accurately assess the vocabulary of native speakers of English, then you would know that using the test with individuals who do not fit that description would be inappropriate. However, as many tests that are developed for English speakers have not been modified for ELLs, it might be necessary to use this test and recognize that the results obtained are negatively biased against the individual, even though some useful information can be gained by examining the test results.

Sometimes there is a potential bias present in the test administration context related to differences in perceptions of status. Many times when administering an assessment test, a clinician will show the client a set of pictures and ask the client to answer some questions about the pictures. Often the clinician and client can both see the pictures. If the client views the clinician as a person of higher status, the client may believe that it would be inappropriate to tell the clinician something that the clinician already knows. One might envision a test situation where both the test taker and the test administrator can see a picture of a boy hiding behind a tree. The clinician states, "Show me the picture of the boy hiding behind the tree," and the client might hesitate during his response. Although some clinicians might view this hesitation as an indication of a client's lack of knowledge, a clinician who is aware of cultural differences might interpret the hesitation to be the client's respect for the clinician's unstated knowledge. However, it wouldn't be hard to imagine a clinician misinterpreting the client's response.

Many of the tests we use, especially those used with younger clients, contain pictures, objects, or tasks that are unfamiliar to clients from nonmajority cultures. For example, test materials that are filled with vocabulary items common to children growing up in cities (e.g., *turnstile*, *skyscraper*) may be unfamiliar to children growing up in rural areas (who would be more familiar with items like *combine*, *herd*) and vice versa.

Another major difference that affects the success of test taking is the assumption, which is often typical of the majority culture, that test takers are members of a low-context culture. Low-context cultures rely on linguistic information for problem solving, but in a high-context culture, the reliance is on world knowledge and observation (Lynch, 2004). So, in low-context cultures it is common to find mathematical problems that are linguistically based, for example, "Let's assume the United States is 3,000 miles wide from one coast to the other coast. If one train left San Francisco traveling 100 miles per hour heading east and another train left New York City traveling west at 200 miles per hour, how many hours would it take for the two trains to cross?" The individual from a low-context culture would probably view this as a mathematical problem only, but an individual from a high-context culture might view this as a problem that made little sense because of the relative speed of railroad travel and the possibility of two trains going in opposite directions being at the same place at the same time. As a result, the person with the low-context perspective is used to not being bothered by facts taken out of context (decontextualized), but the person with the high-context perspective tends to be bothered by the conflicts brought about by world knowledge. When a person administering a

IN THE CLINIC

According to the American Speech-Language-Hearing Association, service providers (SLPs and audiologists) must be aware of any cultural and/or linguistic differences that could stand in the way of providing services that are both appropriate and effective (ASHA, 2010c). As a bilingual (English/Spanish) speech–language pathologist working in a university clinic, I am able to provide speech and language services to the bilingual population within our community. In addition, I am able to assist the audiologists when dealing with a bilingual client or family. Within our clinic we recognize the cultural differences and strive to be culturally sensitive in our service delivery process.

We are going to discuss José, a client who benefited from the collaborative effort of speech–language pathology and audiology. José was from a primarily Spanish-speaking home. His parents spoke no English, and his parents had limited education. José was initially seen by the audiologist because of family concerns about his hearing. José's hearing evaluation revealed that in both ears he had impacted wax (cerumen) that needed to be removed. José was then referred to me by the audiologist to have a bilingual speech and language evaluation because of concerns about his speech and language development.

A few weeks later, José was evaluated and it was determined that he had a significant speech and language delay. He was unintelligible and had reduced receptive and expressive language skills. José relied on gestures, acting out, and pointing to communicate with familiar and unfamiliar listeners. We believed that the blockage in José's ears played a major role in his speech and language delay.

We recommended that José be evaluated by an ear, nose, and throat physician (ENT) to deal with his impacted wax. As we followed up with the parents, we recognized that the parents were inconsistently bringing their son to the ENT and when they were scheduled to attend, we often had to phone to remind them and then provide directions so they could find the office. The physician was able to remove the wax in two visits and recommended surgery to remove José's tonsils and adenoids and insert pressure equalizing (PE) tubes to prevent additional middle-ear problems. The family accepted the recommendation when in the doctor's office but failed to follow up with the ENT appointment because of their disagreement with the plan for surgery.

As the semester progressed, we learned that the family had difficulty with many of the recommendations that were provided. Although the mom was supportive of the recommendations, the dad believed that José would simply grow out of the problem, seeing that a paternal uncle had similar problems and eventually learned to "talk right."

Because of the parents' reluctance to have their child attend therapy and get surgery to improve his condition, we started each therapy session with a counseling session for the mom in which I helped to interpret information that the audiologist provided to the parents. However, the mom always deferred to her husband, the household authority figure, and explained that she would share the information with him as no decision was to be made without his final approval. Although speech and language sessions were typically attended on a regular basis, the family had difficulty arriving on time and with increased needs of other family members, José's problems sometimes became secondary to other family issues.

As José was now about to turn 5 years of age, he was enrolled in kindergarten for the following fall semester. After the second week in therapy and José's second week in school, the dad came back to report that José had been having a lot of challenges in school and was beginning to act out. Because the family viewed education as very important and had now seen the adverse effects of José's hearing and speech delay on his academics, the family followed up with the ENT's recommendation regarding the possibility of wax reoccurring in his ears and the impact of the PE tubes. . . . It was quite gratifying to witness the proactive advocacy from the father and outcomes from our continued interactions with the parents. Cultural sensitivity, cultural awareness, and family education were keys toward providing José with the best possible clinical services. Through the team collaboration, José is now on a positive journey.

Contributed by Elia Olivares, MS, Clinical Faculty, Northern Illinois University.

test is aware of potential bias and works to reduce or eliminate some of these issues, interpretation of test results can more accurately reflect the client's real abilities so that an accurate determination of the presence of a language disorder or difference can be made.

TREATMENT OF SPEECH AND LANGUAGE DIFFERENCES

Speech and language differences are not disorders, and because of this, it would be inappropriate for speech–language pathologists to treat people who use a nonstandard dialect. Intervention for a speech disorder is focused on teaching the client to replace an incorrect way of speaking with a correct way of speaking. In the case of a language difference, remember that there is nothing incorrect to change. However, occasionally parents may ask a speech–language pathologist to provide therapy to teach their child how to move between the version of the language they use at home and the standard version of the language. In this case, the clinician's job would not be replacing the nonstandard aspects of language with the standard language, but instead focusing on teaching the child to "translate" between the two according to the speaking context. The child would be taught to produce equivalent sentences in both dialects so that he or she could successfully communicate in contexts like school where it would be more likely that the standard dialect would be spoken. The following illustrates this point: A student is a speaker of African

American English. When a speech–language pathologist asks him how his best friend gets to school, the student responds, "He *walk* to school." The speech–language pathologist, modeling Standard English, says, "Yes, that's how you tell me that information in 'home talk.' In 'school talk' you can say, 'He *walks* to school.' Now I want you to tell me how you would say this in home talk: 'She sings in the choir.'" The student responds, "She sing in the choir."

The teaching model that was described is called *contrastive analysis* and it is very common in the field of linguistics. Note that the difference between home talk and school talk is not represented as a difference between unacceptable and acceptable, but rather as a choice between equivalent forms that are more communicative and appropriate depending on speaking context. Taylor (1986) provides several excellent examples of how this type of teaching can be employed. Basically, the SLP is teaching code switching, a term discussed in an earlier section, The Role of Communication Within the Culture, of this chapter (p. 125). That is, the speaker needs to determine which dialect is a better fit for the communication context.

TREATMENT OF TRUE SPEECH AND LANGUAGE DISORDERS IN AN L₁ OTHER THAN ENGLISH

One of the challenges to speech–language pathologists that has already been mentioned is accurately making the distinction between speech and language differences versus speech and language disorders. If a true speech and language disorder has been diagnosed, then the speech–language pathologist has at least another two major decisions to make: (1) Which language or dialect will be the language or dialect of the therapy provided? and (2) Who is best equipped to provide the therapy? ASHA has developed practice guidelines to assist professionals in answering these questions. These guidelines are part of a series of best practices documents that can be retrieved by ASHA and National Student Speech, Language, and Hearing Association members from ASHA's Web site (http://www.asha.org). The two documents in question are titled "Clinical Management of Communicatively Handicapped Minority Language Populations" (American Speech-Language-Hearing Association, 1985) and "American English Dialects" (American Speech-Language-Hearing Association, 2003).

One major decision for speech–language pathologists to make is to determine the client's dominant language. If there is true language disorder, it will be evident in the dominant language and that should be the language of therapy. Dominant languages are usually the same language or dialect of language used in the home. This is the language in which the child receives the most input and is usually the language used by one or both parents and the majority of extended family members. Research has shown that it is much easier for children to generalize what they have learned to L_2 if they are provided therapy in their L_1 (Hammer & Rodriguez, 2009). The reverse approach does not work as well. This factor is extremely critical in fostering correct decision making concerning providing children who are ELLs with access to academic training in their L_1. Contrary to some commonly held beliefs by the public at large, denial of L_1 is not the most expedient way to teach English as a second language.

Quiz on the Fly 6.2

1. Eye contact is one type of _____ communication that may represent different meanings across cultures.

2. In the majority culture, having a child who is a late talker may be viewed by parents as more of a problem than in a minority culture because _____ is prized in the majority culture.

3. When two languages are learned at the same time, the learner is said to be _____ bilingual.

4. Differences between standard and nonstandard dialects may be found in the following areas of language: phonology, _____, syntax, pragmatics, and _____.

5. If a speech–language pathologist provides "therapy" for a student who can speak a nonstandard dialect only, the speech–language pathologist's job is not to replace the nonstandard dialect with the standard but to teach _____.

SUMMARY AND REVIEW

Because of the evidence of ongoing changes in the makeup of the American population it is imperative that individuals who are trained as speech–language pathologists and audiologists are cross-culturally competent. These professionals must be able to provide evaluation and treatment services in an unbiased manner, taking into consideration the cultural differences that may impact appropriate service delivery to all of their clients and patients.

This chapter introduced the definition of culture and showed how different sets of cultural values and beliefs can impact attitudes about communication disorders. Culturally based differences in how families perceive their role in their children's language learning, as well as how they incorporate their children into conversations, were also discussed. At all times, respect for differences, whether in parenting style or learning style, was stressed. The point of view that differences are not synonymous with disorders is a critical first step in ensuring that professionals will not make incorrect assumptions about the presence or absence of communication disorders. Specific suggestions for how to reduce bias in assessment were presented. Distinctions between a person's first or dominant language (L_1) and the learning of additional languages (L$_2$) were made because they are relevant to the choice of the appropriate language for assessment as well as selection of a language for therapy purposes.

Culture

What is culture and cultural identification?

A person's culture relates to a set of beliefs and values about his or her place in the world. Cultural identification helps an individual to identify and participate as a member of a specific group. Cultural identification will influence a person's view of the family, a supreme being, and birth and death, and may be shaped by a number of factors including, but not limited to, religion, languages spoken, age, level of education, race, gender, and sexual orientation. Most people will identify with more than one cultural group.

Cultural Competence is Important

How can cultural competence assist a practicing clinician?

Cultural competence is an awareness and understanding of differences among cultural groups. When a clinician is culturally competent, he or she can provide treatment in an objective manner while being sensitive to cultural differences associated with the person with whom they are interacting.

Culture and the Changing Face of the Population

What is acculturation and the three models used to describe it?

When an individual tries to fit in or become part of a group, it refers to acculturation. Acculturation is adopting the social or cultural characteristics of that group. The three models of acculturation are the Anglo-conformity model, the melting pot model, and the cultural pluralism model.

Quiz on the Fly 6.2 Answers

1. Eye contact is one type of **nonverbal** communication that may represent different meanings across cultures. **2.** In the majority culture, having a child who is a late talker may be viewed by parents as more of a problem than in a minority culture because **precocious (early) language** is prized in the majority culture. **3.** When two languages are learned at the same time, the learner is said to be **simultaneously** bilingual. **4.** Differences between standard and nonstandard dialects may be found in the following areas of language: phonology, **semantics**, syntax, pragmatics, and **morphology**. **5.** If a speech–language pathologist provides "therapy" for a student who can speak a nonstandard dialect only, the speech–language pathologist's job is not to replace the nonstandard dialect with the standard but to teach **the contexts where the standard may be preferred**.

The Characteristics of Culture

What are some characteristics of culture?

For the purposes of our discussion, we first examined an individual's role within a family or group and noted that many families may be extended families rather than nuclear families. We then discussed the caregiver, recognizing that in many families, a caregiver may not be a parent. Finally we discussed the perception of the professional by persons within a cultural group and noted that just because a person is educated and has a number of degrees does not automatically make that person trustworthy in the view of a person from another culture.

The Role of Communication within the Culture

What is the relationship between communication and culture?

Individual cultures often have their own language that helps to bind a group together. However, even when members of a group speak the same language, it is common for specific groups of individuals to have unique vocabulary that gives those group members a method of separating themselves from the larger group. Additionally a professional needs to be aware of differences that might exist with nonverbal communication (e.g., eye contact, gestures) when dealing with persons from the nonmajority culture. Inappropriate assumptions based on majority beliefs can often lead to a breakdown in communication and problems between the professional and the person or families he or she is attempting to help.

Do all cultures view communication in the same way?

We have tried to help you understand that, although communication might be an important focus for the traditional American family, communication may take a lesser role when dealing with persons from other cultures. It would not be unusual for a family to focus more on a child's motor development and coordination while communication plays a lesser role within that family. As a result, when dealing with these families, an inability to identify specific milestones regarding speech and language development does not mean that the family is not concerned. It just suggests that within the culture of the family, different aspects of development receive more attention.

Speech and Language Differences Versus Disorders

What is a speech and language difference?

A dialect is a rule-governed variant of the language and everyone who speaks the language actually speaks a dialect of that language. A dialect that is used by an individual would be viewed as a speech and language difference. The rules used by the majority of individuals who speak a language are called the standard dialect, and those who use a minimally different set of language features are using a nonstandard dialect. In most cases, persons who speak a language's nonstandard dialect can understand the standard dialect of that language and vice versa. There is nothing inherently better or more correct about a standard dialect when compared with a nonstandard dialect.

Assessment of Speech and Language with Cultural Awareness

What is test bias and what factors should be examined regarding cultural differences?

Test bias has been described as external variables that may unduly influence the results of the test. It is important for clinicians to determine the target audience for a test being administered, the test taker's perception of status with regards to the test administrator, and the test taker's familiarity with objects and tasks associated with the majority culture. Without this culture awareness, interpretation of test results can be seriously impacted by these external variables.

Treatment of Speech and Language Differences

How are speech and language differences managed?

Speech and language differences are not disorders. Therapy is typically not provided for the majority of children and adults who exhibit these differences. However, parents might recognize that their child needs to possess the pragmatic skill that enables the child to use both nonstandard and standard dialects within the community environment and at school or at work. As a result, an SLP might provide treatment that teaches clients to switch their speech and language skills according to the environment context in which they need to communicate.

Treatment of True Speech and Language Disorders in an L_1 Other Than English

How are speech and language services provided for a child whose first language is not English?

When a child exhibits a language disorder, it is going to be present in the child's dominant language and in his attempts at learning English. The dominant language is the language that the child most often uses at home. Because this is the child's primary language, therapy should be provided in the child's dominant language. Research has shown that therapy provided in the dominant language will also assist in learning the second language. However, the reverse is not true and providing therapy in the second language will have less of an impact on the child's dominant language.

WEB SITES OF INTEREST

Bilingual Therapies
http://www.bilingualtherapies.com/

The Early Childhood Research Institute at the University of Illinois
http://www.clas.uiuc.edu/

Helping English Language Learners
http://www.colorincolorado.org/about/

The Office of Multicultural Affairs of the American Speech-Language-Hearing Association
http://www.asha.org/about/leadership-projects/multicultural/

7

Neurological Impairment: Speech and Language Disorders in Adults

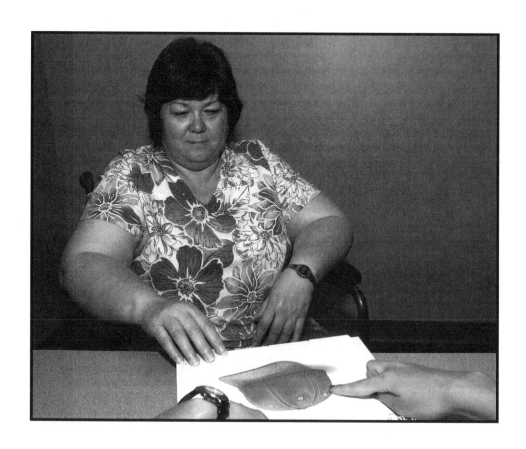

The focus of this chapter will be a discussion of language and speech problems associated with neurological impairment. It is important to note that our discussion will include both language and speech issues, recognizing that these two issues are not synonymous. Patients with neurological impairment exhibit a variety of different symptoms depending upon the location and degree of neurological damage. We will begin our discussion with a review of the brain anatomy as it relates to speech and language skills, and briefly examine the causes of neurological speech and language problems. We will continue with a discussion of the language problems associated with neurological impairment and the various manifestations of that language impairment. Our discussion will then be directed toward damage to the right side of the brain and examine the various disorders associated with this type of damage. As part of this discussion, we will examine methods for evaluating and treating these problems. We will then focus our attention on speech disorders associated with brain damage and describe the various characteristics associated with these speech impairments. We will conclude with discussions of dementia and the treatment of motor speech disorders.

BRAIN ANATOMY ASSOCIATED WITH SPEECH AND LANGUAGE DISORDERS

In general, specific areas of the brain are associated with specific functions. For example, handedness (dominant left or right hand) is associated with a specific cerebral hemisphere. The majority of people are right handed and this is often associated with dominance of their left cerebral hemisphere. Historically, handedness has been assumed to predict localization of language within the brain. It was first speculated that right-handed people would exhibit language dominance in their left cortex, and left-handed people would exhibit language dominance in their right cortex. However, this simple method of examining language localization has not been validated. In fact, it is generally accepted that for the majority of the population, left handed or right handed, language is located on the left side of the brain (Knect et al., 2000).

The two major brain areas that we will use to anchor our discussion of language and speech are Wernicke's area and Broca's area (see Figure 7.1). As noted in our anatomy chapter, Wernicke's area is located in the temporal lobe, and Broca's area is found within the frontal lobe, at the bottom and anterior to the primary motor strip. Wernicke's area is believed to be primarily responsible for the

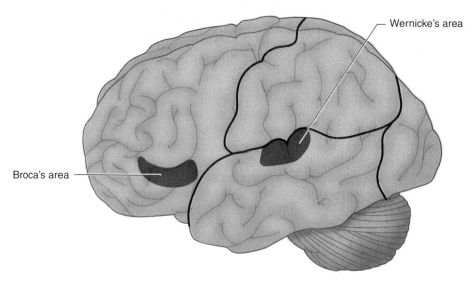

FIGURE 7.1
Broca's and Wernicke's areas of the brain.

comprehension of speech and language and the formulation of language concepts. In contrast, Broca's area is related to linguistic programming, speech motor programming, and the production of expressive speech and language. As you might expect, there are strong connections between Wernicke's area and Broca's area. It is these connections that enable a person to take language that has been formulated in Wernicke's area and transmit it forward to Broca's area, where it is programmed and transmitted to the muscles responsible for speech production. The connection between Wernicke's area and Broca's area is called the *arcuate fasciculus*. Although we can talk in generalities about areas of the brain associated with language and speech, it is important to recognize that there is a great deal of variability across individuals.

LANGUAGE DISORDERS ASSOCIATED WITH NEUROLOGICAL IMPAIRMENT

Aphasia is the loss of the ability to comprehend or formulate language and is typically associated with neurological damage. Although aphasia may be caused by a number of different neurological conditions, the most typical cause of aphasia in adults is a stroke. Strokes occur when there is a blockage in a blood vessel supplying blood to the brain or when there is bleeding in or around the brain. When the brain is deprived of oxygen and nutrients because of this blockage or when there is bleeding in and around the brain, brain cells die. According to the Internet Stroke Center (http://www.strokecenter.org), strokes are "the leading cause of serious, long-term disability in the United States." It has been estimated that about 80,000 persons become aphasic each year in the United States.

There is no one method of classifying the language deficits associated with aphasia. If you question a physician, the physician might view the problem from an anatomical perspective, and a speech–language pathologist (SLP) might view the problem from a communicative perspective and describe the patient's strengths and weaknesses as they relate to language functioning. Very often the language skills exhibited by the patient are described as fluent or nonfluent, and these terms often relate to the areas of the brain that have been affected. *Fluent aphasias* have normal rate and rhythm of speech but lack meaningful content. On the other hand, *nonfluent aphasia* is often characterized by difficulty initiating speech and choppy short utterances with some articulatory difficulty.

Deficits of Expressive Language

To begin our discussion of aphasia, it is important to note that there are a variety of deficits that a patient may exhibit, and these will be characterized as components of aphasia, although they are not exhibited by every patient. The list of deficits is quite extensive and goes well beyond the scope of this book. However, it may be helpful to describe a few of the problems by first examining those deficits associated with spoken language. Imagine running into a former high school friend, recognizing that friend, and not being able to recall his name. Although most people experience this "tip of the tongue" phenomenon, persons with aphasia often have this difficulty but in a more extreme fashion where recalling the name of objects, people, and words is difficult to impossible. A patient is asked to name his favorite food, and he sits and stares and is unable to come up with the word *pizza*. When the patient is asked to name the object on his wrist, he states, "It's a . . . you know, it's used to tell time, it's a clock, no, not a clock it's a. . . ." This patient is unable to verbally identify his watch. *Anomia* is difficulty with retrieving and producing words.

Have you ever called from one room to another looking for your brother but in your hurried attempt to call your brother, you called your dog's name? This type of substitution can also be seen in the speech and language of an aphasic patient. During a conversation with some aphasic patients, they might want to reference their wife but refer to their daughter. This patient might want you to hand him his watch but asks you to "give me the clock." *Paraphasias* are sound and word substitutions that are often found in the speech of aphasic patients whose speech and language is fluent and grammatically correct. Paraphasic substitutions may be associated with word similarities (e.g., *watch* and *clock*) or sound similarities (e.g., *tar* and *bar*). On some occasions a patient will create a new word and use it as if it was part of everyone's vocabulary. For example, a patient might say, "Can you hand me that *gobo*?" when the patient is asking for his or her glasses. These made-up words are called *neologisms*.

For readers who are skilled at texting on their mobile phones, it's not hard to recall that responding to the text message as fast as possible enables you and your friend to maintain communication while proceeding with some other task. To make your texting more efficient, you often leave out the small words that fill out our traditional written correspondence but just get in the way when trying to return the message. For example, you might receive a text from a friend on vacation. *Long flight, no sleep, arrived late, slept till noon* instead of *The trip was really long and I didn't get any sleep. The plane arrived late and then I slept until noon.* For some people with aphasia, their speech is quite similar to the text message. It is not unusual to hear a nonfluent message that does not contain articles and conjunctions, although the crux of the message remains intact. For example, a patient wants to get out of the hospital and go home. He expresses to his wife and doctor, "I go home," rather than saying, "I want to go home now." *Agrammatism* is the deficit exhibited by these patients where articles, conjunctions, and even grammatical morphemes might be left out. The patient typically speaks with a lot of effort, using short sentences. To the untrained observer, this speaker appears to have lost control of his or her speech, but the speech–language pathologist recognizes that the problem is language related.

For some types of aphasia it is very common for the patient to use normal intonation, prosody, and fluent speech and language while stringing together a series of meaningless words that don't make sense to the listener. This verbal deficit of aphasic patients is called *jargon*. Jargon may simultaneously include appropriate English words and neologisms. For example, a patient was asked what type of work he does and he replied, "My very going, *gillies* want and always *mumbub*." If the listener is not listening closely, the rate and intonation of this sentence sounds very much like normal speech and language. However, when the listener makes any attempt at comprehension, it is impossible.

Deficits of Comprehension

Auditory comprehension requires that the patient understands the meaning of the words being spoken and the grammar associated with the utterance. Like expressive language deficits, auditory comprehension problems vary across individuals and may range from difficulty understanding specific vocabulary to a total inability to understand any of the words being spoken. For example, a speech–language pathologist has been informed by a patient's family that his language comprehension is improving because he is now responding to questions. When the grandson walks into the room and asks, "Grandpa, how are you feeling today?" the grandfather replies, "Fine." The family watches as a physician attempts to assess the patient's comprehension by extending his own hand and saying, "Mr. Ryan, give me your hand." The family members observe that the patient extends his hand. To these family members, the patient's language comprehension is improving. As a result, the family members ask the speech–language pathologist to conduct a bedside evaluation to see if the patient has improved. During many of these scenarios, the speech–language pathologist understands the family's strong desire for their relative to get better while recognizing that automatic speech like "I'm fine" or "How are you doing" often occurs with little conscious effort and may not reflect improvement in language functioning. When the speech–language pathologist sees the patient at bedside, she says to Mr. Ryan, "Give me your hand," and she does not extend her hand as a visual clue. Mr. Ryan stares at the speech–language pathologist and does not respond. The speech–language pathologist then places a pencil, paper, and coin on the patient's table and says, "Mr. Ryan, give me the quarter, pick up the pencil, and write your name." Mr. Ryan responds by handing the quarter to the speech–language pathologist and then stares at her while waiting for another command. To the speech–language pathologist it appears that Mr. Ryan is able to understand some simple commands, but as the commands get more complex and require more short-term memory, Mr. Ryan has difficulty. It will be the responsibility of the speech–language pathologist to document the nature of Mr. Ryan's difficulties, develop a management plan for the patient, and then counsel the family regarding the nature of their relative's problem and how they can assist in his path to recovery.

Comprehension of language can take a variety of forms. In the previous examples, the patient was able to comprehend some degree of language but this was often affected by the patient's memory abilities and visual information that was provided. In addition to aphasia, a patient may experience damage in the sensory areas of the brain that results in a variety of disorders. *Agnosia* is difficulty identifying sensory information. We recognize that this patient can perceive a sensation (e.g., hearing) but is unable to make the connection in his brain to identify the nature of sensory information. For example, in the most extreme case, a patient may experience verbal agnosia, or word deafness. As a result of all testing, it is shown that the patient has normal hearing and is able to speak, read, and write, but when asked a question, the patient is unable to comprehend it. In many cases, the same question presented in written format will result in a verbal response from the patient.

When a patient experiences *visual agnosia,* he or she is able to easily read aloud from a book or newspaper but is unable to explain or even know what information has been read. Other forms of visual agnosia may make it difficult for a patient to remember the faces of familiar individuals, know the name of familiar objects, or even recall colors. As you might conclude, agnosias have the potential to seriously impact the life of the patient and the patient's family. These patients and family members will require a lot of support, counseling, and training for teaching the patient methods for dealing with his or her deficits.

Deficits in Reading and Writing

In addition to language difficulties associated with the comprehension and expression of oral language, aphasic language problems may also be associated with the patient's writing and reading skills. Just as oral language requires the use of symbols in the form of sounds to communicate, writing involves the patient's ability to take previous knowledge of letters and numbers and combine these in a meaningful way to form words and sentences. For many patients, *agraphia*, or the inability to write, is a problem that is associated with their aphasia. This inability is not due to a weakness in the patient's arm or hand, but is related to the patient's inability to connect the language areas of the brain with the areas that control the ability to write words. The speech–language pathologist asks the patient to write his or her name and it comes out as a series of scratches and scribbles. The patient believes that he or she has complied with the request but on paper the writing is illegible. These writing difficulties, just like spoken-language difficulties, will depend upon the degree of language difficulty the patient is exhibiting.

Problems associated with reading are called *alexia.* You are probably familiar with the term *developmental dyslexia* that describes a child's reading difficulties that are present from birth and continue into adulthood. In contrast, a patient with alexia had normal reading abilities at one time and now, as a result of a neurological deficit, may experience mild to severe reading difficulties. In its most extreme form, alexia would be classified as a visual agnosia, or word blindness. As alexia is often associated with aphasia, the degree of language impairment and the location of the brain damage will relate to the reading difficulties exhibited by the patient.

Quiz on the Fly 7.1

1. The _____ connects Broca's area to Wernicke's area.
2. Difficulty retrieving and producing words is called _____.
3. "I wanted to *blobo* but I couldn't." *Blobo* is an example of a _____.
4. Difficulty identifying sensory information is called _____.
5. Reading problems acquired following a stroke are called _____.

APHASIA CLASSIFICATION

Although we have already emphasized the variability associated with aphasia, it might be helpful to examine a classification for aphasia that examines typical characteristics of the problem as they are related to the location of the neurological damage, as well as the associated speech and language characteristics associated with this type of neurological damage.

Broca's Aphasia

Lesions that occur in the anterior part of the brain, usually anterior to the lower portion of the motor area, result in *Broca's aphasia*. Broca's aphasia is characterized by nonfluent speech and language. A patient with this type of aphasia often produces sentences that primarily contain nouns, verbs, and occasionally an adjective. In many patients with Broca's aphasia, conversational comprehension appears to be intact but when more complex comprehension is required, the patient has difficulty comprehending the same syntactical relationships that are difficult during expressive output. For example, if a patient with Broca's aphasia is asked, "Do birds fly?" it is likely that the patient would reply, "Yes." However, if the patient is given a statement like "The zebra was killed by the lion," and is asked the question, "What animal was killed?" the patient would have difficulty answering the question because this type of aphasia affects the patient's ability to use and comprehend complex syntactical relationships. Patients with Broca's aphasia also exhibit problems with *confrontational naming*. This task requires the patient to produce the name of an object in a relatively rapid manner. Patients with Broca's aphasia also exhibit difficulty with oral reading and sometimes reading comprehension, although these abilities vary according to the size and location of the lesion. Broca's aphasia is viewed as a disorder of expressive output.

Wernicke's Aphasia

Lesions that occur in the upper portion of the temporal lobe (Wernicke's area) typically result in *Wernicke's aphasia*. This is viewed as a fluent aphasia, with the patient exhibiting difficulty with language comprehension. Patients with Wernicke's aphasia often produce fluent-sounding speech but the content of this speech is often incomprehensible. Family members might listen to the patient's speech and comment that, "It sounds like he's trying to tell us something," when in reality the content of his speech is meaningless. Patients with Wernicke's aphasia often exhibit paraphasias and neologisms when attempting oral communication. Many Wernicke's patients have significant comprehension problems to the point that they don't understand spoken language. When viewed in conjunction with the lack of content exhibited in their expressive output, Wernicke's patients often exhibit nonfunctional comprehension and expression of language. As these individuals have significant language difficulties, reading is also impaired.

Global Aphasia

Global aphasia affects most language areas and is more severe than Wernicke's aphasia. A patient with global aphasia typically has nonfunctional language skills in both receptive and expressive areas. Expressively, patients will produce stereotypical expressions (e.g., "I'm fine") in response to any question that is asked. Patients will also use jargon to produce meaningless utterances and often repeat jargon or phrases multiple times. These multiple iterations of a response (e.g., *blaga, blaga, blaga, blaga*) are called *perseverations* or *perseverative behavior*.

Anomic Aphasia

Anomic aphasia is a common type of language problem associated with neurological deficits. This type of problem is classified as a fluent aphasia. Patients exhibit problems recalling words when attempting to name objects. While word finding may be a characteristic of a variety of different types of aphasia, a patient with anomic aphasia often exhibits normal to mildly impaired language comprehension abilities and word finding is the patient's primary problem. In addition, some patients may exhibit a significant number of receptive and expressive language issues immediately following their brain injury, and it is not uncommon for many of these issues to resolve, leaving the patient with an anomic aphasia.

ASSESSMENT OF LANGUAGE DISORDERS ASSOCIATED WITH NEUROLOGICAL IMPAIRMENT

Anne is a speech–language pathologist assigned to the acute-care wing of a large hospital. When a patient is admitted for a stroke and there are questions regarding the patient's communication, Anne typically receives a referral to evaluate this patient. The evaluation of a patient with a communicative disorder associated with a neurological problem often involves a number of stages that typically begin at the patient's bedside. Prior to conducting the bedside evaluation, the speech–language pathologist will review the patient's hospital chart to determine the medical nature of the patient's problem and view the results of any other evaluations (e.g., physical therapy, occupational therapy, brain scan) that may have been completed. At bedside, the speech–language pathologist is going to do some informal evaluation to determine the patient's ability to comprehend language and then use this language in a meaningful way. The patient may be asked questions that relate to orientation, such as "Where are you now?" The speech–language pathologist may then focus on the patient's memory by showing the patient three objects and then asking the patient about those objects after a 5-minute period of time. Additional questions will relate to language comprehension and expression. A patient may be asked to follow multistage commands such as, "Touch your nose, blink your eyes, and give me your hand." Is the patient able to read printed commands, write simple sentences, and follow yes/no questions? The results of this bedside testing will reveal important information that can be shared with the other professionals interacting with the patient and, more important, used to document the patient's progress as some of the medical issues resolve.

It is important to note that upon admission to the hospital, a patient with recent neurological damage may exhibit complications associated with the trauma that may resolve as the patient medically improves. As these complications improve, the patient often exhibits improvements in awareness, attention, and communication. The improvement that occurs without any direct treatment is known as *spontaneous recovery.* By completing a bedside evaluation, the speech–language pathologist will establish a baseline of communicative functioning. This baseline will be used during subsequent days by the speech–language pathologist and other professionals to determine whether the patient has improved. It is for these reasons that the speech–language pathologist may visit the patient at bedside on multiple occasions to document the changes that occur as the patient's medical problems improve. It is not unusual for a patient to be minimally responsive to questions immediately following a stroke but then, in a couple of days, easily respond to simple questions.

Quiz on the Fly 7.1 Answers

1. The **arcuate fasciculus** connects Broca's area to Wernicke's area. **2.** Difficulty retrieving and producing words is called **anomia**. **3.** "I wanted to *blobo* but I couldn't." *Blobo* is an example of a **neologism**. **4.** Difficulty identifying sensory information is called **agnosia**. **5.** Reading problems acquired following a stroke are called **alexia**.

Depending upon the medical and communicative status of the patient following admission, the speech–language pathologist may schedule more formal testing using any number of standardized tests. Some of the more common tests include the Boston Diagnostic Aphasia Examination (Goodglass, Kaplan, & Barresi, 2001) and the Western Aphasia Examination (Kertesz, 1982). Although the content of these exams will vary, the examiner is attempting to determine the nature of the patient's receptive and expressive language impairment. These exams will help the examiner explore the fluency of the patient's verbal output, ability to comprehend oral and written language, and ability to produce extended monologues, conversation, and written expression.

The clinician conducting testing of the neurologically impaired patient recognizes that although textbooks describe clear distinctions between disorders such as Broca's aphasia and Wernicke's aphasia, most patients exhibit symptoms that might characterize a variety of different labels. In addition, results of formalized tests need to be examined as they relate to the environments in which the patient will be placed. The speech–language pathologist will examine a patient's strengths and weaknesses as determined by formalized tests and then use these results to further test the patient within a more functional communicative environment. For example, it might be determined through formal tests that the patient has memory problems and difficulty following commands. As a follow-up to these test results, the clinician might visit the patient during an occupational or physical therapy session and further assess the patient's ability to follow commands within this unique communicative environment. On some occasions the patient may perform better than expected as a result of familiarity with the routine. In some circumstances the patient's ability to make use of visual information and visual clues provided by the therapist will also help the patient to complete the task. Making use of visual information in addition to auditory information can be an extremely useful strategy for compensating for language deficits. On other occasions it may become evident that within the limited and restricted environment of the therapy room, a patient is able to complete many of the tasks with little or no difficulty. However, when placed in an environment outside of the therapy room, the patient has to deal with a lot more stimulation and distractions and still maintain good language skills.

Once the patient becomes medically stable, the patient's physician will consult with the speech–language pathologist, physical therapist, and occupational therapist in an attempt to determine the next stage in the patient's rehabilitation. Options can include a rehabilitation hospital that might be part of the acute-care setting where the patient is presently being treated. Therapies within this rehabilitation setting are usually short term until future decisions can be made. Depending upon the patient's physical, cognitive, and communicative status, rehabilitation options can include a residential long-term rehabilitation center, home health care by which the patient will receive therapy at home, a community-based private clinic, a nursing home for those patients who require more medical attention and closer supervision, and university clinics where a patient can receive outpatient services.

I CAN'T DO THIS ALONE

Jennifer Heinisch, a speech–language pathologist who works in an outpatient community reentry rehabilitation program, described her experiences working with other professionals:

The majority of my clients are adults who had experienced neurological impairments as a result of strokes and brain injuries. I collaborate on a daily basis with physical and occupational therapists to help clients achieve their functional goals such as returning to independent living at home, being able to drive a car, returning to work, and sometimes returning to school. One focus of our treatment program is outings in the community. These activities provide the client with an opportunity to test out those skills that they have learned or relearned in the therapy room during real-life functional activities. For example, a physical therapist and I had planned an outing to a grocery store with one of our clients. While I was using this outing as an opportunity to work on strategies to compensate for reduced reading comprehension, memory, organization, and math, the physical therapist was also using the outing as an opportunity to address how increased environmental distractions impact the client's safety when moving through the store with a walker. To make this shopping opportunity meaningful to the client, we met with the client and her family to discuss where the family shopped and the types of products that are typically purchased. This outing allowed us to view the client as a functioning individual rather than a client within the therapy room. We wanted to determine how the demands of a real-world situation would impact the client's ability to be independent.

During our therapy sessions, the client had done very well with structured, clinic-based tasks that involved reading and comprehending labels on food and household products, remembering items on a "to-do" list (with visual aids), and organizing tasks in an efficient order. However, when these same skills were targeted in the grocery outing, the client also had to focus on maneuvering her walker around various obstacles and deal with the many distractions within the store. When we observed our client, we noted that her overall cognitive performance was adversely affected by all of the stimulation and demands of the task. The client was not able to appropriately use her shopping list to accurately obtain all the items that she needed, and she was not able to focus on the specific details on product labels to allow her to purchase the items that she wanted. This outing allowed us to further develop therapy strategies to help the client work on functional skills. During a subsequent outing following a period of additional therapy, the client's independence improved remarkably. Had we not included the first outing as part of this client's treatment plan and collaborated with the client, client's family, and the physical therapist, we would have failed to maximize this client's functional progress toward her cognitive–communicative goals.

———————

Contributed by Jennifer Heinisch, MA, CCC-SLP.

TREATMENT OF LANGUAGE DISORDERS ASSOCIATED WITH NEUROLOGICAL IMPAIRMENT

Language treatment programs for individuals with neurological impairment are as varied as the symptoms exhibited by the patient. However, all treatment is focused on one goal; helping the patient return to a level of functional communication. This includes making his or her needs known, requesting assistance with activities of daily living, and trying to communicate at levels similar to those prior to the patient's medical problem. Of course, functionality is related to the environment in which the patient will be placed and this will help to determine the focus of language treatment. In addition, family involvement should be a strong consideration when implementing this language treatment program.

As with most communicative disorders, the results of the diagnostic evaluation should serve as the foundation for treatment planning. The SLP is going to note the patient's strengths and weaknesses and then design a program to meet the patient's needs. A typical approach to treatment will focus on the patient and the patient's family and environment in which the patient will function. Treatment can be focused on three different but related areas. The clinician can work on stimulating those functions that have been impacted by the trauma and helping the brain to reorganize functions. As a result, we might observe Michael, a speech–language pathologist, working in a rehab setting with a patient, Mrs. Green, who has difficulty naming objects. During therapy Michael might recognize that Mrs. Green has difficulty naming common household objects. As a result, Michael would design a language activity with related objects such as a fork, spoon, and knife, and develop various comprehension and expressive tasks in which Mrs. Green is encouraged to name the objects in response to sentences like "We cut with a _____?" while the clinician holds up a knife. This task might be followed by the sentence "We eat with a _____?" while the clinician holds up a fork. The speech–language pathologist is working to help stimulate the patient's language abilities by working with similar objects that might be found at a common location within the home. In addition, the speech–language pathologist is addressing both the client's strength, receptive language, and the client's weaker area, expressive language, at the same time using visual stimulation to help the client to name the object.

Secondly, the patient can be taught a variety of compensatory strategies that are directly related to those functions that might be impaired. For example, a patient may have difficultly requesting specific objects. During therapy the clinician might work with this patient and also include family members to demonstrate the use of less specific but descriptive language to identify the object that is requested. As the patient, Jerry, is getting dressed, he wants to put on his watch but is unable to locate it. Jerry says to his wife, "Where is my . . . the thing I use to tell time?" In this example Jerry is able to effectively communicate to his wife despite the fact that he cannot specifically say the word *watch*. When the patient has difficulty coming up with the name for the object he wants, or the date of a family event, or the name of the family pet, the clinician would encourage the patient to describe the characteristics of the object or where the event might be located so that he would be able to communicate but not be impeded by his inability to come up with a specific word. A third component of treatment includes family members and friends in an attempt to help the patient maintain a satisfactory quality of life outside of the hospital or therapy room. In order for a patient to succeed outside of the therapy room, it will be important for family members to be willing participants in the patient's therapy and make necessary adjustments at home so that the patient will be able to function better with any limitations associated with the disability. Family members will need to be educated about the nature of the patient's problems and provided with strategies for dealing with the patient's difficulties. By observing and interacting with the clinician, family members can learn what skills need to be emphasized outside of the therapy room. It would not be unusual for a spouse of the patient or children of the patient to sit in on therapy and observe the clinician working with the patient. In addition, family members may meet separately with the clinician to learn how to modify their own communication when interacting with their spouse or learn suggestions that can be provided to other family members during larger family events. Because communication is impaired, patients may consciously isolate themselves from friends and relatives. When family members recognize this type of behavior, they can make an effort to create situations at home that encourage communication or even consider family participation in a local stroke club where family members and patients get together on a regular basis to socialize, discuss common problems, and gather additional objective information from professionals who might participate in the group.

IN THE CLINIC

Sarah Reed is a speech–language pathologist working in the acute-care wing of a large city hospital. Sarah is often called on to evaluate patients within a few days of being admitted into the hospital. During a recent visit to see Mr. Garcia, a patient who experienced a stroke in his right cerebral hemisphere, Mrs. Garcia calls Sarah aside and explains, "My husband's speech sounds like it always did and he also seems to understand everything that I'm saying; however when the kids are around and we're all talking, my husband is always interrupting and won't let anyone finish." Mrs. Garcia sighs in frustration and says, "He's just not the same." Sarah explains that the right-hemisphere damage that Mr. Garcia experienced has caused some subtle changes in his brain, resulting in behavioral changes. Through therapy that includes counseling, the Garcias will have to learn to deal with these changes, while at the same time Mr. Garcia may have to be instructed in the changes perceived by family members so that acceptable adjustments can be made within the family structure.

RIGHT-HEMISPHERE BRAIN DAMAGE AND COMMUNICATIVE DISORDERS

Prior to this point, we have focused on language problems associated with damage to the left cerebral hemisphere. However, *right-hemisphere brain damage* (RHD) often results in a variety of language-related and non-language-related problems.

However, unlike the language disorders associated with damage to the left cerebral hemisphere, RHD often results in less specific and more diffuse types of problems. In fact, many of the deficits that are noted may be found within the general population, and although these might be looked at as odd and even sometimes inappropriate, they are characteristics of many people. The big difference is that for the patient with RHD, these problems did not exist prior to the stroke or head injury. We often refer to these problems as *cognitive–communicative problems*.

It is common for the patient with RHD to exhibit language difficulties associated with pragmatics, maintaining attention, problem solving, reasoning, and organization. As we described with Mr. Garcia, he lacks the ability to monitor his own speech and fails to respond appropriately during conversational interaction with a number of individuals.

In general, patients with RHD appear to have difficulties in three areas that we can describe as being distinctive, but in reality these deficits often overlap and interact with one another. These categories are communication, attention and perception, and cognition (Blake, 2005). Examples of communication problems noted in patients with RHD include difficulties with idioms and making inferences. Mrs. Weinstein has just returned home from the hospital and is scheduled for speech therapy for RHD. Mr. Weinstein tells his wife that he's just received a bill from the hospital and there's a problem; however, "I don't want to rock the boat until you begin your therapy." Mrs. Weinstein replies that she "didn't know that they owned a boat." In this case, the patient with RHD has trouble with the meaning of the idiom and takes a literal interpretation. Communication problems also arise relative to the pragmatics of languages. Adults with RHD take fewer turns during conversation and often talk more about themselves when compared to typical, healthy adults. Subtle aspects of language will also be affected. Individuals with RHD will have trouble understanding jokes but will have no difficulty with physical or slapstick humor. Aspects of language like sarcasm and identifying a lie may also be difficult for the patient with RHD.

In addition to communication problems, patients with RHD often experience difficulties with attention and perception. Our ability to focus on a specific task and filter out unnecessary distractions is called *attention*. As attention serves as the background behavior that enables us to focus on a communicative situation to comprehend language and ultimately communicate with other individuals, a deficit in attention is going to also impact our ability to communicate. Patients who are easily distracted may have difficulty with a variety of different tasks. A very common deficit of attention in patients with RHD is *left neglect*. As attention requires the person to pay attention to sensory stimuli in the form of vision, hearing, taste, and touch, any damage that prevents the brain from processing this sensory information can lead to left neglect. Neglect typically affects the side of the body that is opposite to the site of the brain damage, and left neglect is a common problem associated with RHD. For example, a patient with RHD may experience sensory neglect on the left side of his or her body. One of the more common types of neglect has to do with the visual system. Patients with neglect may ignore writing that appears in their left visual field as their brain is not interpreting the information. In a similar manner a patient may not be aware that a family member is in the room when that family member is standing or sitting to the left side of the patient. Perceptual problems associated with RHD damage are often associated with reading and writing. Patients may have difficulty correctly perceiving letters and words, may exhibit organizational problems while writing, and may misperceive or misinterpret objects within a picture.

The third category that is affected by RHD is *cognition.* Cognition tends to include a person's ability to sequence, reason, and solve problems. You will recognize that the tasks associated with cognition are integral to our previous discussions of language impairment, attention, and perception. As a result, it is difficult to talk about cognitive deficits without including other aspects of the patient's problem. When we ask a patient to follow a multistage command and the patient has difficulty, the problem might be a combination of language comprehension, memory deficits, and organizational deficits. As most SLPs will attempt to determine the patient's communicative abilities, attempts to isolate cognitive impairment from language impairment is typically not done. The clinician will attempt to determine a patient's overall level of functioning and then develop a plan of treatment to improve the patient's functional skills.

TRAUMATIC BRAIN INJURY

Traumatic brain injury (TBI) has also been called acquired brain injury or simply head injury. These type of problems occur as a result of a sudden trauma (e.g., falling off a skateboard and hitting your head on the pavement) or the piercing of the skull by a foreign object (e.g., a gunshot). We typically note TBI associated with motor-vehicle accidents, professional football, war injuries, and a number of other traumas. Summary statistics regarding TBI are given in Table 7.1.

Persons with mild TBI sometimes lose consciousness and may experience confusion and disorientation. In the past, this injury was often referred to as a concussion. For many patients with mild TBI, symptoms are often transient and recovery is complete, with little effect noted following the injury. However, there is some growing concern regarding the cumulative effects of concussion and its long-term impact on the patient's memory, attention, and ability to concentrate. Patients with more severe TBI may experience medical symptoms for a year following the injury that include headaches, fatigue, sleep disturbances, and memory loss.

TABLE 7.1
Facts about traumatic brain injury

---

1. Traumatic brain injury is the leading cause of death and disability in children and adults from ages 1 to 44.
2. Brain injuries are most often caused by motor vehicle crashes, sports injuries, or even simple falls on the playground, at work, or in the home.
3. Blasts are a leading cause of TBI among active-duty military personnel in war zones.
4. An estimated 1.6 million to 3.8 million sports-related TBIs occur each year.
5. Veterans' advocates believe that between 10% and 20% of Iraq veterans, or between 150,000 and 300,000 service members, have some level of TBI.

Source: Statistics retrieved from the Brain Trauma Foundation's Web site, https://www.braintrauma .org/tbi-faqs/tbi-statistics, on December 1, 2010.

In addition, patients with more severe TBI may exhibit aphasia and problems with memory, cognition, and attention.

Common causes of TBI include falls and motor-vehicle crashes. In a typical crash, the head is thrust forward and stopped suddenly by the dashboard or windshield, resulting in damage to the brain. In the case of gunshots and direct trauma to the skull, problems arise because of direct damage to a specific area of the brain. This type of injury is very similar to those previously described with patients who have experienced strokes. However, for the majority of people with TBI, the associated injuries are diffuse and often affect a variety of language and cognitive functions.

It is often easier to grasp the idea of a direct trauma to the brain resulting in aphasia, as diffuse problems (e.g., attention or memory) associated with many traumatic injuries are much more difficult to explain. It is likely that the presence of these diffuse problems will affect a person's attention, information, and cognition (Adamovitch, 2005). However, our ability to identify the nature of the problems comes about when a patient cannot complete an activity that was routine prior to the injury. If we examine the real-life example in the example to follow, we will note how diffuse problems might be identified and treated.

I CAN'T DO THIS ALONE

Matt is a Marine sergeant who has recently returned from Iraq after his truck hit a roadside explosive device. While Matt did not sustain any loss of limbs, he did suffer a head injury that left him hospitalized for a number of months. One of Matt's nurses, Nicole, noted that Matt seemed to have intact language skills but had difficulty getting dressed. As activities of daily living are often dealt with by the occupational therapist, Matt was referred for occupational therapy. Corey, the occupational therapist, noted that Matt understood the need to get dressed, and also had the physical abilities to get dressed. However, Matt was still unable to complete this important activity. As a result, Matt was referred to Lilli, the speech–language pathologist who deals with patients who experience traumatic brain injury. Through testing, Lilli determined that Matt exhibited organizational difficulties that prevented him from getting dressed and completing many other activities that required memory and sequencing. As Lilli realized that many of these activities were functional skills that Matt would have to acquire before being discharged from the hospital, she discussed these issues with Corey to develop a plan to help Matt learn to compensate for his difficulties. Lilli developed a number of sequential activity cards that listed written instructions and small photographs so that Matt could use these visual references to deal with his deficits. Lilli shared these cards with Corey, who was helping to retrain Matt regarding many of the activities of daily living that required sequencing and organizational skills. In this example, the nursing staff was the front line for helping to identify the patient's problem while the speech–language pathologist worked closely with the occupational therapist to help the patient learn to compensate for his difficulties.

Patients with TBI often exhibit a wide range of deficits, from those that minimally affect their day-to-day functioning to severe deficits that make functioning very difficult. A patient with TBI may receive therapy from a number of professionals including occupational therapists, physical therapists, speech–language pathologists, and psychologists. As the deficits associated with TBI often require lifestyle modifications the patient, in conjunction with his or her therapists, learns to deal with the problem and attempts to move forward with life.

DEMENTIA

According to the American Psychiatric Association (2000), dementia is defined as an impairment of short- and long-term memory with related changes in abstract thinking, judgment, and personality that causes significant social and occupational impairment. It is known that dementia may be caused by a variety of chronic disorders of the brain. These can include Alzheimer's disease, Pick's disease (shrinking of the frontal and temporal lobes of the brain), multiple strokes, and other brain disorders such as TBI. Dementia may also be caused by endocrine disorders such as diabetes. When symptoms related to impaired language, memory, cognition, and even personality changes first appear, these might be associated with a variety of

I CAN'T DO THIS ALONE

Eric received a long distance call one day that his father, Larry, who lived alone, had not arrived at work. Eric thought that his father was experiencing some memory loss but assumed that this was a normal part of aging. Eric routinely spoke on a weekly basis with his father, but these conversations generally focused on social conversation, the weather, and his father's health. As Eric had not visited his father in a while, he decided that a plane trip was necessary. When Eric arrived at his father's condo, he noticed that food was not being put away in the refrigerator, garbage was not being removed, and his father's personal hygiene had deteriorated. When discussing these issues with his father, Eric's dad was unaware that anything had changed and didn't think there was a problem. When Eric questioned his dad regarding getting lost on the way to work, his dad was unable to remember a problem. As Eric began wondering about his dad's memory and language skills, he started asking his dad some questions. He asked his dad where he had grown up, where he went to high school, and what he did during World War II. Larry was able to answer these questions with no problem. When Eric asked his father what he had eaten for dinner, Larry was unable to respond. When Eric asked his father to tell him why Eric was in the condo, Larry was unable to respond. As it was obvious that Larry was exhibiting early signs of dementia, Eric decided that he needed to have his father evaluated so that management plans could be made to ensure that Larry did not make decisions that would negatively affect his well-being.

conditions that might not be dementia. When it is determined that the symptoms exhibited a gradual onset, it is likely that the patient's problems are dementia related. The sudden onsets of a patient's problems are more typically associated with strokes or sudden brain injuries. For the physician, discussions with speech–language pathologists, occupational therapists, and physical therapists and conversations with family members can provide important details regarding the nature of the patient's problem.

MOTOR SPEECH DISORDERS

Although neurological impairment of the brain can result in a variety of language disorders, it is important to recognize that neurological impairment can also result in damage to those areas of the central nervous system or peripheral nervous system that are associated with speech production. Neurological impairment that affects the muscles responsible for speech production or the areas of the brain responsible for speech programming (e.g., Broca's area) results in a *motor speech disorder* and affects the patient's ability to verbally communicate.

Dysarthria

Dysarthria is a motor speech disorder resulting from paralysis, weakness, or incoordination of the speech musculature that is of neurological origin (Darley, Aronson, & Brown, 1969). As you might imagine, when a patient's ability to transmit movement information to any of the three systems involved in speech production is impaired, a breakdown in speech production will occur. It is not hard to imagine that the patient who has weakness in his right arm and right leg will also have right-sided muscular weakness in the articulators, as well as laryngeal and respiratory muscles. As a result, we are going to see patients who have difficulty providing respiratory support for speech, or difficulty articulating sounds and words, or difficulty coordinating the articulators, resulting in slurred and hypernasal speech.

For many patients with damage in their language-dominant hemisphere, it is very common to also have dysarthria that is characterized by continuously contracted muscles. *Spastic dysarthria* results in slurred speech, a slower speech rate, hypernasality, and a strained or strangled vocal quality. In contrast, a patient with muscular dystrophy (a progressive degenerative disease) will have weak and flabby muscle tone that affects the three systems required for speech, resulting in a flaccid dysarthria. Damage to the cerebellum often results in muscular weakness and difficulty with coordination. The speech of a person with cerebellar problems is called *ataxic dysarthria* and is characterized by vowel distortions and irregular articulatory breakdowns. As the cerebellum contributes to a patient's ability to coordinate his or her muscles, it is not surprising to see these irregular articulatory breakdowns. The patient may also exhibit a slower rate of speech. In addition, the patient may put excessive stress on specific words in a sentence and these may not always be appropriate.

There are a number of disorders where excessive movement may be observed. Chorea is a disorder of excessive movement; a major disease group is called Huntington's chorea. You may recall that the famed folk singer and activist Woody Guthrie ("This land is your land") died from complications associated with Huntington's chorea. A patient with chorea exhibits frequent irregular rapid movements that may affect the speech muscles, limbs, or the entire body. *Hyperkinetic dysarthria* is the speech disorder associated with chorea. In contrast to hyperkinetic dysarthria, a patient who exhibits slower movements or lack of appropriate movement due to muscle rigidity and stiffness will probably exhibit *hypokinetic dysarthria*. Parkinson's disease results in muscle rigidity, stiffness, and an inability to move quickly. The reader may be familiar with the former heavyweight boxing champion Muhammad Ali or noted actor Michael J. Fox as two individuals with Parkinson's disease. As Parkinson's disease is progressive, the speech characteristics of these patients change as the disease changes. These patients often exhibit a hoarse vocal quality and may demonstrate a tremor in their voice. Maintaining vocal intensity is an issue and the patient may also exhibit a fast speaking rate. Finally, it is also possible for a patient to exhibit characteristics of both flaccid and spastic dysarthria, which results in *mixed dysarthria*. In a disease like amyotrophic lateral sclerosis (ALS), commonly referred to as Lou Gehrig's disease (Lou Gehrig was a famous baseball player who died from complications of the disease), patients often exhibit characteristics of both flaccid and spastic dysarthria because the disease attacks the body in a way that results in weakened flaccid muscles in one system while causing spasticity in another system. Noted mathematician and physicist Stephen Hawking (http://www.hawking.org.uk/index.php/disability) has ALS and at this time is unable to verbally communicate.

Apraxia of Speech

Apraxia of speech is a disorder that results in a patient's difficulty or inability to produce learned speech movements. This difficulty occurs in the absence of weakness or paralysis of the speech muscles. Verbal apraxia has been called a disorder of motor planning or programming. The patient may look like he has been physically unaffected by the neurological problem; however, when he attempts to speak, the production of words and sentences may be difficult. The characteristics of apraxia may include difficulty initiating speech and, in extreme cases, difficulty phonating. In addition, these patients have difficulty imitating movements such as protruding their tongue. A speech–language pathologist may ask the patient to lick his lips and the patient fails to respond. However, when a dab of peanut butter is placed on the patient's lips, he licks it off with no problem. The difficulty is associated with initiating and programming the muscles. Additional speech problems include a slow speech rate, distortions of sounds, and inconsistent sound errors. To the observer, the speech of these patients will appear hesitant, interrupted, and not fluent. For these patients, longer words are usually more difficult to produce than shorter words. The patient may have difficulty initiating the word *where* when asking a question and yet 5 minutes later be able to say the word with no difficulty.

> *Quiz on the Fly 7.2*
>
> 1. Hitting your head against a car dashboard or being knocked unconscious during a football game often results in _____.
> 2. Impairment of short- and long-term memory with related changes in abstract thinking, judgment, and personality is _____.
> 3. What is a motor speech disorder with symptoms that include slurred speech and hypernasality? _____
> 4. Low muscle tone is often associated with which motor speech disorder? _____
> 5. What is a motor speech disorder that causes speech motor planning or programming difficulties? _____

TREATMENT OF MOTOR SPEECH DISORDERS

Although the symptoms of motor speech disorders are quite varied, the goal of any treatment program is going to be achieving functional communication. For many clients, the speech–language pathologist will work with the patient to help restore some of the functions that were lost because of the neurological problems. As dysarthria is a weakness in the muscles responsible for speech, the clinicians will work on a variety of activities to help the patient to restore some of the strength in those weakened muscles. You can easily imagine a physical therapist working with a stroke patient to lift weights to strengthen arm muscles, but you may wonder how the speech–language pathologist helps the patient with dysarthria. The answer is not attaching weights to the patient's tongue or lips to increase strength. The speech–language pathologist will design a number of speech production tasks that begin with simple requirements like naming pictures from a magazine or family photo album. In this way, the clinician is trying to help the patient to reestablish communication from the brain to the speech muscles and improve the strength of those muscles. Obviously, the more opportunities that the patient has to repeat words, the better chance the patient has for speech improvement.

For the apraxic patient, the clinician will work on repetition of words in an effort to help the patient overcome or compensate for the deficits in speech motor programming. Remember that these patients do not have muscular weakness; the goal of therapy is not to strengthen speech muscles but to reestablish the patient's ability to more easily initiate sentence production and more fluently produce sentences. However, it is also recognized by the clinician that, depending upon the nature of the neurological impairment, some patients may exhibit limited success in therapy, but other patients will be extremely successful and appear to fully restore their speech to previous levels. For patients whose restoration of speech is extremely limited, other forms of communication may be necessary; the speech–language pathologist may decide to recommend augmentative or alternative communication systems. These systems can range from low-tech use of pictures and symbols to represent objects or patient's needs to voice output devices and computer programs that can be programmed to talk for the patient.

SUMMARY AND REVIEW

The focus of this chapter has been an examination of speech and language disorders associated with neurological impairment. We began our discussion with an examination of the brain anatomy associated with speech and language production. After completing our discussion of the neurological anatomy required for normal speech and language functioning, we examined language deficits associated with neurological impairment. As part of this discussion we examined assessment and treatment of these language deficits. In addition to a discussion of language deficits that typically result from damage to the left side of the brain, we discussed language and cognitive deficits associated with right-hemisphere damage and TBI. This was followed by a discussion of dementia and motor speech disorders associated with neurological impairment. We explored a variety of different types of dysarthria and finished with a discussion of speech motor planning or programming problems associated with verbal apraxia. We concluded this chapter with a section on the treatment of motor speech disorders.

Brain Anatomy Associated with Speech and Language Disorders

What are the major language areas and major speech areas of the brain?

For the majority of the population, the major language centers can be found within the left cerebral hemisphere. The major language area of the brain, Wernicke's area, can be found in the temporal lobe and is primarily responsible for language comprehension and the formulation of language concepts. The major speech area of the brain, Broca's area, is located in the frontal lobe, at the bottom and anterior to the primary motor strip. Broca's area is related to speech motor programming and the production of expressive speech and language.

Quiz on the Fly 7.2 Answers

1. Hitting your head against a car dashboard or being knocked unconscious during a football game often results in **traumatic brain injury**. **2.** Impairment of short- and long-term memory with related changes in abstract thinking, judgment, and personality is **dementia**. **3.** What is a motor speech disorder with symptoms that include slurred speech and hypernasality? **spastic dysarthria 4.** Low muscle tone is often associated with which motor speech disorder? **flaccid dysarthria 5.** What is a motor speech disorder that causes speech motor planning or programming difficulties? **verbal apraxia**

Language Disorders Associated with Neurological Impairment

What is a language disorder that occurs as a result of neurological impairment?

Aphasia is the loss of the ability to comprehend or formulate language following neurological impairment. Individuals with aphasia may exhibit problems with understanding language, producing language, or both areas. Deficits are not only restricted to oral language but may be found in writing and reading as well.

Aphasia Classification

What are some classifications for aphasia?

A patient with aphasia may exhibit expressive speech and language that is viewed to be nonfluent or fluent. Broca's aphasia results in nonfluent speech that often lacks the language structures that enable the sentence to sound complete. Wernicke's aphasia is viewed to be a fluent aphasia as the prosody, rate, and rhythm of speech remain intact, although the content of the patient's language is often significantly impaired.

Assessment of Language Disorders Associated with Neurological Impairment

What is the focus of an assessment for a patient with a neurologically related language disorder?

The focus of this assessment is to determine the patient's strengths and weaknesses so that a management and treatment program can be developed. The assessment process begins at the patient's bedside to first establish a baseline of performance, and then further testing will be completed to determine the patient's receptive and expressive language skills, including reading and writing. The examination will also focus on the patient's speech skills to determine the presence of any motor speech disorders.

Treatment of Language Disorders Associated with Neurological Impairment

What is the focus of treatment for a patient with a neurologically related language disorder?

The focus of language therapy is to help the patient return to a level of functional communication and reestablish damaged neural pathways. Patients are taught compensatory strategies to help overcome some of their deficits, and family members are included in the process so that improvements in communication can take place both within the therapy room and at home.

Right-Hemisphere Brain Damage and Communicative Disorders

What are the problems associated with right-hemisphere damage (RHD)?

Right-hemisphere damage often results in less specific and more diffuse types of language difficulties and other types of difficulties that are different from those associated with damage to the language areas. Patients with RHD may exhibit difficulties in communication, attention and perception, and cognition. Subtle changes during conversational interaction may be observed. These patients may lose some of their ability to concentrate on a specific task for a period of time and often show signs of visual or sensory neglect. Problem solving and decreased organizational skills might also characterize these patients.

Traumatic Brain Injury

What is traumatic brain injury and what are its symptoms?

A sudden trauma to the head or the piercing of the skull by a foreign object results in a traumatic brain injury. These traumas are associated with sports injuries, accidents, and gunshot wounds. While many of these patients may experience aphasia, it is more likely that these patients experience more diffuse problems with attention, information, and cognition.

Dementia

What are the characteristics of dementia and what can cause it?

Dementia has been defined as memory impairment with related changes in abstract thinking, judgment, and personality. Disorders such as Alzheimer's disease, Pick's disease, multiple strokes, TBI, and endocrine disorders such as diabetes can result in dementia.

Motor Speech Disorders

What is a motor speech disorder?

Neurological impairment that affects the muscles responsible for speech production or the areas of the brain responsible for speech programming results in a motor speech disorder. *Dysarthria* is a motor speech disorder resulting from paralysis, weakness, or incoordination of the speech musculature that is of neurological origin. Depending upon the nature of the neurological impairment, a patient may exhibit a variety of different speech symptoms that range from slurred or imprecise consonant production to hypernasality to impaired respiratory support for phonation. Apraxia of speech is a motor speech disorder that results in a patient's difficulty or inability to produce learned speech movements.

Treatment of Motor Speech Disorders

What is the goal of treatment for motor speech disorders?

The goal of treatment is to help the patient to develop functional communication skills by working with the client to increase strength to those weakened speech muscles, teaching the client how to improve sound and word production, and teaching the client how to compensate for deficits that have occurred.

WEB SITES OF INTEREST

BrainLine
http://www.BrainLine.org

Brain Trauma Foundation
http://www.braintrauma.org

Internet Stroke Center
Washington University, St. Louis
http://www.strokecenter.org

National Institute on Aging
Progress Report on Alzheimer's Disease 2009
http://www.nia.nih.gov/Alzheimers/Publications/ADProgress2009/

NINDS Traumatic Brain Injury Information Page
http://www.ninds.nih.gov/disorders/tbi/tbi.htm

Stephen Hawking Discussing His Disability
http://www.hawking.org.uk/index.php/disability

8

Voice Disorders

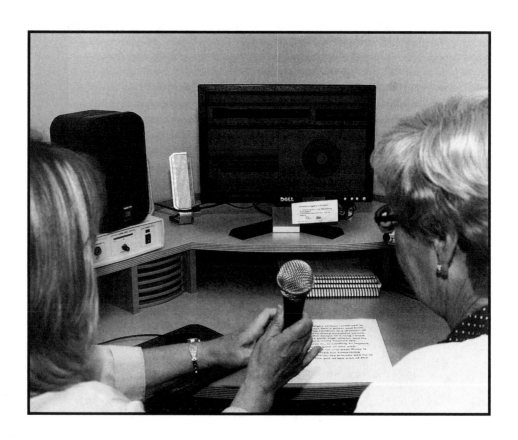

While many lay people are aware that speech–language pathologists work with children who misarticulate sounds and adults who have lost their language because of strokes, fewer people are aware that speech–language pathologists work with children and adults who experience problems with their vocal mechanism. This chapter will focus on reintroducing the reader to the voice production mechanism, including the workings of the vocal folds. With this knowledge, we will move on to discuss the characteristics of normal voice production. Having this background in normal functioning, we will then explore voice disorders associated with tissue changes to the larynx, voice disorders associated with neurological problems, and voice problems associated with laryngeal cancer. The next sections will focus on a discussion of voice evaluations conducted by an *otolaryngologist* (a doctor who specializes in the ear [oto-] and the larynx [-laryngologist]) and speech–language pathologist, including a discussion on viewing the larynx. The last section of this chapter will focus on voice therapy, specifically on treating persons who frequently use their voice (e.g., teachers) and a second discussion on treating persons who have had their larynx removed because of cancer.

ANATOMY OF VOICE PRODUCTION

In our discussion of the anatomy of phonation in chapter 2, we described the cartilaginous structures of the larynx. In the front of the body we have the large *thyroid* cartilage that sits atop the *cricoid* cartilage (see Figure 8.1A). At the back of the larynx we find the *arytenoid* cartilages sitting upon the cricoid cartilage (see Figure 8.1B). The cartilaginous structures serve to protect the vocal folds and serve as anchor points for the origin and insertion of the muscles responsible for producing sound. The vocal folds, which are actually the thyroarytenoid muscle, attach to the backside of the thyroid cartilage (located facing the front of your body). Toward the back of your body, the vocal folds attach to two protrusions on the arytenoid cartilages (see Figure 8.1B). As we have previously discussed, the vocal folds open and close as we breathe and produce sound. These same vocal folds rapidly vibrate when producing voiced sounds.

The complex structure of our vocal folds enables us to make a variety of vocal changes. Have you considered that within a short period of time you can go from singing "Happy Birthday" to talking with your colleagues to imitating your family dog, all by changing the shape and tension of your vocal folds? In addition, to best understand the breakdowns that occur within the voice production system, we first need to examine the complex structure of the vocal folds. The vocal folds are actually a multilayered structure. As can be seen in Figure 8.2, these layers include an

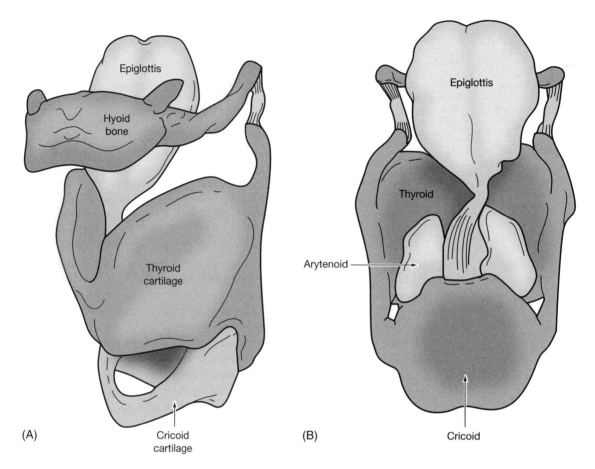

FIGURE 8.1
(A) Anterior view of the laryngeal cartilages and (B) posterior view of the laryngeal cartilages.

outside layer like the skin inside of your mouth (epithelial layer). The middle structures consist of a Jell-O-like layer, a rubber-band layer, and a cotton-string layer
(also known as the Lamina Propria). Finally the bulk of the vocal folds is made up
of the thyroarytenoid muscle. It is the relationship between the outer layers of the
vocal folds, the cover (epithelial layer, Jell-O-like, rubber-band layer) interacting
with the cotton-string layer, and the thyroarytenoid muscle (the body) that enables
us to produce our normal-sounding voice. When changes occur to these structures,
we first perceive a difference in the person's voice and then perhaps the presence
of a problem. In the next section, we will examine the characteristics of the normal
voice and then move on to a discussion of different types of voice problems.

CHARACTERISTICS OF VOICE PRODUCTION

In order for us to describe the characteristics of an abnormal voice, we first have to
identify those characteristics of a normal voice. When we describe a person's voice,
we can examine vocal characteristics on a perceptual level and relate these

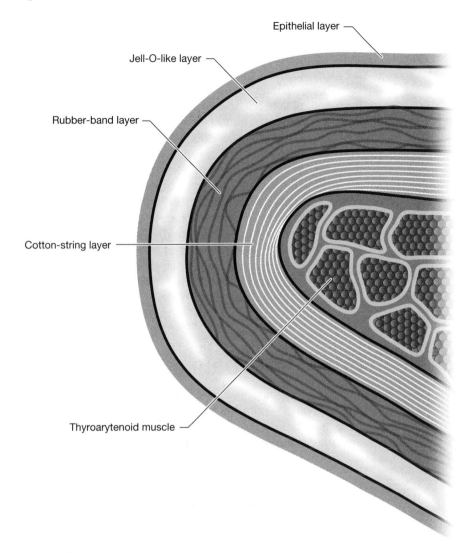

Epithelial layer

Jell-O-like layer

Rubber-band layer

Cotton-string layer

Thyroarytenoid muscle

FIGURE 8.2
The complex, multilayered vocal folds.

characteristics to the underlying physiological properties that are required to produce voice. The first characteristic that we will describe is *pitch*. Pitch is related to the number of vocal-fold vibrations produced within a given period of time. If we asked an individual to take a breath and sustain the /ɑ/ sound, we could use a computer program to calculate the average number of times that the person's vocal folds vibrated per second. This figure varies from individual to individual and is known as *fundamental frequency*. Fundamental frequency varies as a function of vocal-fold thickness and length. As described in chapter 2, a male has an average fundamental frequency of vibration of 125 cycles per second (Hertz, or Hz, is used to identify cycles per second), females average 225 Hz to 250 Hz, and children produce sounds as fast as 400 Hz.

When individuals have problems with their voice, we may characterize their pitch as too low or too high. The second characteristic of the voice is *loudness*. Like pitch, loudness is a perceptual characteristic of an underlying physiological property. Intensity is the physiological property, and it is associated with the amount of subglottal air pressure that is built up prior to producing sounds, the degree of vocal-fold tensing, and the length of time associated with vocal-fold adduction. For some persons we might describe their voice as too loud or too soft. The third characteristic of the voice is *resonance*. Resonance is associated with how the sound produced by the vocal folds vibrates in the pharyngeal, oral, and nasal cavities. Depending upon where the sounds resonate, we might describe a person's voice as nasal; hypernasal (too much resonance in the nose); or we might say, "He sounds like he has a cold" (denasal, or hyponasal), suggesting that there is not enough resonance associated with his voice. The fourth characteristic of the voice is *vocal quality*. Vocal quality is associated with resonance and laryngeal tension. When a person uses his or her voice with too much laryngeal tension, we might say that person's voice is rough or breathy. It is often excessive use of the voice and associated tension that result in changes in vocal quality. Given these descriptions of the normal characteristics of voice, we can begin our examination of voice disorders.

DEFINITIONS AND PREVALENCE OF VOICE DISORDERS

To begin our discussion of voice disorders, we have to recognize that voice disorders are perceptual events that are identified by a speech–language pathologist or an ear, nose, and throat (ENT) specialist (otolaryngologist). While it is possible to measure the frequency of vocal-fold vibration or the intensity of the vocal output, the determination of normal versus abnormal voice is made when all of the perceptual factors come together to produce the unique vocal characteristics of the individual. Upon hearing the person's voice, the listener makes a determination regarding the person's voice. As a result, we have a number of definitions of voice disorders that relate to our perception of the characteristics of the individual voice. Aronson (1985, p. 7) reported that "a voice disorder exists when quality, pitch, loudness or flexibility differs from the voices of others of similar age, sex, and cultural group." Boone, McFarlane, and Von Berg (2005) stated that voice disorders result from faulty processes of respiration, phonation, or resonance, and, like Aronson, stated that when one or more aspects of voice such as loudness, pitch, quality, or resonance are outside of the normal range for the age, gender, or geographic background of the speaker, we say a voice disorder exists. According to ASHA (1993), "a voice disorder is characterized by the abnormal production and/or absences of vocal quality, pitch, loudness, resonance, and/or duration, which is inappropriate for an individual's age and/or sex."

Voice disorders occur across the life span, affecting children and adults, and are often related to occupations and gender. Ramig and Verdolini (1998) summarized a number of studies of voice disorders and reported that in school-age children, 3% to 6% exhibited voice disorders. According to these same authors, 3% to 9% of the entire population have a voice disorder. The *prevalence* (how many people exhibit the problem at any one time) of voice disorders among teachers has been investigated, and teachers exhibited almost double the number of voice problems compared to nonteachers, both at the specific time of testing and during the course of their lifetime. It was also determined in the same study that women exhibited greater numbers of voice problems compared to men. Ramig and Verdolini (1998), quoting statistics from the National Center on Voice, reported that 24% of the U.S. population have jobs that "critically require" voice use. Given these statistics, we begin to recognize that, for many people, a healthy voice has economic and communicative implications. In the section to follow we will examine how voice disorders are classified and begin to examine these disorders.

Quiz on the Fly 8.1

1. The physiological correlate of intensity is _____.
2. The perceptual correlate of fundamental frequency is _____.
3. The three major cartilages of the larynx are _____, _____, and _____.
4. The number of people who exhibit a problem at a specific time is called _____.
5. The innermost layer of the vocal folds is the _____ muscle.

CLASSIFYING VOICE DISORDERS

In this section we are going to divide voice disorders according to etiology, or causation. We are going to use three umbrella categories to identify these voice problems and then describe the problem within the context of its etiology. The three etiological classifications are: (1) *phonotrauma* (Verdolini, 1999), or disorders associated with misusing and overusing the vocal mechanism; (2) neurological disorders; and (3) organic disease, or problems originating within the body resulting in structural changes to tissue and organs.

Phonotrauma

The frequency and intensity with which a person uses his or her voice has a direct impact on the occurrence of voice problems. However, it is important to recognize that there is a lot of variability from person to person, and this variability can result in a voice problem for one person but not a second person, even if he or she exhibits many of the same behaviors. The problems we will discuss not only relate to the behaviors exhibited by the individual but also the person's biological makeup.

The term *phonotrauma* suggests a relationship between vocal behavior, changes in laryngeal tissue, and the resulting voice problems that some people may experience. Traditionally, terms like *vocal misuse* and *vocal abuse* have been used to describe these relationships, although the use of phonotrauma better describes changes that occur to the larynx as a result of the person's behavior. When we discuss the results of phonotrauma, we will see that the inappropriate vocal behaviors that are exhibited are often lead to changes in laryngeal tissue that will be perceived as changes in the person's voice.

Phonotrauma is an umbrella term that encompasses a lot of different types of vocal behaviors. As previously noted, many individuals may exhibit inappropriate vocal behaviors that have no effect on voice production. However, for some individuals, these inappropriate behaviors will ultimately result in vocal-fold tissue changes and a subsequent change in their voice. A classroom teacher may exhibit abrupt, hard starts to her speech, especially when initiating vowel sounds. This type of behavior has been termed *hard glottal attack* and can lead to changes in laryngeal tissue and more chronic problems. *Puberphonia* has been noted in some males who have gone through puberty but continue to use their higher pitched voice. The problem has been related to both emotional and physical issues. *Persistent glottal fry* is a vocal behavior exhibited by some individuals and has been described as the sound of corn popping or the sound of a motorboat engine. Although most speakers will on some occasion exhibit vocal fry, this behavior is viewed to be an inappropriate vocal quality when the speaker is using this behavior all of the time. Although glottal fry is occasionally heard as part of normal voice production, some individuals consistently use this mode of voice and often complain about vocal fatigue and a monotone voice. For some individuals, it is possible to talk continuously for 3 hours on their mobile phone with little to no impact on their vocal mechanism. For others, 3 hours of continuous talking results in vocal fatigue, a rough or hoarse vocal quality, or even a weaker voice. In many individuals, *excessive talking* results in changes in voice production.

In the section to follow, many of the behaviors that will be described will be labeled vocal abuse because of the manner in which the individual uses his or her vocal mechanism. Excessive and prolonged loudness of the voice is often associated with a number of jobs and activities. Teachers are often faced with classroom situations where they need to get the attention of a student or a group of students. Instead of walking up to the student and speaking at a normal loudness level, the teacher chooses to yell across the room to get the student's attention. An aerobics instructor is conducting a step class but the microphone is not working properly, so the instructor decides to lead the class while attempting to talk louder than the music. Individuals who work in noisy environments or environments that require loud voices include factory workers, teachers, sports coaches, clergy, and aerobics instructors. To produce this loud voice, individuals have to increase the tension in their vocal folds, increase subglottal air pressure, and more forcefully explode the vocal folds. Maintaining loudness for an extended period of time can have a detrimental effect on vocal-fold functioning. In addition to excessive loudness, there are a number of other behaviors that are viewed to be abusive to the vocal mechanism, as illustrated by the

---

Quiz on the Fly 8.1 Answers

1. The physiological correlate of intensity is **loudness**. **2.** The perceptual correlate of fundamental frequency is **pitch**. **3.** The three major cartilages of the larynx are **thyroid**, **cricoid**, and **arytenoid**. **4.** The number of people who exhibit a problem at a specific time is called **prevalence**. **5.** The innermost layer of the vocal folds is the **thyroarytenoid** muscle.

following: children who scream excessively, people who attend sporting events who yell and scream for their favorite team, some individuals who participate in sporting events and yell to their teammates, and those individuals who experience some mild form of hoarseness who believe that it's necessary to talk louder to compensate for their weakened voice. As a result of the aforementioned behaviors, individuals often experience vocal-fold tissue changes in association with these behaviors. In the section to follow, the changes that can occur will be described.

Phonotrauma and Changes in Laryngeal Tissue

Traumatic Laryngitis

Imagine the following scenario: It's a Saturday afternoon on campus and everyone is going to the football game because it's homecoming weekend. The score is close and every time your team is close to scoring, you're screaming and yelling and hoping for a touchdown. When the game is over, you begin to notice a hoarse quality to your voice and it's more difficult for you to make sounds. However, there isn't a lot of pain associated with this lack of voicing and as everyone is headed for pizza, you go along. The pizza place is noisy because everyone is talking about the game and trying to be heard above the music. After a couple of hours you decide to head back to your apartment and notice that not only is your voice hoarse, but occasionally your voice breaks up and it's hard to get your vocal cords to work. What you are experiencing is *traumatic laryngitis*. This condition has resulted from the screaming, yelling, and loud talking during the day. If we visually examine your vocal folds, we would see that they are red and swollen, and not vibrating as efficiently as they typically function. Because the tissues are swollen with fluid, they don't vibrate as fast and you sound like you have a lower pitched voice. Traumatic laryngitis can also occur as a result of excessive smoking and drinking. What many individuals fail to recognize is that when a person consumes alcohol, the alcohol is absorbed into the bloodstream and exhaled via the lungs. As the alcohol is exhaled during respiration, it has the potential to dry out the vocal folds, which leads to further laryngeal irritation. When consumed over the long term, alcohol has the potential to cause permanent tissue changes within the larynx. Getting back to the student who yelled and screamed during homecoming, she's not worried because she has lost her voice before and it has always come back the next day. For most cases of traumatic laryngitis, the vocal folds will return to normal given a period of vocal rest.

When an individual does not rest his or her voice, this traumatic laryngitis can become a more persistent or chronic condition. Depending upon the individual, the swelling of the vocal folds can lead to more serious conditions like vocal nodules.

Vocal Nodules

Vocal nodules have been described as benign, or noncancerous, growths on the vocal folds. It is believed that these nodules come about as a result of vocal abuse. It appears that when the vocal folds are swollen, the normal pattern of vocal-fold vibration is disrupted, and the vocal folds do not move in the same wavelike manner as do normally functioning vocal folds. As a result, localized swelling occurs on the vocal folds about a third of the way from their attachment in the front. These early swellings are often soft and pliable. However, with continued trauma, the swellings

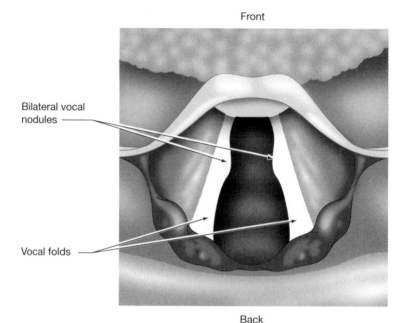

Front

Bilateral vocal nodules

Vocal folds

Back

FIGURE 8.3
Bilateral vocal nodules.

become hard and fibrous in a manner similar to the development of a callus on your finger. Vocal nodules can be on one vocal fold (*unilateral*) but most chronic vocal nodules appear *bilaterally*, or on both vocal folds (see Figure 8.3). It is very common for individuals to try to compensate for their breathy and hoarse voice by increasing their loudness and increasing the muscular tension in the larynx. While these behaviors may help to compensate during the short term, they cause further strain on the vocal mechanism, resulting in further development of the problem.

Treatment for vocal nodules continues to be a controversial issue. Speech–language pathologists argue for behavioral therapy to teach the client good vocal hygiene and modification of laryngeal behaviors in an effort to eliminate vocal nodules. For the otolaryngologist, the course of treatment is often surgery to remove the nodules. Although surgical treatment removes the nodule, there is potential for the development of scar tissue on the vocal fold. In addition, if the person does not modify the laryngeal behavior that originally caused the problem, there is the potential for further trauma and the return of the vocal nodules. Boone et al. (2005, p. 70) reported that "it is not unusual clinically for new nodules to reappear several weeks after surgical removal of nodules in both children and adults. Unless the underlying hyperfunctional vocal behaviors are identified and reduced, vocal nodules have a stubborn way of reappearing." Pannbacker (1999), in an article reviewing the results of many studies that examined the benefits of voice therapy and surgery, concluded that at the time of her review there were too few studies to decide whether one course of treatment was better than the other.

Vocal Polyps

Like vocal nodules, vocal polyps are benign laryngeal growths that often occur in the same location, about one third of the way up on the fold. In contrast to vocal nodules, vocal polyps often occur on one vocal fold (unilateral) and remain soft and pliable. Vocal polyps often occur as a result of a single laryngeal event such as loud yelling at a concert or a scream during a horror movie. As a result of this trauma, some small blood vessels may break on the surface of the vocal fold at the point where the folds make frequent contact. The broken blood vessels are surrounded by bodily fluids and encapsulate to form this growth. As the vocal folds continue to vibrate, this will cause further irritation of the polyp resulting in further growth. For some individuals, the polyps cause a desire to cough and clear their throats, which further add to the trauma. As the polyp prevents the vocal folds from making good contact, the person's voice is often perceived as breathy and hoarse. In some cases, these patients may exhibit two voices, or *diplophonia* ("double voice"), which occurs when "the vocal folds are under differing degrees of tension or mass and each vibrates at a different frequency" (Colton, Casper, & Leonard, 2006, p. 20). Voice therapy can be successful at eliminating vocal polyps for many clients. For clients who require surgery, a period of voice therapy prior to surgery may help to make the client more aware of the behaviors that caused the problem in the first place and the need for continued voice therapy following surgery to prevent any recurrence of the problem.

Neurological Disorders

The majority of the muscles of the larynx that are responsible for laryngeal abduction and adduction receive information from cranial nerve X, the vagus nerve. When an individual experiences a neurological disorder, it has the potential to affect laryngeal opening and closing and the person's ability to phonate, or produce sound. Most of these disorders are beyond the scope of this text. However, we will address two neurological conditions that are associated with voice problems. These are vocal-fold paralysis and spasmodic dysphonia.

Vocal-Fold Paralysis

As the vocal folds open and close, it is possible that some disease process will prevent the vocal folds from completing their function. If we examine the functioning of both vocal folds, we note that some individuals will be unable to close their vocal folds. *Bilateral adductor paralysis* results in an inability to close the vocal folds. As you might imagine, bilateral paralysis is often a life-threatening issue, with voice production secondary to the medical needs of the patient. A person with bilateral adductor paralysis cannot produce sound; more importantly, the person is at risk for aspiration, or sucking or inhaling a fluid or food into their lungs, which in turn can lead to pneumonia and death. *Bilateral abductor paralysis* results in an inability to open the vocal folds. For this person, respiration is the primary concern and the person often has to have a *tracheotomy*, in which an opening is created in their trachea, or windpipe, so that breathing can occur. In both types of bilateral vocal-fold paralysis, treating voice and speech production plays a secondary role to maintaining normal body activities.

The most common type of vocal-fold paralysis is *unilateral vocal-fold paralysis*, which is often associated with trauma or disease. The left recurrent laryngeal nerve is part of the peripheral nervous system. This nerve is the final pathway from the brain to muscles responsible for laryngeal adduction. As the path of this nerve involves a trip into the chest and around the main artery of the heart (aorta), it is common for this nerve to be damaged in patients undergoing heart surgery or other types of chest surgery. The patient is often left with vocal folds in a position that is neither completely open nor completely closed. The resulting voice is often hoarse, breathy, and decreased in loudness.

In some individuals, unilateral vocal-fold paralysis is a result of a trauma to the chest or laryngeal area. It is interesting to note that the design of baseball catchers' masks and hockey goalie masks have changed in recent years. Old masks were rounded and only covered the face and chin area. If you take a look at modern masks, you will note that they extend to provide protection for the laryngeal areas so that a baseball catcher is protected from the 95-mile-an-hour fastball that is foul-tipped and a hockey goalie is protected from stopping a puck with his throat. These new designs help to cut down on the number of traumatic injuries associated with blows to the laryngeal area.

Spasmodic Dysphonia

Historically, *spasmodic dysphonia* was thought to be psychological in nature, but more recently the problem has been seen as a neurological problem characterized by excessive laryngeal adduction. The vocal characteristics are consistent with a spasm of the muscles. The patient exhibits a lot of struggle and strain when attempting to talk and occasional stoppages of the voice are noted (Aronson, 1985). Some patients exhibit a choked voice quality or a voice that sounds as if it is squeezed. Interestingly, during nonphonatory activities like whispering, the symptoms are absent or minimal. Treatments have included unilateral severing of the recurrent laryngeal nerve and injections of Botox (a highly purified preparation of botulinum toxin that is used to treat muscle spasms) to provide symptom relief. However, there continue to be questions regarding these treatments as symptoms often return following a period of time.

Organic Disease

Our focus for this section will be medical conditions including those caused by complications from surgery that have an impact on voice production. We will discuss laryngeal granulomas, papilloma, and cancer of the larynx.

Granulomas

An inflammation in the body caused by tissue irritation is called a *granuloma*. One type of inflammation that is associated with voice problems can be caused by the tube that is inserted into the lungs to administer anesthesia during surgery. The tube rubs against the arytenoid cartilage, causing inflammation and the development of a laryngeal granuloma. The laryngeal granuloma may prevent normal movement of laryngeal cartilages, resulting in a breathy and hoarse vocal quality. In most cases, the condition will resolve without any treatment providing that the patient does not try to compensate for his or her weaker voice by using excessive laryngeal tension. In some cases surgery to remove the granuloma and/or voice therapy may be necessary to prevent the patient from using excessive effort to compensate for decreased vocal abilities. A vocal-process granuloma, or contact ulcer, is another type of granuloma that affects voice production. Historically, contact ulcers were believed to be a function of a patient's behavior. This problem was thought to be associated with middle-aged men who aggressively used their voices in a forceful manner to communicate. In recent years, vocal-process granulomas have been associated with gastroesophageal reflux disease (GERD). As the esophagus is in close proximity to the vocal mechanism, when stomach acid backs up because of reflux, it frequently results in inflammation of the vocal processes of the arytenoid cartilage and the development of a granuloma. Patients with vocal-process granulomas exhibit low pitch, vocal fatigue, and frequent throat clearing. Treatment for this problem has included surgery for the patient's GERD, which has resulted in the elimination of the vocal-process granuloma (Deveney, Benner, & Cohen, 1993).

Papilloma

Papilloma has been described as a wartlike growth, caused by a virus, that can result in obstruction of the airway. Juvenile papilloma has been identified as the most common form of laryngeal tumor in children, with 75% of the cases identified before the age of 5 (Sinal & Woods, 2005). Papillomas are typically removed by surgery, although they tend to reoccur and may require additional surgery. While multiple surgeries may be necessary to save the life of the patient, it is not unusual for scar tissue to develop on the vocal folds, resulting in voice changes. These voice changes may include hoarseness, low pitch, and breathiness. Many children, as they get older, can develop a resistance to the virus and the problem no longer reoccurs. However, given the number of surgeries and location of the papilloma, the patient may be left with a permanent voice problem.

Carcinoma (Cancer)

According to the American Cancer Society, one of the early warning signs of laryngeal cancer is persistent hoarseness for more than 2 weeks. Cancer often occurs within the vocal tract but more specifically on one or both vocal folds. If left untreated, the disease becomes life threatening. Cancer of the larynx has been associated with smoking, environmental irritants, metabolic disturbances, and other unknown causes. According to the Office of the Surgeon General (2004), the combination of smoking and alcohol consumption caused most laryngeal cancer cases. In 2003, an estimated 3,899 deaths occurred from laryngeal cancer. Although the primary symptom of laryngeal cancer is hoarseness, other symptoms include a lump in the neck, tenderness in the neck, and swallowing problems. Treatments for laryngeal cancer include chemotherapy, laryngeal radiation, and partial or complete *laryngectomy*. A laryngectomy involves the removal of laryngeal structures affected by the cancer. As the result of a laryngectomy, the trachea will be redirected and an opening (*stoma*) created in the patient's neck, thus enabling the patient to breathe through this opening. As the person no longer has vocal folds to create sound, alternate methods of communication need to be learned. Speaking without a larynx is termed *alaryngeal communication* and will be discussed later in this chapter.

Quiz on the Fly 8.2

1. Voice disorders associated with misusing and overusing the vocal mechanism are called _____.
2. A disorder that affects one side of a structure is called _____.
3. A laryngeal growth that usually occurs following a single traumatic event is a _____.
4. A wartlike growth that occurs within the vocal tract and obstructs breathing is a _____.
5. The removal of the larynx because of cancer is called a _____.

ASSESSMENT OF VOICE DISORDERS

The assessment of voice disorders needs to be accomplished by a speech–language pathologist working closely with an otolaryngologist. In many locations, the person with a voice disorder will be evaluated by both professionals during the same visit. A voice evaluation includes an extensive case history and client interview, observation of laryngeal functioning, and acoustic and physiological testing. In this section, we will briefly describe the voice evaluation process.

Interviewing the Client

We begin the interview by asking the person to describe the problem. If the patient has already been to see the otolaryngologist, they might respond, "I have vocal nodules." In this case, the speech–language pathologist might ask, "What does it mean if you have vocal nodules?" By asking this question, the interviewer can determine the person's level of understanding regarding the problem. If the speech–language pathologist has the first contact with the patient, the person might say, "I've had a hoarse voice for a couple of weeks." The clinician would then begin to ask additional questions to determine the nature of the person's problem. The clinician would ask the client for a description of the problem ("Tell me how your voice sounds"), how the problem developed ("Did your problem begin suddenly after a specific event, or did it begin in a gradual manner?"), and if there are any associated symptoms (e.g., pain in the neck). It will also be important to determine the consistency of the voice problem and how long the person has experienced the problem. Questions like "How long have you had the problem?" and "Is the problem always there, or does it come and go?" will enable the interviewer to make important decisions for both diagnosis and treatment. It will also be important for the clinician to determine the effect of the voice problem on the person's day-to-day functioning: "Does your voice problem prevent you from completing any activities?" or "Do you have to change your daily routine because of your voice problem?"

By collecting all of this valuable information, the clinician can start to develop a mental picture of this person, the person's voice, and the impact of the voice problem on the person's communication. It is important to recognize that we view our patients as people before we think of their disorders. As a result, our interview always requires that we examine the patient's voice problem in the context of their daily lives. To that end, we will also obtain information regarding the person's medical history, including medications being taken, job history and relationship between the work environment and vocal use, family constellation, academic history, and any other information that will provide a more rounded picture of the person being evaluated. In addition to the interview, observation of the larynx will be an important component of the voice evaluation.

Viewing the Larynx

Our ability to view the larynx is another important component of the voice evaluation. There are a number of methods used to view the larynx, and we will discuss each option. We will first explore a method of viewing the larynx that is typically associated with obtaining tissue samples to test for cancer. This section will be followed by a detailed description of viewing the larynx using relatively low-tech methods and progressing to more advanced methods.

Direct Laryngoscopy

One method of directly viewing the larynx involves a procedure that is usually done in a hospital after the patient has been put to sleep. This procedure is *invasive* (requiring entry into the body), and is usually completed so that the physician can take a tissue sample (biopsy) to determine the nature of a growth within the laryngeal area. As the patient is sleeping during this procedure, it is impossible to assess the active functioning of the vocal mechanism.

Indirect Laryngoscopy

Historically the most common method for viewing the larynx used a light source, a mirror worn by the physician, and a dental mirror. To view the larynx or vocal folds in this manner, the doctor positions a light source behind the patient while he or she sits in front of the patient. As the doctor is wearing a circular mirror on his or her forehead, the circular mirror directs the light toward a dental mirror that he or she has positioned at the back of the patient's throat. The light is reflected off the mirror to the dental mirror that reflects the light down the patient's throat toward the vocal folds. During this process, the patient is holding his or her tongue with gauze to pull the tongue and epiglottis forward, making it easier for the physician to view the vocal folds. Because the patient's tongue is somewhat immobile and the dental mirror is resting on the person's tongue, the doctor can only ask the patient to say "a" and prolong the sound while attempting to view the movement of the vocal folds. Most other speech activities would be difficult to accomplish. Although the physician can view vocal-fold movement, the amount of time available is relatively short as the patient may gag from the presence of the laryngeal mirror, the mirror

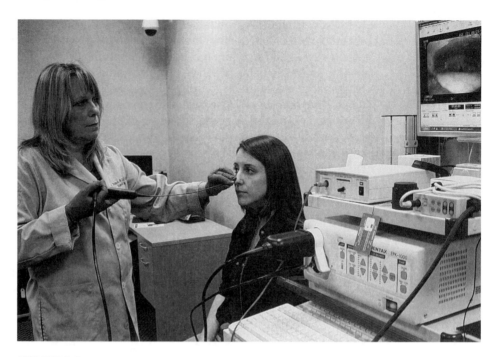

FIGURE 8.4
Examining the larynx using a flexible fiberscope.

may fog up as the person breathes, and it is not easy for the patient to hold his or her tongue for any extended period of time. However, for years this method of evaluation was the most efficient method of viewing the vocal folds without having to anesthetize the patient to gain a more direct view of the larynx.

During the past 30 years, technology has been developed that enables physicians and speech–language pathologists to view the larynx during periods of quiet breathing, singing, continuous phonation of sounds, and conversational interaction. Using a flexible *fiber-optic nasolaryngoscope*, or *fiberscope* (see Figure 8.4), the examiner is able to directly view the opening and closing movements of the vocal folds as well as determine the presence or absence of laryngeal pathology. The fiberscope is a flexible bundle of glass fibers that has an eyepiece or camera on one end, and is typically attached to a cold light source (light produced by a gas so that there is little heat generated) and a television or computer monitor. The end of the fiberscope that

---

Quiz on the Fly 8.2 Answers

1. Voice disorders associated with misusing and overusing the vocal mechanism are called **phonotrauma**. **2.** A disorder that affects one side of a structure is called **unilateral**. **3.** A laryngeal growth that usually occurs following a single traumatic event is a **vocal polyp**. **4.** A wartlike growth that occurs within the vocal tract and obstructs breathing is a **papilloma**. **5.** The removal of the larynx because of cancer is called a **laryngectomy**.

is inserted into the body contains a camera lens that allows the viewing of the larynx. Because the fibers are flexible and can transmit light, this fiberscope can be inserted into the patient's nasal passage, pass over his or her soft palate, and then move down the back of the throat so that the patient's vocal folds can be seen. While this procedure may be a little uncomfortable for the patient, he or she is able to talk, sing, and communicate with the examiner while the movements of the vocal folds are watched. The observer is able to note the opening and closing movements of the vocal folds, the color of the tissue, and the presence of any vocal pathology but cannot view the individual cycles of vocal-fold vibration as they occur too quickly to view without special equipment.

To view the cycle-to-cycle opening and closing of the vocal folds, an examiner might use a video strobe light (*stroboscopy*) that can be set to pulse at a variety of frequencies. Many of you may remember a trip to a local dance club where video strobe lights were used to make the dancers look like they were moving in slow motion. In a similar manner, a strobe light can be directed through the fiberscope so that the vocal folds appear to move in slow motion, and the physician and speech–language pathologist can obtain a more comprehensive view of the client's vocal-fold movements to make a more effective diagnosis of the patient's problem. While stroboscopy can be done with a flexible fiberscope, many examiners report better results with a *rigid fiberscope* (see Figure 8.5) that resembles a small telescope. The fiber-optic fibers are encased by a rigid tube. In a manner similar to the

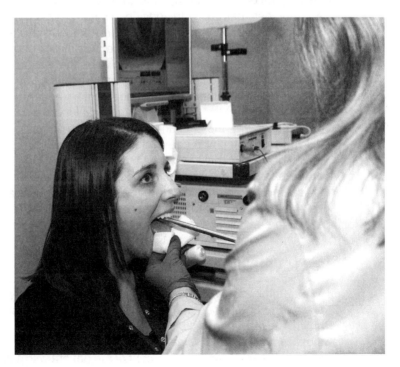

FIGURE 8.5
The rigid fiberscope.

FIGURE 8.6
The larynx viewed through the rigid fiberscope.

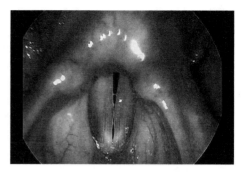

flexible scope, the rigid scope transmits light and helps to record video signals of vocal-fold movement. Because of the rigid nature of the scope, it is inserted in the mouth with the light directed down the pharynx toward the vocal folds. Excellent images of vocal-fold movement can be obtained in this manner (see Figure 8.6).

Acoustic and Physiological Measures of Voice

During laryngoscopy, the physician and speech–language pathologist attempt to determine the patient's ability to move the vocal folds while at the same time observing the characteristics of the laryngeal tissue and determining the presence of any laryngeal pathology. In addition to these direct observations, the examiners will ask the patient to complete a number of vocal activities like raising and lowering pitch, producing a loud and soft voice, sustaining phonation, and producing conversational speech. During these activities the examiners will record the person's speech so that the acoustic signal can be analyzed by special computer programs that will determine the person's fundamental frequency, variations in the frequency of vocal-fold vibration, ability to vary vocal loudness, and other vocal characteristics. Additionally, the examiners can use equipment to measure the physiological activity associated with vocal-fold opening and closing and respiration. When all of these measurements have been completed, the examiners will evaluate the results of the patient interview, the laryngeal examination, and the acoustic and physiological measurements to determine the nature of the patient's problem and potential management strategies. When all of this information has been evaluated, the examiners will sit down with the patient and discuss a management plan.

TREATING VOICE DISORDERS

The treatment of voice disorders is covered extensively in a number of books that are referenced throughout this chapter. In the discussion that follows we will examine the treatment of voice disorders associated with phonotrauma as this is the most common type of voice problem that we encounter. The second part of this discussion will examine the treatment of the patient with a laryngectomy and focus on the various types of therapy provided to assist the patient who has lost his or her larynx.

I CAN'T DO THIS ALONE

Dr. Michael Karnell, director, Speech & Swallowing Service, University of Iowa Hospitals, describes the services provided within his department:

The voice clinic at the University of Iowa is an interdisciplinary service staffed by an otolaryngologist and a speech pathologist who both specialize in the area of voice disorders.

My role is to objectively characterize the patient's perceptions of the problem and to characterize the perceptual characteristics of the voice problem from the speech pathologist's perspective. In addition, we use current technology to measure acoustic stability of the patient's voice, other functional vocal capabilities, and to complete a videostroboscopic examination of laryngeal function.

The role of the otolaryngologist is to identify medical and/or surgical problems that impact the voice. A detailed medical history is taken and a thorough physical examination of the patient's head and neck is performed, including indirect laryngoscopy.

After the physician and speech pathologist have completed their examinations, the findings are reviewed with the patient and recommendations are considered. Recommendations may include medical intervention (prescription or nonprescription medications), surgical intervention (altering laryngeal structures to eliminate disease or improve function), and voice therapy. These results are shared with the client so that all of the potential benefits and detriments can be evaluated. Ultimately, the patient chooses the course of action. The otolaryngologist dictates his results in front of the patient and includes a summary of the voice clinic findings and recommendations, referencing the findings of the speech pathologist. The speech pathologist produces a written report describing the perceptual, acoustic, and stroboscopic findings. This report is included in the medical record as an attachment to the physician's report. Follow-up assessment and recommendations are scheduled as needed and performed with special consideration of previous findings and recommendations.

Contributed by Michael Karnell, PhD, University of Iowa, Department of Otolaryngology-Head and Neck Surgery.

Phonotrauma

As voice disorders vary according to the patient's age and sex, as well as the type of disorder exhibited, treatments often vary according to the individual. However, Colton et al. (2006, p. 321) tell us that "the goal of voice therapy is to restore the best voice possible, a voice that will be functional for purposes of employment and general communication." Because voice disorders often involve a breakdown in the voice production system, a major focus of therapy is teaching the individual how the system works and the effects of excessive behaviors upon the system. While many individuals will approach voice therapy in the same manner that they approach their physician, by saying, "Make me better, give me a pill so I can get rid of this problem," voice therapy involves a commitment by patients to understand the nature of their voice production system and the effects of excessive behaviors on voice production. In many cases, and in particular those problems that arise from disease or tumors, the primary focus of treatment is going to be medical and often involves surgery. However, for the largest group of voice problems, those associated with vocal misuse, abuse, and phonotrauma, the treatment approach is going to involve increasing the client's awareness of their inappropriate vocal behaviors, educating the client regarding the changes necessary to help to improve their voice, and encouraging the client to make these changes so that their voices improve and they are able to maintain a more appropriate voice. A major part of therapy involves working closely with the speech–language pathologist so that behaviors can be modified and the patient can learn to accept greater responsibility toward making those changes. Consider the patient whose voice is their career. Although you might immediately think about a professional singer, we are really addressing teachers, salespeople, clergy, or anyone who uses their voice as part of their job. Without a healthy voice, communication will be impaired and the person may not be able to fulfill their job responsibilities.

For the frequent vocal user, and in particular the classroom teacher, is it going to be reasonable for the speech–language pathologist to suggest complete vocal rest? This suggestion would seem to be quite unreasonable given the daily responsibilities of the job. However, the speech–language pathologist and patient will sit down and discuss all of the vocal behaviors that occur during the day. Perhaps the teacher enjoys singing on her way to school and then joins her colleagues in the teacher's lounge where there is a lively discussion about salary negotiations. This discussion is followed by eight periods of teaching, including lunch duty. At the end of the day, the teacher may participate in another activity that involves a lot of vocal use (for example, coaching, tutoring, participating on a sports team), and when she returns home, there are children to care for and family interactions that also require a lot of communication. When all of these activities are discussed, is it any wonder that so many teachers experience voice problems? The speech–language pathologist and teacher will begin to explore potential modifications to the daily schedule that may provide opportunities for vocal rest so that the teacher's voice production system can recuperate from the intense workout it receives throughout the day. It will not be realistic to suggest that the teacher give up any of her teaching schedule as this is the main component of her job responsibility. As a result, a discussion will ensue to investigate potential modifications that can be made in the teacher's schedule. It might be suggested that singing in the car and loud interactions in the teacher's lounge be eliminated for a period of time so that the teacher has not fatigued her voice before the day has even begun. Some teachers have recognized that using a microphone connected to a small amplifier and speaker reduces vocal effort and causes less vocal fatigue. Other suggestions include vocal rest between class periods, using a lunch break or free period to rest her voice, and increasing her awareness of how often and how loudly she is talking in class. Does the teacher walk to the back of the classroom to get the students' attention or does she yell at them to pay attention? Sometimes, a few behavioral modifications can

MAKING A DIFFERENCE

Lisa was an elementary school teacher who complained of a voice problem that had been getting worse for several years. Lisa stated that her voice was "good" in the early morning but by the middle of the day, she was hoarse, had pain in her throat, and could not be adequately heard by her students. The hoarseness and pain continued in the evening and progressed in severity throughout the week. This condition was affecting Lisa's ability to care for her own children because she did not want to speak at all after returning home from work. Lisa stated that she was frightened that she would need to resign from her teaching position.

Lisa was evaluated by an otolaryngologist (ENT) who diagnosed a left vocal-fold polyp and muscle tension dysphonia. The ENT recommended speech therapy before and after surgery for removal of the polyp. The speech–language pathologist assisted Lisa in understanding how her voice is produced and how removal of the polyp would not likely result in the outcome she desired unless speaking behaviors were modified. During speech therapy sessions, Lisa learned how to care for her voice and how to utilize her voice in an efficient manner to reduce vocal strain. She reported that she never realized how she exhibited tension in her voice and used speaking patterns that added to her hoarseness. After several weeks of therapy, Lisa reported that she was able to teach for an entire week and care for her family without hoarseness. Lisa told her therapist, "Thank you for giving me back my voice."

Contributed by Cynthia Hildner, MS, clinical faculty member, Northern Illinois University.

have a significant impact on the quality of the teacher's voice. This is not an easy process and involves the active participation of both clinician and teacher. As previously stated, it is unrealistic to think that behavioral change is going to occur without the active commitment and participation of the client. For additional information on vocal hygiene and helping teachers to understand voice disorders, the reader is directed to an excellent Web site developed by the National Center for Voice and Speech with support from the Department of Speech Pathology and Audiology at the University of Iowa (http://www.uiowa.edu/~shcvoice/).

Alaryngeal Communication

Alaryngeal is a term that means without a larynx. As previously discussed, some people have cancer of the larynx and it becomes necessary to remove that structure and surrounding structures affected by the cancer. When a person has their larynx removed, their trachea is repositioned and a stoma is created that enables the person to breathe through this opening. As the patient no longer has vocal folds, another source of vibration must be found to produce speech.

Depending upon the patient and their emotional outlook and willingness to attend therapy, there are three options available for therapy. An *artificial larynx*, sometimes referred to as an *electrolarynx* (see Figure 8.7), provides a source of vibration. The patient can place this device on his or her neck (see Figure 8.7A) or in his or her mouth (see Figure 8.7B) and this will cause the air in the vocal tract to vibrate. The patient can then use his or her articulators to shape these vibrations into recognizable speech. This device does not require extensive training and is relatively easy to use. The drawback to this device is the monotone quality of the patient's voice, which often sounds robotic in nature. The second type of alaryngeal communication is called esophageal speech. Esophageal speech uses the esophagus, or tube to the stomach, as the sound source for the voice. A patient is instructed in methods for injecting or trapping air with the tongue and capturing this air at the top of the esophagus. In more practical terms, the patient is taught to create sounds with a burp. The burping sound creates air that vibrates in the vocal tract and these vibrations are shaped by the articulators. For many patients this technique was difficult to master and often resulted in stomach distress. More recently, a procedure called a tracheoesophageal puncture has been used to help the patient to direct air from

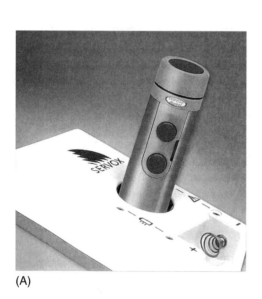

(A)

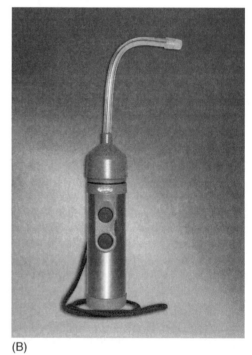

(B)

FIGURE 8.7
(A) Servox electrolarynx and (B) Servox electrolarynx with speaking tube. (Reprinted with permission of Servona GmbH, Troisdorf, Germany)

the trachea to the esophagus so that sound is produced in an easier and more efficient manner. With this method, the patient is able to put his or her finger over the stoma which forces the air back through a special tube into the esophagus. This procedure is often done at the same time as the laryngectomy so that therapy can be initiated as soon as possible. While having the larynx removed is very traumatic for most patients, knowing that different forms of therapy are available to restore their voice can be a positive experience for many patients.

I CAN'T DO THIS ALONE

Advances in the rehabilitative care provided to people with head and neck cancer are quite extraordinary when one considers the history of postlaryngectomy care. As this subspecialty progresses, clinicians would do well to be aware of the practice standards, particularly with regard to the scope of practice (see http://www.asha .org for the scope of practice).

A mere 30 years ago, many speech pathologists could not fathom one of their colleagues placing a prosthetic into a tracheoesophageal puncture site, inserting a catheter into the aerodigestive tract, or otherwise invading another person's body. None of these advances in voice restoration would have been possible without the collaboration of surgeons and speech pathologists. Many speech pathologists, blending their foundational knowledge of speech science with their clinical and personal acumen, develop solid interdependent relationships with surgeons. To do so requires setting aside issues of ego and "turf" and focusing substantial energies on the person for whom we are caring.

As we, speech pathologists, stretch our practice domain, boundaries need to be respected. One day, a man who had been fit recently with a tracheoesophageal prosthesis came into the clinic because his prosthesis was not working. It was apparent that the prosthesis had extruded from the common wall puncture site. I was experienced at dilating the site and, by doing so, was able to reinsert the prosthesis. However, given that the patient lived alone and a several-hour drive from the clinic, I was concerned that the prosthesis might be coughed out and aspirated, or coughed out leaving the puncture to close. I called the surgeon at his office in an adjacent hospital and explained the situation. He promptly declared that the gentleman needed "a quick suture" to anchor the prosthesis to his neck. I concurred. "Okay, let me know if anything else comes up," I heard the surgeon say. For all of our collaboration, he expected me to stitch the prosthesis into place. I begged off and walked the gentleman to the surgeon's office. There, I was content to have the need resolved by someone with the proper training and credentials. At the same time, I was grateful to know that I had earned the surgeon's confidence.

Contributed by Peter Feudo, ScD, dual-certified speech–language pathologist and audiologist.

SUMMARY AND REVIEW

The focus of this chapter was examination of the anatomy and physiology of normal voice production, the characteristics of the normal voice, and a detailed description of vocal pathologies, assessment, and treatment. We first reviewed laryngeal anatomy and followed this discussion with the characteristics of a normal voice. We continued by examining voice disorders in three different categories: phonotrauma, neurological disorders, and organic disease. With our background completed on the classification of voice disorders, we went on to discuss an interdisciplinary approach to voice evaluation, and concluded with a discussion of voice therapy, with specific focus on phonotrauma and therapy for patients with laryngectomies.

Anatomy of Voice Production

What is the structure of the vocal folds and how is a normal-sounding voice produced?

The vocal folds are a multilayered structure that include an epithelial layer, three middle layers (Lamina Propria), and the large thyroarytenoid muscle. It is the interaction between the cover (epithelial layer, Jell-O-like layer, rubber-band layer) and the inner layers (cotton-string layer and thyroarytenoid muscle) that enable us to produce a normal-sounding voice.

Characteristics of Voice Production

What are the characteristics of a normal voice?

A normal voice can be characterized by a physiological characteristic and its perceptual correlate. The frequency of vocal-fold vibration can be quantified by measuring a person's pitch. Intensity is a measurable characteristic of voice and we note a person's loudness. Resonance relates to where sounds vibrate within the vocal tract and we note a voice as being normal, nasal, hypernasal, or hyponasal. The fourth characteristic is vocal quality, which relates to resonance and laryngeal tension.

Definitions and Prevalence of Voice Disorders

What is a voice disorder?

According to ASHA, a voice disorder is characterized by the abnormal production and/or absences of vocal quality, pitch, loudness, resonance, and/or duration, which is inappropriate for an individual's age and/or sex.

Classifying Voice Disorders

What are some categories of voice disorders?

Phonotrauma is one category that results from misusing and overusing the vocal mechanism. The resultant problems include traumatic laryngitis, vocal nodules, and vocal polyps. A second category of voice disorders relates to neurological conditions and includes vocal-fold paralysis and spasmodic dysphonia. A third category of voice disorder is associated with organic conditions, or conditions that arise within the body. These include papilloma and carcinoma.

Assessment of Voice Disorders

What are the components of a comprehensive assessment of voice?

A voice assessment will include an in-depth interview of the client, some type of laryngeal exam that will enable the otolaryngologist and speech–language pathologist to view the laryngeal mechanism, and various acoustic and physiological measures of voice production.

Treating Voice Disorders

What type of therapy is provided for a patient who experiences phonotrauma?

The goal of therapy is to help to restore the best voice possible for the patient in order for the person to be able to effectively communicate. Therapy for phonotrauma includes patient education regarding the anatomy and physiology of voice production, counseling regarding the identification and modification of behaviors associated with the phonotrauma, and instruction in good vocal hygiene aimed at the reduction of vocal behaviors that lead to the problem.

WEB SITES OF INTEREST

International Association of Laryngectomees
http://www.theial.com/

National Center for Voice and Speech
http://www.ncvs.org/

National Spasmodic Dysphonia Association
http://www.spasmodic-dysphonia-support.org/

The Voice Academy
http://www.uiowa.edu/~shcvoice/

9

Swallowing Disorders

Cynthia D. Hildner, MS
Northern Illinois University

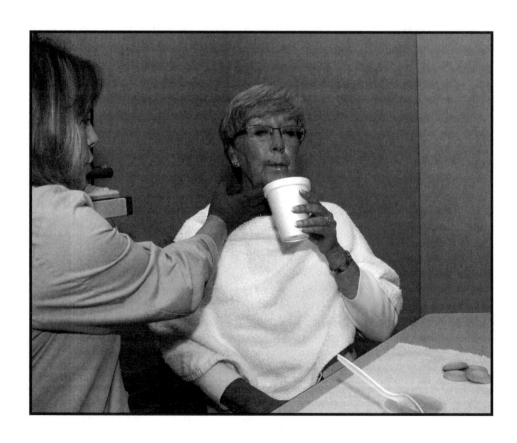

In the present chapter we will focus on the normal process of *deglutition* (swallowing) and then examine the same process when the system is impaired. We will begin our discussion by describing the phases of normal swallowing and explaining the nature of swallowing problems (*dysphagia*) at each phase in the process.

Dysphagia (dis-FAY-juh) can be defined as difficulty moving food from the mouth to the stomach (Logemann, 1998). This can encompass a wide variety of symptoms such as difficulty controlling food or saliva within the mouth; coughing before, during, or after swallowing; and a sensation that food is sticking in the throat or is unable to be swallowed. In addition to discussing the problems associated with the phases of swallowing, we will examine a number of pathological conditions and describe their impact on a person's health and ability to swallow normally. When we have completed our discussion of swallowing difficulties, we will describe the processes involved in evaluating swallowing, followed by how we manage and provide therapeutic treatment for individuals who exhibit dysphagia. Additionally, we will briefly discuss the variations in swallowing found across the life span from birth to advanced age.

You may be interested to know that the evaluation and treatment of swallowing disorders by speech–language pathologists is a relatively new job responsibility. It was during the late 1970s and early 1980s that swallowing began to receive attention among speech–language pathologists. Until this point, treatment of swallowing disorders was often completed by physical therapists, respiratory therapists, or nurses within medical centers. However, because speech–language pathologists focus on learning the structures and functions of the oral, vocal, and respiratory systems, it made logical sense for this clinical specialty to incorporate the diagnosis and treatment of swallowing into their scope of practice. Speech pathologists have since taken a leading role in research into understanding the complex function of swallowing and the methods of evaluating and providing treatment for individuals with dysphagia. Before we begin our examination of the phases of swallowing, it is important to ask two questions: (1) Why do we need to evaluate and treat swallowing disorders? and (2) What is the impact on the patient? You are encouraged to read the I Can't Do This Alone feature to see how the physician and SLP work together to deal with dysphagia.

To better understand swallowing disorders, it is important for you to first understand the anatomy of the deglutition system and the multiple-stage process that makes up normal swallowing.

I CAN'T DO THIS ALONE

Ralph and Frank were watching the Chicago Bears on television. As Frank got up to leave the room, he noticed that his brother appeared to be somewhat dazed and the right side of his face looked different from the left side. When Frank called to his brother, Ralph did not respond. Frank was pretty sure that something was wrong with his brother and it was probably a stroke. Frank called emergency services to transport Ralph to the hospital. As Frank's mother had suffered a stroke years before, Frank was somewhat ready when Dr. Singh indicated that Ralph's speech was slurred, he was confused, and they were unsure about Ralph's ability to understand conversation. Dr. Singh indicated that he would send a request for a consultation by the speech pathology program to have Ralph evaluated. In addition, Dr. Singh explained to Frank that because Ralph's muscles in his face, tongue, jaw, and voice box were weakened by the stroke, it was likely that Ralph would have swallowing and feeding problems as well. Dr Singh explained, "Before I can prescribe a diet for your brother, the speech pathologist in conjunction with the radiologist will evaluate your brother's swallowing because we want to make sure that no food or liquids get into his lungs. When people get liquids and food in their lungs, this can cause serious medical problems." Frank was pleased that Dr. Singh was so thorough in taking care of his brother and somewhat surprised that a speech–language pathologist would do a swallowing evaluation as he thought that speech pathologists only helped stroke patients to learn how to communicate following a stroke.

ANATOMY AND PHYSIOLOGY OF SWALLOWING

The act of swallowing requires the complex integration of areas of the brain cortex, the brain stem, peripheral nerves, and over 25 pairs of muscles. Knowledge of the structure and functioning of the mouth (oral cavity), the throat (pharyngeal and laryngeal cavity), the respiratory system (trachea, bronchi, and lungs), and the esophagus (tube to the stomach) is essential for understanding the swallowing process. The key structures in the oral cavity include the lips, teeth, cheeks, tongue, hard palate, and soft palate, which are important for preparation of the foods and liquids for swallowing. Additionally, within the oral cavity are the ducts of the salivary glands, which provide moisture for the mouth.

The *epiglottis*, found within the pharyngeal cavity, is attached to the back of the tongue and is a cartilage that flips downward during the swallow to cover and protect the opening of the larynx. Within the pharyngeal cavity we can find pockets, or *pharyngeal recesses*, called the *valleculae* and the *pyriform sinuses*. These pharyngeal recesses are important for providing a safety net that helps to prevent foods and liquids from entering the larynx. However, in some patients, ingested materials can fall and get trapped within this area. At the juncture between the base of the pharynx and the top of the esophagus is an important muscle called the *cricopharyngeus*

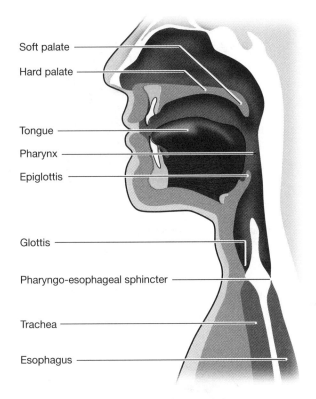

Soft palate

Hard palate

Tongue

Pharynx

Epiglottis

Glottis

Pharyngo-esophageal sphincter

Trachea

Esophagus

FIGURE 9.1
Lateral view of the vocal tract.

muscle. The cricopharyngeus remains closed until swallowing occurs to prevent air or refluxed stomach contents from entering the pharynx. You will be aware of the tightness and subsequent opening of this muscle when you feel the need to burp.

As previously discussed, the laryngeal system is involved with breathing and the production of sound. The larynx is closed during swallowing to provide further protection against food or liquids entering the trachea and lungs. To refresh your memory, we have included a lateral view of the vocal tract so that you can view important structures associated with swallowing (see Figure 9.1).

PHASES OF NORMAL SWALLOWING

Swallowing includes two distinct functions: airway protection and the movement of foods and liquids from the oral cavity to the stomach. When an individual swallows, the goal is to direct the ingested material toward the stomach in a timely and efficient manner while at the same time protecting the respiratory system. To understand these actions we can examine normal swallowing as a four-phase process (see Figure 9.2), which will be described in the following sections. These phases of

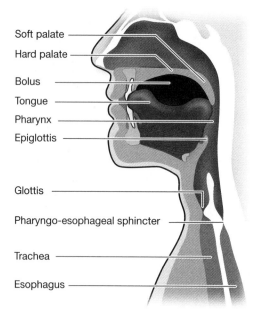

Soft palate

Hard palate

Bolus

Tongue

Pharynx

Epiglottis

Glottis

Pharyngo-esophageal sphincter

Trachea

Esophagus

(A) Oral preparatory phase.

(B) Oral phase.

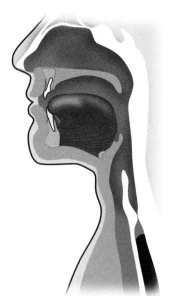

(C) Pharyngeal phase.

(D) Esophageal phase.

FIGURE 9.2
The four phases of swallowing.

swallowing are the oral preparatory phase, the oral phase, the pharyngeal phase, and finally the esophageal phase.

Oral Preparatory Phase

The focus of the oral preparatory phase of swallowing is to prepare solids and liquids for the subsequent stages of swallowing (see Figure 9.2A). Both solids and liquids need to be manipulated in such a way as to form a ball, or *bolus*. The bolus is formed when the lips are closed and a person chews the solid food and mixes it with saliva to change it into a manageable form for swallowing. During bolus preparation, the soft palate lowers and the tongue is used to gather all of the material in the oral cavity. Although liquids do not typically require chewing, they do require containment in the mouth using the same process involving the lips, soft palate, and tongue. During bolus formation for liquids and solids, respiration continues through the nasal cavity. As you might expect, the oral preparation of liquids is faster than solids as less preparation is required, and the speed of transport will be critical to prevent leakage and possible misdirection of the liquid toward the lungs.

Oral Phase

Once the bolus is formed, the individual must move the bolus to the back of the mouth in preparation for swallowing (see Figure 9.2B). The oral phase of swallowing is focused on the posterior, or backward, movement of the bolus. This is accomplished when the tongue elevates, pushing against the hard palate, and moves in a posterior manner to push the bolus to the rear of the mouth. As a simple exercise, you might take your favorite cookie, chew it (oral preparation), and focus on the movements accomplished to move that cookie to the back of your throat (oral phase). The time for the oral phase is typically 1 to 1.5 seconds (Logemann, 1998), depending upon the thickness of the bolus. In a manner similar to the oral preparatory phase, the lips are closed during this phase, and respiration continues with the lowering of the soft palate and breathing through the nose.

Pharyngeal Phase

The pharyngeal phase of swallowing involves movement of the bolus from the back of the oral cavity through the pharynx to the opening of the esophagus (see Figure 9.2C). The triggering of the pharyngeal swallow occurs as a function of sensory receptors in different anatomical structures that appear to be related to the patient's chronological age. For younger individuals, the pharyngeal swallow is triggered as the bolus passes by the posterior lateral walls of the oral cavity. In older individuals (over age 60) with normal swallowing, the pharyngeal swallow appears to be triggered as the bolus passes the base of the tongue, a structure that is further along in the pharynx. During the pharyngeal swallow, a number of anatomical activities take place. The nasal cavity is closed off from the oral cavity when the velum is elevated and retracted, the larynx is raised and moved slightly forward, and the vocal folds close to ensure that no food or liquid is able to pass into the airway. As the bolus passes into the pharynx, the tongue works in conjunction with the muscular walls of the pharynx and contracts to propel the bolus toward the esophagus.

It only takes about 1 second for the bolus to move from the top of the pharynx, where the pharyngeal swallow response is triggered, to where it enters the esophagus. The movement of the bolus is continuous and smooth, with no delay in its movement. The anterior movement and elevation of the larynx combined with downward tipping of the epiglottal cartilage appears to direct the food around the laryngeal airway so that it reaches the esophagus without food or liquid entering the trachea.

Esophageal Phase

The esophagus is an 18- to 25-cm muscular tube that lies immediately behind the trachea. Unlike the pharynx that is open at rest to allow for air to enter the respiratory system, the esophagus is a flattened (collapsed) tube at rest. Movement of the bolus into the esophagus occurs when the *upper esophageal sphincter* (a closed muscular ring), which joins the pharynx and esophagus, opens (see Figure 9.2D). It is important to know that the opening of the upper esophageal sphincter is tied directly to the pharyngeal stage of swallowing. The upper esophageal sphincter is a normally closed sphincter. During swallowing it relaxes and, because of the connection of muscle to the larynx, is pulled open as the larynx moves up and forward during swallowing. You can feel the movement of the larynx during swallowing by gently feeling your Adam's apple move upward and forward as you swallow. It is also interesting to note that the width and duration of opening of the upper esophageal sphincter is modified and adjusted according to the size and consistency of the food bolus. We are aware of this when we struggle to swallow a large pill or a large bite of pizza. The bolus then passes through the esophagus because of sequentially timed muscular contractions called *peristalsis*. Peristalsis begins as the bolus enters the esophagus and continues until the food passes the sphincter at the junction of the stomach (lower esophageal sphincter) and enters the stomach. The movement of the bolus from esophageal opening to stomach typically takes 8 to 20 seconds.

DISORDERED SWALLOWING

As mentioned at the outset of this chapter, disordered swallowing is termed dysphagia. Although dysphagia may result from a variety of different disorders, the physician and speech–language pathologist are most concerned with the complications that can result from dysphagia. These complications can include malnutrition, dehydration, and respiratory conditions such as aspiration pneumonia. A diagnosis of dysphagia indicates that there is evidence of impaired efficiency of bolus transit or evidence of bolus misdirection. Specifically, during the swallowing evaluation, conditions may be observed that indicate reduced swallowing efficiency, including slowed movement of food or liquid through the oral cavity or pharynx. Remaining food or liquid, referred to as *residue,* may be present in the mouth or throat, resulting in greater time required for eating to maintain nutritional needs. Of critical importance is the identification of bolus misdirection that results in *laryngeal penetration* and *aspiration.* Laryngeal penetration occurs when the patient attempts to swallow but the bolus or residue from prior swallows enters the laryngeal area above the vocal folds. Penetration of a large piece of food in the laryngeal airway can cause the person to choke, requiring forceful coughing or the Heimlich maneuver to remove the food. Smaller amounts of foods or liquids may penetrate into the laryngeal airway that do not result in choking but may lead to coughing when the material reaches the vocal folds or, eventually, the entrance into the trachea. Laryngeal penetration below the level of the vocal folds into the trachea is defined as aspiration. *Aspiration pneumonia* occurs when food or liquid enters the bronchi of the lungs, resulting in an infection. As you might suspect, when food or liquid enters the laryngeal airway or lungs, there is a high risk of infection. These infections result in fever, fatigue, coughing, lung discharge, or even death.

Swallowing disorders will be examined to determine the breakdowns that occur during the four phases of swallowing and how these breakdowns relate to the symptoms of a specific pathology. In the section to follow, we will discuss swallowing disorders as they relate to swallowing phases and various pathologies.

Swallowing Phases and Dysphagia

In general, any condition that is going to affect the oral and laryngeal musculature has the potential to disrupt swallowing. As we previously discussed, the oral preparation phase is focused on breaking down food, mixing it with saliva, and forming the bolus. The bolus is formed in the oral cavity, and any difficulties experienced by the patient relative to oral cavity structures (e.g., lips, jaw, tongue) have the potential to affect the oral preparation phase. Patients may have food fall from the mouth, have difficulty forming the bolus, or have liquids and solids prematurely enter the pharynx, causing laryngeal penetration and possibly aspiration. During the oral phase of deglutition, the bolus is transported toward the back of the tongue so that the pharyngeal swallow can be triggered. It is not unusual for a patient to exhibit a significant delay in moving the bolus from the oral cavity to the back of the mouth. These delays might be related to muscular weakness, inability to initiate motor movements following a command, or decreased oral sensation. For patients exhibiting difficulty during the oral phase of deglutition, the bolus may break apart, dispersing food throughout the oral cavity, or food may become lodged between the cheeks and teeth or under the patient's tongue. During this stage, as in the previous stage, some of these delays can result in food falling into the pharyngeal cavity, triggering coughing and gagging.

During the pharyngeal stage of deglutition the bolus triggers the pharyngeal swallow so that it can be moved from the base of the tongue to the esophagus. When a delay in triggering the swallow occurs, the bolus can arrive in the pharynx before the swallow has been initiated, resulting in coughing, choking, and potential for aspiration. Many patients who exhibit a delay in initiating the pharyngeal swallow indicate problems with swallowing liquids. In our previous discussion we also noted that the velum closes during this stage. On some occasions, when the timing of velopharyngeal closure is delayed, some patients may experience nasal backflow as the food and liquid are forced back into the nasal cavity. Additionally, some patients may exhibit esophageal backflow from food or liquid that has entered the esophagus.

It might be helpful to think of the swallowing mechanism as a system of tubes and valves (Logemann, 1998) as in your home. The tubes (oral cavity, pharyngeal cavity, and esophagus) are passageways for the bolus to flow, just as the pipes transport water into and through your home. The valves (lips, tongue, velum, base of tongue to pharyngeal wall, larynx, upper esophageal sphincter) open and close, controlling the flow of food and liquids. These valves allow for adjustments in the system so that foods and liquids are directed in the correct manner.

SWALLOWING DISORDERS ASSOCIATED WITH VARIOUS ORGANIC CONDITIONS

It is not surprising to learn that any neurological disorder that impacts the sensory and motor activities within the oral, pharyngeal, and laryngeal systems has the potential to cause swallowing problems. These breakdowns typically occur between the oral and pharyngeal phases of swallowing and may have a gradual or sudden onset. In this section we will briefly highlight a number of neurological conditions and cancers, and discuss the swallowing difficulties associated with these disorders.

Cerebrovascular Accidents

Cerebrovascular accidents (CVAs), or strokes, are the most common cause of neurogenic swallowing difficulties. It has been reported that 30% to 40% of stroke victims will exhibit dysphagia, 20% of these individuals will die of aspiration pneumonia in the year following their stroke, and of those individuals who survive their first year after a stroke, 10% to 15% will also die of aspiration pneumonia (Murry & Carrau, 2006). As a result, the identification and treatment of dysphagia associated with neurological problems becomes a critical role for the speech–language pathologist within a medical setting. Most common CVAs occur unilaterally. A right-hemispheric stroke affects the left side of the patient's body and often results in dysphagia, characterized by lengthened time for food to move through the pharynx, and greater occurrence of laryngeal penetration and aspiration of liquids when compared to patients with left-hemispheric strokes. Patients with left-hemispheric strokes show weakness on the right side of their body and are more likely to exhibit oral-stage swallowing problems that have been correlated with the presence of apraxia (inability to carry out purposeful movements in the absence of paralysis). It has been demonstrated that early identification, management, and treatment of stroke patients with swallowing problems can significantly reduce the risk of aspiration pneumonia.

Traumatic Brain Injury

Traumatic brain injury (TBI), as previously described in chapter 7, is an acquired brain injury that can be associated with a sudden trauma like a car accident or a gunshot wound. Because people with TBI often exhibit rapid changes in their neurological and cognitive state, it is necessary to closely monitor these patients and perform multiple swallowing evaluations as the patient's status changes. Patients with TBI will often exhibit delayed or absent pharyngeal responses and aspiration during and after a swallow. Because these patients will exhibit attention problems, cognitive problems, and memory problems, their judgment regarding what food is safe to select and the amount to choose needs to be closely monitored.

Amyotrophic Lateral Sclerosis

Amyotrophic lateral sclerosis (ALS) is a neurological disease of unknown etiology that results in weakness, paralysis, and degeneration throughout the brain and spinal cord. In more than half of the cases, the problem begins as a painless weakness in the hand, foot, arm, or leg. Early symptoms of ALS often include speech, walking, and swallowing difficulty. Although some cases begin to appear in individuals in their 40s, the majority of cases have an onset in people who are 60 years old or older. As this disease attacks the motor neurons, causing the muscles to gradually weaken and atrophy (waste away), paralysis occurs, affecting both sides of the body, including the muscles necessary for chewing and swallowing. Thus, a high percentage of ALS patients will exhibit dysphagia. ALS is a progressive disease that will require continual monitoring by the patient's physician and speech–language pathologist. Patients will exhibit difficulty with drooling, chewing, and swallowing, with aspiration of saliva and food compounded by a poor ability to cough with sufficient strength to clear the airway. The progressive decline in swallowing ability may ultimately lead to the need for medical management to maintain nutrition and respiration.

Parkinson's Disease

Parkinson's disease is a progressive neurological disorder that results from a loss of the neurotransmitter dopamine. Patients with Parkinson's exhibit muscular rigidity and tremors. Two of the more famous people who have Parkinson's disease are the former world heavyweight boxing champion Muhammad Ali and the actor Michael J. Fox (*Back to the Future*). Patients with Parkinson's disease often exhibit difficulty with the oral phase of swallowing, showing particular difficulty with solid food. Because of the difficulties these patients have with motor movements, dysphagia problems can be found during all of the swallowing phases. During the pharyngeal phase of swallowing, there is often a delay, resulting in aspiration before the swallow. One of the most common causes of death in patients with Parkinson's disease is pneumonia.

Head and Neck Cancers

Head and neck cancers, including those of the tongue, larynx, or pharynx, and esophageal cancers frequently affect swallowing. For example, the most common symptom associated with esophageal cancer is dysphagia; in many cases, it is the first symptom that is identified by the patient. Depending upon the size and location of the lesion, the movement of food toward the stomach might be obstructed by the lesion or the muscles involved in the peristaltic movement of the esophagus might be impaired. Treatments to remove or treat the tumor, such as radiation therapy, also have the potential to impact the patient's ability to swallow. It is easy to understand how surgical removal of a head or neck tumor located in the tongue, pharynx, or larynx could result in difficulty with chewing and swallowing. Further, radiation treatments for head or neck cancer often result in changes to saliva production, causing a dry mouth referred to as *xerostomia*.

Quiz on the Fly 9.1

1. "Difficulty moving food from the mouth to the stomach" is a definition of _____.
2. The phases of swallowing are referred to as the _____, _____, _____, and _____ phases.
3. Misdirection of food or liquids into the larynx below the level of the vocal folds is called _____.
4. The most common neurologic disorder that causes difficulty with swallowing is _____, or _____.
5. Radiation treatments for head and neck cancers may result in a dry mouth due to changes to saliva production, which is referred to as _____.

THE MULTIDISCIPLINARY DYSPHAGIA TEAM

Although the speech–language pathologist provides expertise in identifying the features of the swallowing disorder and development of the therapeutic treatment plan, a team of medical professionals must work together because of the complexities of managing the care for a person with a swallowing disorder. The medical team consists of physicians, radiologists, nurses, dieticians, respiratory therapists, and social workers.

The speech–language pathologist receives a physician's order to evaluate the person with a suspected swallowing difficulty. This order may be sent to the speech pathologist during the person's stay as a patient in the hospital or may occur when the person is residing at home or in a nursing home. The individual's primary physician, as well as physicians from other medical specialties such as gastroenterology,

MAKING A DIFFERENCE

Michael, a 35-year-old attorney, was diagnosed with a rare tumor on one of the key nerves controlling swallowing. Following complex surgery to remove the cancer, Michael was able to talk, remember, and reason as before but was not able to swallow foods, liquids, or his own saliva. A feeding tube was placed directly into Michael's stomach to provide his needs for nutrition. Michael was evaluated by a speech–language pathologist who developed a treatment program including exercises for the tongue, throat, and swallowing stimulation. After 6 weeks of dysphagia therapy, Michael was able to swallow very small amounts of food and liquid on a specially designed dysphagia diet while utilizing swallowing compensatory strategies and swallow maneuvers. After several months of therapy, Michael was able to resume safe eating by mouth and had the feeding tube removed. Michael expressed his gratitude to his speech–language pathologist by stating, "Before my illness, I took swallowing for granted. No one can understand how important it is to be able to drink a cool glass of liquid until you have lost your ability to swallow. Thank you for guiding me through my swallowing recovery and encouraging me to continue with the exercises and treatments."

otolaryngology, surgery, or neurology may write the order for a swallowing evaluation, depending on the nature of the person's underlying medical diagnoses. The physician will provide detailed information regarding the person's medical history and information regarding the reason for the order, such as symptoms reported by the person or findings from test results, such as aspiration pneumonia, malnutrition, or dehydration. The speech–language pathologist will share test results from the swallowing evaluations and therapy progress with the physician, often via written reports.

While in the hospital or receiving medical care at home or in a nursing home, the patient's nurse is also an important member of the dysphagia team. Because the nursing staff will be responsible for the patient's care on a daily basis, the nurse will be a key contact person, providing information about any swallowing difficulties that are noted during meal times and any medical concerns that may be affecting swallowing. For example, the person may have difficulty with memory or communication and not be able to report difficulties with swallowing that occurred during meals since the last visit from the speech–language pathologist. Additionally, the patient may have required medications that caused excessive sleepiness or confusion that interfered with his or her ability to eat. Although the nurses will be responsible for the patient's daily medical care, the speech–language pathologist will often communicate regularly with the nursing staff to coordinate care for the person's eating. The speech–language pathologist will regularly communicate with the clinical dieticians when the person is hospitalized, and on a less frequent basis when the person leaves the hospital and returns to his or her primary living site. This coordination of services will be critical if the person is having difficulty maintaining weight or hydration or has a feeding tube (more discussion of feeding tubes will follow later in this chapter in the section Nonoral Feeding Considerations).

Depending on the patient's other medical conditions, it might be necessary for the speech–language pathologist to interact with the respiratory therapist. For example, if the person requires assistance for breathing care because of a tracheostomy breathing tube or respiratory diseases, the speech–language pathologist will coordinate care for the person's respiratory system with the respiratory therapists to provide suctioning of the airway, if needed. The social worker may be contacted to ensure that carryover of the plan for dysphagia management is continued once the person leaves the hospital. This might include continued speech therapy services after hospital discharge and extra assistance for the person during meals to ensure safe swallowing. Critical to the dysphagia team is inclusion of the patient with dysphagia and their family in the treatment planning and decision making. This will be discussed later in the Education and Training section of this chapter.

EVALUATING SWALLOWING

The process of evaluating swallowing involves a number of distinct steps. The first step involves screening the patient for the presence of a potential swallowing disorder. This screening is followed by a clinical evaluation that focuses on the patient's medical history, current status, and nutritional needs and helps the speech–language pathologist recommend the most appropriate instrumental tests that will more accurately determine the patient's abilities. The third component of this evaluation is an instrumental evaluation of swallowing.

Screening Swallowing

Screening procedures are methods for determining the presence or absence of a problem without identifying the specifics involved in the breakdown. Screening for a swallowing disorder might include chart review, discussions with the nursing staff, or brief observation of the patient who is being fed. As described by Logemann (1998), screening should be quick, low risk, and low cost. The purpose of screening is to identify those patients who will require a more in-depth evaluation. A good screening measure clearly differentiates those individuals with signs or symptoms of dysphagia from those without signs or symptoms. However, it is not unusual to identify patients who appear to have risk factors for dysphagia but later on are identified as not

---

Quiz on the Fly 9.1 Answers

1. "Difficulty moving food from the mouth to the stomach" is a definition of **dysphagia**. **2.** The phases of swallowing are referred to as the **oral preparatory, oral, pharyngeal,** and **esophageal** phases. **3.** Misdirection of food or liquids into the larynx below the level of the vocal folds is called **aspiration**. **4.** The most common neurologic disorder that causes difficulty with swallowing is **stroke,** or **CVA**. **5.** Radiation treatments for head and neck cancers may result in a dry mouth due to changes to saliva production, which is referred to as **xerostomia**.

exhibiting dysphagia. Likewise, we might identify patients who appear to have a normal swallow during screening but later are determined to have dysphagia. Obviously, minimizing the number of false positives and false negatives should be a goal of any screening measure. Given the large number of patients who might be referred to a speech–language pathologist in a hospital or other medical setting, and the need to provide early identification of dysphagia to prevent related medical complications, a dysphagia screening is the first step toward identifying the specific swallowing-related needs of the patient and planning appropriate management. During the screening, the speech–language pathologist will look for a number of behavioral signs that suggest the presence of dysphagia. These include reports of coughing, choking, drooling, a history of frequent bouts of pneumonia or upper respiratory problems, the presence of a tracheostomy tube, or symptoms such as patient complaints of difficulty swallowing or taking excessive time to complete meals.

Clinical Assessment of Swallowing

The speech–language pathologist completing the clinical evaluation of swallowing (bedside swallowing evaluation) will need to follow a number of basic steps as part of this evaluation process. These steps include obtaining and reviewing case history information, obtaining information from the immediate family and relatives, and directly assessing the patient's ability to eat and drink.

When obtaining and reviewing the case history information, the speech–language pathologist attempts to determine the exact nature of the complaint as it relates to the patient's swallowing. For example, a patient might report coughing every time when trying to swallow medication or choking when attempting to drink some juice. In addition, the clinician needs a detailed picture of the patient's past and present medical conditions so that an appropriate management plan can be developed. The clinician will ask about the type of nutrition the patient is receiving. Does the patient receive an oral diet (food and liquid by mouth), a nonoral diet (nutrition provided via a feeding tube), or a combination of both? The clinician will need to determine the patient's respiratory status to determine if the patient has pneumonia, receives supplemental oxygen, or has a tube in their trachea (tracheostomy tube) to receive oxygen. The clinician will try to determine whether the patient had a prior history of swallowing difficulties and whether the patient had problems maintaining nutritional health when eating by mouth. The prior history information may be documented in the patient's medical chart or obtained directly from the patient or patient's family. By compiling all of this information prior to evaluating a patient's ability to swallow, the speech–language pathologist can better plan the evaluation, with a goal to limit risks related to laryngeal penetration and aspiration during the evaluation. Additionally, the speech–language pathologist will note precautions listed by the medical team regarding infectious diseases or mobility restrictions. It will also be important to note the patient's general alertness and ability to adequately understand directions so that he or she can participate in the clinical swallowing evaluation. For treatment planning, the clinician needs to know the patient's ability to comprehend information and swallow prior to this hospitalization and the nature of the patient's current living situation.

The clinical evaluation of swallowing is viewed as the first step toward developing a comprehensive swallowing therapy program. The clinician will complete a visual examination of various oral structures such as the lips, tongue, and velum, as well as an examination of the patient's gag reflex, ability to cough, and characteristics of the patient's voice. During this examination the clinician will assess the strength, range of motion, and accuracy of movement of the oral structures, as well as their sensory capabilities for touch, temperature, and taste. The clinician will then check for the timing of the swallow response and any indicators of aspiration.

The speech–language pathologist begins by assessing the patient's ability to produce a saliva swallow, which if completed without significant difficulty will allow progression to careful introduction of liquids, pureed foods, and finally solid foods requiring *mastication* (chewing). The speech–language pathologist is always cautious during this evaluation and, to ensure patient safety, presents the liquids to the patient starting with very small amounts (1/2 teaspoon) and then gradually progressing to larger amounts from a spoon, cup, and straw. In a similar manner, solid foods are presented in small amounts beginning with pureed consistencies like pudding and moving toward larger amounts of foods requiring mastication. Attention is focused on how the patient prepares and controls the bolus; swallowing efficiency, including delays in transit through the oral cavity; and timing of the swallowing response. In addition, the clinician is also looking for signs or symptoms of aspiration. If at any time during the progression with food or liquid, the patient demonstrates signs or symptoms of aspiration such as coughing, throat clearing, wet-sounding "gurgly" vocal quality, changes in breathing pattern, or complaint of discomfort, the evaluation is modified to prevent further occurrences of that symptom. The results of these measures will reveal strengths and weaknesses that the patient exhibits within his or her swallowing system so that additional tests can be scheduled.

Having detailed the steps involved in the bedside evaluation, it is important for you to note that this bedside evaluation is not always predictive of laryngeal penetration and aspiration. Research has shown that even experienced clinicians occasionally have difficulty detecting aspiration during this clinical swallowing evaluation (Splaingard, Hutchins, Sulton, & Chaudhuri, 1988). Later research studies have further replicated this finding, noting the clinical swallowing evaluation was inadequate for detecting aspiration that occurred without a cough response, referred to as *silent aspiration*. Thus in most medical settings, additional instrumental testing procedures are completed by the Department of Radiology, often in conjunction with the Department of Speech–Language Pathology, to help to document the patient's swallowing abilities and the potential for, and existence of, aspiration.

Instrumental Evaluations of Swallowing

In addition to the bedside evaluation, the speech–language pathologist can take advantage of technologies available within a medical setting to further evaluate the swallowing abilities of patients. Two instrumental examinations can be used to further evaluate swallowing, and these are the *videofluoroscopic swallow study* (VFSS) and the *fiber-optic endoscopic evaluation of swallowing* (FEES).

Videofluoroscopic Swallow Study

The VFSS (also called a modified barium swallow) is an X-ray procedure that is completed by the speech pathologist working in conjunction with a *radiologist* (a physician who specializes in using radiation in the diagnosis and treatment of disease). The VFSS procedure is conducted with the patient seated in a chair or, if needed, a specialized wheelchair to provide sufficient postural support. The patient is given an assortment of consistencies of food and liquid containing *barium*. Barium sulfate is a contrast material that is typically used during X-ray procedures of the gastrointestinal tract. However, barium can also be used to visualize the movement of the bolus through the oral and pharyngeal cavities and through the entrance into the esophagus. Visualizing this movement allows the clinician to identify and document disorders of swallowing such as delays in oral or pharyngeal transit, delay in the initiation of the pharyngeal response, and apparent weakness in the muscles of the tongue, pharynx, or larynx as they occur. During this procedure, it is also important to determine if bolus misdirection is occurring. By using barium as a contrast medium, laryngeal penetration and aspiration can be clearly visualized. The speech–language pathologist and radiologist will try to observe if the patient coughs with aspiration or if the patient does not respond with a cough and thus has silent aspiration.

Fiber-Optic Endoscopic Evaluation of Swallowing

As we previously described in chapter 8, a flexible fiber-optic endoscope, or fiberscope, can be used to view the vocal tract, articulators, and the larynx. The FEES examination uses the fiberscope to allow direct visualization of the swallowing process as it occurs. The speech–language pathologist and physician are able to view swallowing functions including oral transit of the bolus into the pharynx, velar closure, pharyngeal muscle squeezing action, closing of the vocal folds, and epiglottal movement. Although the precise moment of the swallow cannot be seen because the light from the endoscope reflects off the closed epiglottis, immediately after the swallow, when the pharyngeal and laryngeal structures return to their resting positions, signs of a dysphagia can be noted. These signs may include food or liquid residue remaining in the pharyngeal cavity or even in the laryngeal entrance to the airway or in the trachea. The FEES evaluation allows for visualizing multiple swallows with a variety of food consistencies, or the completion of a small meal without dangers of lengthy radiation exposure.

During both the VFSS and the FEES evaluations, an important component of the examination is to determine the effectiveness of a number of therapeutic interventions focusing on the safety and efficiency of swallowing. If during the VFSS or FEES the person has aspiration of food or liquid, the speech–language pathologist will introduce a change in the way that the person swallows, referred to as *swallowing compensations*, or a change to the consistency of the food or liquid swallowed, referred to as *diet modification*. For example, if the person aspirates thin liquids, the goal for the speech–language pathologist is to find a swallowing compensation to prevent or minimize the risk of aspiration of thin liquids so that the patient can continue to consume thin liquids such as water. But, if swallowing compensations are found not to be effective, a diet modification to a thicker liquid consistency may be recommended.

IN THE CLINIC

Mrs. Monroe, a 70-year-old woman who was recently diagnosed with Parkinson's disease, reported that she was having difficulty swallowing her medications because of frequent coughing. Her husband reported that she also seemed to cough frequently during meals and thought that she was just "eating too fast." During the videofluoroscopic swallow study (VFSS), the speech–language pathologist was able to determine that Mrs. Monroe was aspirating thin liquids, which triggered a cough response, but she was not found to have difficulty swallowing solid foods. During the VFSS, thickening the barium to a nectar-thick level was found to eliminate aspiration.

The speech–language pathologist reviewed the VFSS results with Mr. and Mrs. Monroe, showing them the aspiration of the thin liquid barium recorded on DVD and the effectiveness of thickening the barium, which resulted in no aspiration. The family was provided with a plan for thickening liquids at home.

Mrs. Monroe stated, "I did not understand how my swallowing has changed from my Parkinson's disease. This test helped me to clearly see why I need to thicken my liquids."

Mr. Anderson, a 70-year-old man, was also recently diagnosed with Parkinson's disease and reported frequent coughing while taking medications and during meals. During his VFSS, the speech–language pathologist was able to determine that Mr. Anderson was aspirating particles of solid foods that had remained in his throat after swallowing. Because Mr. Anderson was not able to feel this residual food in his throat and because of weakness of the pharyngeal muscles, he was given the instruction to take small bites of food and to swallow two times between each bite, using effortful swallows. Thin liquids, when swallowed in small sips, were found to be swallowed safely. The speech–language pathologist reviewed the VFSS recording and results with Mr. Anderson, showing him the pharyngeal residual food and the subsequent aspiration of the food particles contrasted with the safe swallowing when the swallowing compensations were utilized. Mr. Anderson stated, "I did not realize that the coughing was due to difficulty swallowing from my Parkinson's disease. I can see clearly now why I need to follow your recommendations."

DYSPHAGIA TREATMENT

When swallowing is impaired, the clinician develops a plan that is referred to as a dysphagia management plan. This plan takes into account the implementation of therapeutic rehabilitation and consideration for how the patient can safely, efficiently, and effectively maintain a diet to sustain his or her needs for nutrition and hydration. In other words, the speech–language pathologist establishes recommendations for dysphagia treatment that are based on the evaluation results and include methods for eating that may address swallowing compensations, diet modifications, and a program of swallowing exercises. In summary, the development of the complete dysphagia management plan is a challenging puzzle that takes into account the underlying medical disorder that led to the dysphagia, results of the swallowing evaluations, the patient's individual needs, and the input provided by other members of the dysphagia team.

Swallowing Compensations

Swallowing compensations or compensatory strategies are one component of the dysphagia management plan. These swallowing compensations include *postures*, *swallowing maneuvers*, and *diet modification*.

Postures

Variations in the posture of the head and neck are utilized during swallowing therapy to redirect the flow of liquid and food safely through the pharynx. These postures include tucking the chin, turning the head, tilting the head, or even side lying. The patient is encouraged to make these changes prior to swallowing and maintain the posture until all of the food has been completely swallowed. It is important that any postures suggested to a patient are verified for effectiveness and safety, preferably with an instrumental swallowing evaluation.

Swallowing Maneuvers

A second type of compensation is called swallowing "maneuvers," where variations in swallowing produce a more efficient and effective swallow. Swallowing maneuvers require more training and also require that the patient has more memory skills in order to complete this more complex task. The speech–language pathologist will determine if a maneuver is effective during the swallowing evaluation and provide specific instructions during swallowing treatment sessions. One maneuver is called the Mendelsohn maneuver, which is used to increase the pharyngeal opening for passage of the bolus from the pharynx into the esophagus. For this maneuver, the patient is instructed, "When you swallow and you feel your Adam's apple (larynx) lift, do not let it drop. Hold your larynx up with your muscles for 2 seconds and then let it relax." The speech–language pathologist will provide feedback and training to the patient during the therapy session to ensure that the patient is correctly completing this modified swallow pattern and improved swallowing is noted. Patients will practice these maneuvers during treatment sessions and gradually incorporate them into their daily routine during meals.

Diet Modification

A frequently used compensation is the modification of food and liquid consistencies referred to as diet modification. These modifications help to reduce the risk of, or prevent, aspiration and also facilitate the patient's ability to maintain an oral diet. Because a thin liquid can rapidly flow, a person with dysphagia may not be able to start the swallow response quickly enough to allow the airway to close and prevent the thin liquid from being aspirated. Therefore, liquids may be thickened to aid control of the liquid in the mouth and to slow their rate of movement. Liquid thickeners are readily available at pharmacies and have instructions for increasing the level of thickness to the level determined by the speech pathologist. Additionally, food consistencies may be modified to fit the needs of the patient who has difficulty chewing foods, forming solid foods into a bolus in the oral cavity, or efficiently clearing the foods through the pharynx without the risk of choking or aspiration of residual food. Recommendations often stipulate that foods provided to the patient are only a pureed consistency like applesauce or mashed potatoes, or that the foods are ground or diced into small pieces prior to presentation to the patient. Although patients and families can select specific foods that meet the recommendations for diet consistency provided by the speech–language pathologist, a standardized format, called the National Dysphagia Diet (see Table 9.1), was developed by the American Dietetic Association. This plan provides suggestions for foods and texture modifications, including menus for each diet level. It should be noted that the speech–language pathologist will work with the patient to provide training in the compensations and maneuvers until the patient is able to complete them accurately and consistently, without signs or symptoms of aspiration or swallowing difficulty. Additionally, modification of the liquid and solid consistencies may result in the patient being able to continue to eat by mouth without the need for a feeding tube.

TABLE 9.1
National Dysphagia Diet (NDD)

Diet Consistency Levels

    NDD Level 1:
    Pureed (smooth, homogenous, cohesive foods)

    NDD Level 2:
    Mechanically altered (cohesive, moist, soft textured foods requiring minimal chewing)

    NDD Level 3:
    Advanced (moist, soft, bite-size foods that are easy to chew; no crunchy, hard, or sticky foods)

    NDD Level 4:
    Regular diet (all foods allowed)

Liquid Thickness Levels

    Thin:
    water, coffee, juice, anything that will rapidly liquefy in the mouth

    Nectar-like:
    thickened to a consistency that coats the spoon and flows at a slower rate

    Honey-like:
    thickened so liquid slowly drips or flows in a thick ribbon off the spoon like honey

    Spoon thick:
    thickened to a soft pudding consistency

Source: Based on information from *The National Dysphagia Diet: Standardization for Optimal Care.* American Dietetic Association, 2002.

Swallowing Exercises and Sensory Stimulation

Dysphagia treatment also involves exercises that are carefully implemented based on the findings from the bedside swallowing and instrumental evaluations. If during an evaluation the tongue, lips, pharynx, or larynx are found to be weak, limited in range of movement, or reduced in their ability to coordinate, exercises will be recommended to improve those affected muscles.

Other tongue exercises may focus on improving coordination that will result in improved bolus control within the mouth. It is important to note that with any swallowing exercises, caution must be used so that the patient does not choke or aspirate on foods or liquids during the exercises.

Other treatment techniques do not focus on muscle movements but focus instead on *sensory stimulation* to the oral and pharyngeal cavity. These sensory stimulation techniques are designed to heighten awareness in the mouth or to increase the speed of the swallowing response. Sensory stimulation techniques may be used during therapy sessions as well as throughout meals, and may include modification of food textures, introducing specific flavors such as sour lemon, or the addition of carbonated beverages.

Education and Training

A critical part of the dysphagia treatment process involves patient and family education and training regarding the nature of the dysphagia and the treatment plan. Therapy time will be devoted to helping the patient and family understand normal swallowing, the patient's dysphagia, and potential risks due to the dysphagia. The risks that will be discussed include complications that were previously discussed in this chapter, such as pneumonia, malnutrition, or dehydration. The treatment plan including therapy goals will be discussed with special attention given to patient agreement and input into the process. Part of the treatment sessions will involve assessing for patient and family understanding and carryover of the swallowing compensations and bolus medication recommendations.

Nonoral Feeding Considerations

When developing a management plan for a patient with dysphagia, the speech–language pathologist will make recommendations regarding a patient's ability to have an oral diet or whether a feeding tube is required. Sometimes the dysphagia is so severe that the patient cannot swallow, aspiration cannot be prevented, or foods cannot clear the pharynx. In these situations, a feeding tube may be recommended. Feeding tubes can be inserted into the stomach via the nasal passage, pharynx, and esophagus (*nasogastric tube*), or through an incision in the abdominal wall directly entering the stomach (*gastrostomy tube*). The decision regarding the type of feeding tube that is required is made by the physician with input provided by the patient and family. Generally, the nasogastric tube is considered a short-term remedy for feeding, but the gastrostomy tube is used for patients who will require more time and have greater difficulty recovering their ability to swallow

IN THE CLINIC

Mrs. Johnson suffered a stroke to the right side of her brain, causing weakness on the left side of her body. Since the time of her stroke, Mrs. Johnson has had difficulty with eating and swallowing. She has been instructed to eat and drink carefully because she is not able to tightly close her lips on the left side, causing liquids to spill from her mouth. When Mrs. Johnson eats, she has difficulty chewing solid foods such as meats and breads. The nurses note that, after eating, Mrs. Johnson finds that most foods become pocketed in the space between her bottom gums and cheek on the left side of her mouth. The speech–language pathologist noted during the clinical swallowing evaluation that Mrs. Johnson took several seconds to swallow sips of liquids, called a delayed swallow response, and took several swallows for each small bite of food. The speech–language pathologist also noticed that Mrs. Johnson cleared her throat occasionally during the meal, which was a sign of possible aspiration of food or liquid. The speech–language pathologist recommended that Mrs. Johnson be further evaluated with a videofluoroscopic swallow study.

The VFSS revealed no aspiration of food or liquid, but evidence of a delayed swallow response of greater than 2 seconds was revealed. This delay resulted in thin liquids entering the opening of the larynx before the swallow occurred, with eventual penetration to the surface of the vocal folds resulting in throat clearing. Swallowing liquids thickened to a nectar-thick level prevented this laryngeal penetration and potential for aspiration. Additional dysphagia signs included weakness of the left-sided pharyngeal muscles, causing food residue to remain in the pharynx after the swallow. When Mrs. Johnson was asked to turn her head to the left, this action prevented the residue from collecting in the pharyngeal recesses. A recommendation was made for Mrs. Johnson to eat a softer diet, called a Dysphagia 2 diet, with ground meats and no breads, and to have all liquids thickened to nectar thickness. Mrs. Johnson's family members and the nursing staff were instructed to remind her to always use her swallowing compensations that included turning her head to the left while swallowing, to check her mouth for pocketed foods, and to stick with her diet modifications.

and eat. The speech–language pathologist will be an important resource of information for the patient and family when trying to understand the extent of the dysphagia, the rationale for tube feedings, and what situations to anticipate regarding therapy for dysphagia when a person has a feeding tube. It is important for the patient and family to understand that feeding tubes are not always permanent and that dysphagia treatment can usually continue when the patient has the feeding tube. During this process, the speech–language pathologist will work closely with the dietician, nurse, physician, patient, and family to progress toward the goal, if indicated, of resuming a total oral diet.

VARIATIONS IN SWALLOWING ACROSS THE LIFE SPAN

Although the information provided thus far has focused primarily on adults with swallowing disorders, it is important to note that newborns, infants, and children may also have dysphagia. Pediatric dysphagia may result from neurologic disorders such as cerebral palsy; anatomic differences such as cleft palate; chronic diseases; gastroesophageal reflux disease (GERD); respiratory disorders, including those requiring a tracheostomy; or developmental delays and disorders such as autism. Additionally, babies that are born prematurely will likely have feeding difficulties with tasks such as learning to suck from a bottle or breast, and may have specific swallowing deficits in any of the four stages of swallowing. When evaluating an infant or child, swallowing will always be assessed according to developmental milestones, neurologic maturity, and development of the respiratory and gastrointestinal systems. Crucial to the assessment and treatment of feeding and swallowing problems in the pediatric population is the importance of adequate nutrition for growth and development. The speech– language pathologist will work closely with the pediatric medical team and the family to determine the best methods for feeding that allow for the safest and most efficient swallowing.

At the other end of the life-span continuum is the geriatric population. After the age of 60 and through the next decades of life, swallowing changes have been found to occur within the healthy aging population. Swallowing response times slow, tastes change, muscles of the tongue and pharynx become weaker, and swallowing endurance declines. The speech–language pathologist must take into account these normal age-related changes when evaluating swallowing and recognize how these normal changes may predispose an elderly patient to dysphagia when medical conditions occur.

SUMMARY AND REVIEW

The focus of this chapter was an introduction to the phases of normal swallowing and further discussion regarding the evaluation and treatment of dysphagia. You were first introduced to the four phases of swallowing, followed by a discussion of disordered swallowing and the various organic conditions associated with swallowing problems. We then focused on evaluating swallowing where we discussed bedside evaluations and instrumental evaluations of swallowing. The remaining sections of the chapter focused on dysphagia treatment where various compensatory strategies were discussed. These were postures, swallowing maneuvers, and diet modification. Additional discussion focused on swallowing exercises, sensory stimulation, and the very important component of patient and family counseling so that when a patient is finished with therapy, a support system is in place to help the patient to continue to use those skills that were learned in therapy and maximize his or her abilities to maintain an oral diet.

Anatomy and Physiology of Swallowing

What anatomical structures are integral to the process of swallowing?

Swallowing requires the complex integration of areas of the brain cortex, the brain stem, peripheral nerves, and over 25 pairs of muscles. Knowledge of the structure and functioning of the oral cavity, pharyngeal cavity, laryngeal cavity, respiratory system, and the esophagus are essential for understanding the swallowing process.

Phases of Normal Swallowing

What are the four phases of normal swallowing?

The four phases of normal swallowing are the oral preparatory phase, oral phase, pharyngeal phase, and esophageal phase.

Disordered Swallowing

What are laryngeal penetration and aspiration pneumonia?

Laryngeal penetration occurs when the patient attempts to swallow but the bolus or residue from prior swallows enters the laryngeal area above the vocal folds. Aspiration pneumonia occurs when food or liquid enters the bronchi of the lungs, resulting in an infection.

Swallowing Disorders Associated with Various Organic Conditions

What organic conditions might be associated with swallowing disorders?

Any neurological disorder that impacts the sensory and motor activities within the oral, pharyngeal, and laryngeal systems has the potential to cause swallowing problems. These include cerebrovascular accidents, traumatic brain injury, amyotrophic lateral sclerosis, Parkinson's disease, and head and neck cancers.

The Multidisciplinary Dysphagia Team

What professionals might be involved on the dysphagia treatment team?

Treating dysphagia often involves a multidisciplinary approach to care. Professionals involved on the treatment team include the speech–language pathologist, physician, radiologist, nurse, dietician, respiratory therapist, and social worker.

Evaluating Swallowing

What are the components of a swallowing evaluation?

A swallowing evaluation will include a thorough review of the patient's medical record, an interview with the patient, a bedside swallowing exam, and an instrumental evaluation of swallowing that might include a videofluoroscopic swallow study or a fiber-optic endoscopic evaluation of swallowing.

Dysphagia Treatment

What type of therapy is provided for a patient who experiences dysphagia?

Therapy for dysphagia is designed to rehabilitate the swallowing mechanism so that the individual can return to safe oral feeding for nutrition and hydration maintenance. Therapy for dysphagia is focused on patient and caregiver education regarding the anatomy and physiology of normal and disordered swallowing. Patients are instructed in various compensatory techniques to minimize aspiration and laryngeal penetration and facilitate resumption of swallowing necessary for oral intake.

Variations in Swallowing Across the Life Span

Are swallowing problems limited to older persons with neurological problems?

Dysphagia is often a concern for children with neurological problems like cerebral palsy. In addition, conditions like cleft palate, gastroesophageal reflux disease (GERD), and respiratory disorders requiring a tracheostomy may be associated with swallowing difficulties. If we examine healthy individuals over the age of 60, we can also find swallowing problems as some people age. Swallowing response times slow, tastes change, muscles of the tongue and pharynx become weaker, and swallowing endurance declines.

WEB SITES OF INTEREST

ALS Association
http://www.alsa.org/

American Speech-Language-Hearing Association
http://www.asha.org/public/speech/swallowing/

Mayo Clinic
http://www.mayoclinic.org/swallowing-problems/

National Institute of Neurological Disorders and Stroke
http://www.ninds.nih.gov/disorders/swallowing_disorders/swallowing_disorders.htm

National Institute on Deafness and Other Communication Disorders (NIDCD)
http://www.nidcd.nih.gov/health/voice/dysph.htm

National Parkinson Foundation
http://www.parkinson.org

10

Fluency Disorders

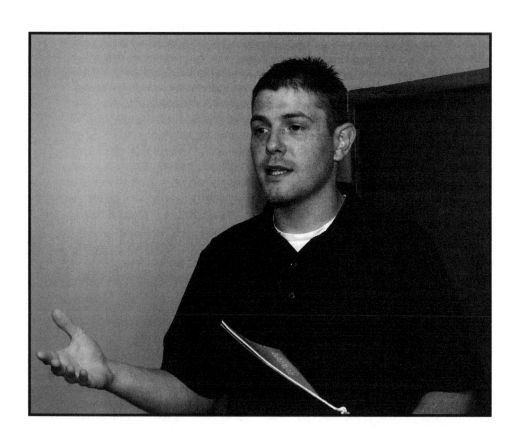

The focus of this chapter will be an examination of breakdowns in the forward flow of speech, known as fluency disorders. Most typically, fluency disorders are associated with the problem of stuttering, which will be the major focus of the present chapter. However, fluency problems are sometimes associated with other types of problems and these will be discussed at the end of the chapter. To begin our discussion we will help you to identify differences between normal, or typical, disfluencies and stuttering. We will follow this discussion by examining stuttering onset and how the problem of stuttering develops. You will then be introduced to various historical and current perspectives regarding stuttering causation. The next part of the discussion will focus on evaluating stuttering so that decisions regarding treatment can be made. Treatment for adults and children will conclude our examination of stuttering. In our final section, we will move from a discussion of stuttering to an examination of other fluency breakdowns—cluttering and those breakdowns associated with neurological problems.

FLUENCY AND STUTTERING

Fluency has been described as the smooth and effortless forward flow of speech. As we are talking about fluency disorders in this chapter, we need to provide a perspective for examining the breakdowns that occur in a speaker's fluency. To begin, we will define disfluency as anything that interrupts the forward flow of speech. You might think of disfluency as a hesitancy to produce a word, a cough that interrupts the flow of speech, or the locking up of the speech muscles so no sound can be produced. As we believe that disfluencies encompass all breakdowns in speech, we would like to suggest that there are two classes of speech disfluency. The disfluencies that occur across word boundaries are generally judged to be normally occurring in the speech of most individuals and are called *between-word*, or normal, disfluencies (Conture, 2001). A second category of speech disfluency breaks up a word, is judged to sound abnormal, and is generally referred to as *within-word disfluency*, or *stuttering* (see Table 10.1).

Normal disfluencies occur in the speech of most individuals. These fluency breakdowns are often used to provide the speaker with enough time to respond or hold his or her place so that the speaker can organize his or her thoughts without losing a turn. You might notice a speaker saying "I was um, um, um going to the movies last night" or a young child verbalizing "Mommy, Mommy, can I, can I go?"

TABLE 10.1
Categorizing disfluency

Disfluency	
Within-Word Disfluency (Stuttering)	**Between-Word Disfluency (Normal Disfluency)**
Sound/syllable repetitions	Phrase repetitions
Monosyllabic whole-word repetitions	Revisions
Audible sound prolongations	Interjections
Inaudible sound prolongations	Multisyllabic whole-word repetitions
Broken words	

Source: Based on *Stuttering* (2nd ed.), by E. G. Conture, 1990, Englewood Cliffs, NJ: Prentice Hall.

To the untrained observer, the use of interjections or phrase repetitions may sound like stuttering. However, these disfluencies typically occur for reasons that are recognized by the speaker (Yairi & Seery, 2011). For example, speakers will use between-word disfluencies when attempting to find a word, when formulating a sentence, or even when distracted during a conversation. In contrast, when a speaker knows the intended word and then has difficulty producing the word, we determine that these disfluencies are stuttering. Although all speakers produce within-word disfluencies, it is the frequency with which these disfluencies occur that result in our diagnosis of stuttering. Stuttering is characterized by sound and syllable repetitions and sound prolongations. Sound and syllable repetitions break up a word so that the first sound or syllable of the word is repeated. A sentence might look like "Can I have an a-a-a-apple?" or "The boy was go-go-going." Sound prolongations tend to be those that you can hear (audible) and those that are silent (block or inaudible). During an audible sound prolongation, the client stretches the sound for an extended period of time as in "He aaaaate an apple." During the production of an inaudible prolongation, the word often begins with a silent pause that can be short duration and not really noticeable to the listener, or longer and more noticeable. A client might try to introduce himself and say "Hi, my name is . . . . Bob," where there might be 1 to 2 seconds of silence before his name is produced. When an inaudible sound prolongation occurs in the middle of a word, this typically results in a broken word. Although these do not occur as frequently as sound/syllable repetitions or sound prolongations at the beginning of words, they do appear to be a strategy used by some persons who stutter.

According to the NIDCD (National Institute on Deafness and Other Communication Disorders, 2010b),

> stuttering is a speech disorder in which sounds, syllables, or words are repeated or prolonged, disrupting the normal flow of speech. These speech disruptions may be accompanied by struggling behaviors, such as rapid eye blinks or tremors of the

TABLE 10.2
Six dimensions of stuttering

1. *Overt Speech Characteristics*—disruptions in the forward flow of speech that include sound and syllable repetitions and sound prolongations. These disruptions occur within the respiratory, phonatory, and articulatory systems but are perceived as stuttering.

2. *Physical Concomitants*—those behaviors that occur in association with stuttering that often signal a person's attempt to deal with their stuttering and move forward with their speech. These behaviors can be seen as tense body movements, eye blinking, and torso movements. The behaviors are not necessary to diagnose the problem but often accompany the stuttering.

3. *Physiological Activity*—nonobservable but measurable behaviors that have been investigated and observed to be associated with stuttering. These include changes in skin reactions, pupil responses, and brain-wave activities.

4. *Affective Features*—strong emotional reactions associated with stuttering for some children and adults who stutter. These reactions may lead to avoidance behaviors, fear, sadness, and frustration that often become the primary features of the person's problem.

5. *Cognitive Process*—the process of planning and producing speech, possibly providing an overload to the speaker's system, resulting in a speech breakdown. In addition, a person's level of awareness; the manner in which they react to this awareness may result in additional reactions to the stuttering.

6. *Social Dynamics*—the manner in which the person's stuttering affects their daily interactions, class participation, social interactions in the workplace, and adjustments to new environments.

Source: Information from *Stuttering: Foundations and Clinical Applications*, by E. Yairi and C. H. Seery, 2011, Upper Saddle River, NJ: Pearson.

lips. Stuttering can make it difficult to communicate with other people, which often affects a person's quality of life.

Symptoms of stuttering can vary significantly throughout a person's day. In general, speaking before a group or talking on the telephone may make a person's stuttering more severe, while singing, reading, or speaking in unison may temporarily reduce stuttering.

There continues to be a lot of controversy amongst those persons who specialize in the area of stuttering. For some, stuttering is seen as a breakdown in speech; as a result, definitions of stuttering will mainly focus on this breakdown. To others stuttering is seen as a multidimensional problem that not only includes the speech breakdown but a number of other dimensions as well. Yairi and Seery (2011) have identified six dimensions to the problem of stuttering (see Table 10.2). Note that when considering the problem of stuttering, it is important to recognize that for one client the speech breakdown might be the primary concern, but for a second client the fear and anxiety associated with the stuttering will dominate the client's perception of the problem. Although further exploration of this controversy is beyond the scope of this text, it is important for you to recognize that the way stuttering is defined has implications for assessment, treatment, and research in the area. It is interesting to note that in a number of countries, the term *stuttering* is referred to as *stammering*. Stammering and stuttering are both used to refer to the unique breakdown in fluency that we have described.

THE ONSET OF STUTTERING

Incidence and Prevalence

Stuttering is a disorder of childhood, with 60% of the cases beginning before the age of 3 and 95% of the cases by 48 months of age. The stuttering we are describing here has been referred to as *developmental stuttering*. The *incidence* of stuttering has been defined as the percentage of the population who has stuttered at some point in their life. In the case of stuttering, this can include the child who reportedly stuttered for 2 weeks but outgrew the problem and the adolescent who is presently stuttering. Incidence of stuttering is reported to be 5% of the population. The *prevalence* of stuttering has been defined as the percentage of the population who presently exhibit the problem. Prevalence of stuttering is reported to be somewhere between 0.7% and 1%. It is interesting to note that although these figures are correct, examination of data for children close to stuttering onset indicates that at stuttering onset, the prevalence is approximately 2.6%, suggesting that stuttering is a more prevalent problem among preschoolers than previously thought (Yairi, 2004).

Incidence and prevalence depend on the gender of the individual. For children close to the onset of the problem, there is an approximate ratio of two males for every female who stutters. Interestingly, as these children get older there are greater differences between males and females, with figures ranging from 4:1 to 5:1 males to females in adolescents and young adults. Speculation and research regarding these gender differences strongly suggests a genetic component to stuttering (Kidd, Kidd, & Records, 1978; Yairi & Ambrose, 2005).

Genetics and Stuttering

We know that stuttering runs in families. Children who stutter have more relatives who stutter when compared with other families where there is no person who stutters. Investigators have attempted to examine the genetics of stuttering by looking for specific genes that may account for the problem. In a recent report from the NIDCD (National Institute on Deafness and Other Communication Disorders, "Researchers Discover," 2010) it was reported that three genes were identified to be the cause of stuttering in subjects from Pakistan, England, and the United States. Research is continuing with examinations of large populations to determine the nature of these gene mutations and the possibilities of new treatments. It is also interesting to note that a number of genetic stuttering studies have been conducted with both identical and fraternal twins. As you might remember, identical twins develop from one fertilized egg and thus carry the same genetic makeup. On the other hand, fraternal twins result from two fertilized eggs and often look and act very differently (see Figure 10.1). The results of these studies suggest that the occurrence of stuttering in identical twins is significantly higher for identical twins than for fraternal twins (e.g., Howie, 1981). We would like to point out that stuttering among the identical twins occurred in approximately two-thirds of the cases. Although this figure is high, it also suggests that if stuttering is purely genetic, all of the twins

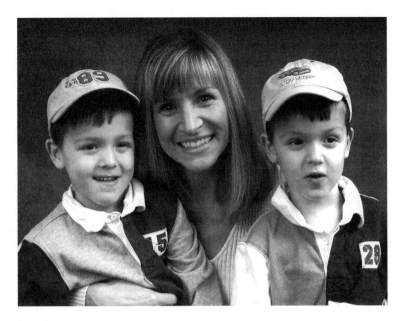

FIGURE 10.1
The incidence of stuttering is higher in identical twins when compared to fraternal twins.

would exhibit stuttering. As a result, one might conclude that other factors like environment may also play some role in the occurrence of stuttering.

Onset: Gradual or Sudden

Historically, stuttering onset has been described as a slow and gradual process in which children often begin stuttering by producing brief and effortless sound and syllable repetitions. This perspective continues with the belief that it is only after a period of time that children begin to produce an increasingly larger number of stutterings with more physical tension (e.g., Johnson et al., 1959). However, more recent findings reported by Yairi and Ambrose (1992) indicated that for a group of 87 children who stuttered, approximately 40% of these children exhibited onsets of the problem within a 3-day period, with some children displaying onsets of the problem within 1 day. In addition, whereas previous onset reports suggested that stuttering evolved from normal or mild repetitions of the problem, the parents in the Yairi and Ambrose study characterized their child's speech problem as moderate to severe and sometimes described the stuttering as being produced with severe physical tension. From a more practical perspective, given the variability of stuttering onset and the potential emotional distress of both parents and young children, the speech–language pathologist needs to be prepared to deal with the parents' concerns and in some cases the moderate-to-severe stuttering symptoms exhibited by these young children. In the section to follow, we will examine the development of the problem and the potential changes that may occur.

I CAN'T DO THIS ALONE

Brad attended stuttering therapy for at least 1 year and shared his observations regarding therapy.

I believe that a speech pathologist can make a huge difference in the quality of life for a person who stutters. Based upon my experience, stuttering impacted all facets of my life. This included communicating with my family and friends and my career. My speech often left me feeling disabled and alone. In addition, I often tried to hide my stuttering and had difficulty sharing my problem with others. Working with a speech pathologist helped me to learn the technical aspects of changing my speech but also helped to break down the barriers that I had built up regarding communication. My speech–language pathologist served a number of roles that included: friend, confidant, coach, and cheerleader during my daily battle to change my speech.

Over the years I have worked hard to hide my problem. Stuttering has been something that I have always been ashamed of and feel has been limiting with respect to my life choices. I have avoided speaking situations, viewing them as opportunities to stutter, with little upside and a huge downside. I think back to my college fraternity days and remember that never once over the 4 years did I speak up and share my opinions in chapter meetings for fear of stuttering and embarrassing myself in front of my brothers. It was the same way in high school and college classes. I just refused to take the risk to talk in class or any other situation that presented itself as I feared that I would stutter and would embarrass myself in front of my classmates. I even remember a class in graduate school where 25% of the grade was based on classroom participation and I still refused to speak up and participate, and my grade suffered as a result. I was just too fearful of what might happen and what people would think if I did stutter.

Recently I have started working again with a speech pathologist and he has provided me with the encouragement that I needed to try some new speaking situations. In this regard I have agreed to participate in some speaking situations at my church that in the past would have been easy to turn down. One is related to playing Martin Luther in a large speaking role in front of the 500-member congregation. During this speaking situation, my speech was excellent and I received a lot of great feedback from the congregation about how powerful I was in the role. These speaking experiences have helped to elevate my self-esteem and have helped me to feel very good about myself, with the courage to tackle future speaking challenges. In addition, these successes have made me a little more adventuresome at work with respect to speaking up and tackling challenging speaking assignments.

The speech pathologist provides a safe environment where the person who stutters can open up (for maybe the first time) and share feelings and experiences related to this problem. As the relationship grows, the speech pathologist can become the friend and confidant of the person who stutters, someone to look forward to seeing and sharing with. A good speech pathologist can also push the person who stutters to dream; and for the first time, that person can see things as possible that not too long ago were viewed as out of reach. My experience is that

(continued)

it can be very powerful to have someone that you trust, who understands your problem, and who you can open up to. The speech pathologist can provide context for the person who stutters and speak to the severity of the problem, based upon other persons who stutter that the speech pathologist has treated. I think that in a lot of cases such a patient may view the stuttering problem as more severe than it really is. The speech pathologist can help that person put situations into perspective and realize that things are not as bad as they seem.

I find that when I meet with my speech pathologist, my speech is very good and for the most part I do not stutter. I like to reflect on this success throughout my week as positive reinforcement in my daily battle. In addition, as I engage in speaking situations I try to imagine myself as talking with my speech pathologist, and I find that this is a good strategy to aid in keeping me somewhat fluent. I also think that my speech pathologist has helped to make me feel more comfortable with my stuttering. One of the ways that he has done this is by providing me with opportunities to speak to his speech pathology classes at the university where he teaches. In the past I never could have imagined myself talking to others about my stuttering, but I have found these experiences to be wonderful confidence builders that have helped me to be more accepting of myself and more open to sharing my experience coping with my stuttering with others.

THE DEVELOPMENT OF STUTTERING

Having discussed the varied onset of stuttering, the question that emerges is what happens once a child exhibits stuttering? A number of early studies reported the development of stuttering as a progression from a series of mild, less physically tense symptoms to more frequent occurrences of stuttering and changes in the physical tension and behaviors associated with the problem. Bluemel (1932) and later Van Riper (1954) talked about the initial development of the problem as *primary stuttering*. Primary stuttering was characterized by easy repetitions of sounds and syllables. This stage was followed by the *secondary stuttering* stage, in which the degree of physical tension increased and the children developed behaviors in association with stuttering as well as fear and avoidance reactions to their speech.

A second well-known developmental sequence of stuttering was proposed by Bloodstein (1960). Bloodstein used a retrospective form of research in which he examined diagnostic reports from a large number of persons who stuttered, and attempted to document a sequence of development based upon the information contained within the diagnostic reports. The results of Bloodstein's investigations led to the development of a four-phase model that appears to be linear in that the phases are associated with the age of the clients. Bloodstein described Phase 1 (ages 2 to 6) as being characterized by repetitions of syllables and words (content and function words) at the beginning of phrases and sentences. Stuttering during Phase 1 was described as episodic with the problem coming and going, and the child having little awareness of the stuttering. During Phase 2 (elementary school age) the problem has become more chronic, the child sees himself/herself as a person who stutters, and yet continues to show little to no concern about the problem.

In Phase 3 (8 years of age to adulthood), the client stutters as a function of specific situations. In addition, various sounds and words are now problematic but there continues to be little to no avoidance of speaking situations. During the final phase, Phase 4 (later adolescence and adulthood), the client fears and anticipates communicative situations, specific words, sounds and situations, and there is avoidance of speech situations and evidence of fear and embarrassment.

In contrast to the methodology used by Bloodstein, Yairi and his colleagues at the University of Illinois conducted a large-scale longitudinal investigation of the development of childhood stuttering. They collected "firsthand objective data" using audio and video recordings (Yairi & Seery, 2011). These investigations examined the frequency of occurrence of stuttering, the types of stuttering produced, and the behaviors produced in association with stuttering. In addition, language, phonology, and many other types of data were also collected. Because these investigations were longitudinal in nature, a child could be identified close to the onset of stuttering and then followed for 4 years or more.

We have known for some time that the majority of children who are identified as stuttering during their preschool years will outgrow the problem, thereby exhibiting *spontaneous* or *natural recovery*. Spontaneous recovery has been associated with a biological or maturational process, but natural recovery also recognizes that parents may modify communicative environments within the home, and this may also account in part for improvement in the child's speech. Results of a number of longitudinal investigations of stuttering (e.g., Månsson, 2000; Yairi & Ambrose, 2005) have reported that a preschooler who has begun to stutter has a 65% to 80% chance of natural recovery by 3 to 5 years following stuttering onset. During the first year of post-stuttering onset, only about 9% of these children naturally recover. The number continues to grow to 22% during the second year after onset, until it reaches 80% by about 5 years after onset. However, it is important for the reader to recognize that 20% of these preschool children will continue to exhibit persistent stuttering and will require some form of intervention.

Given the long recovery time of stuttering and the 20% persistency rate, the question arises regarding what factors might predict recovery or persistency. Biological factors such as gender and family history have been identified as prognostic factors. We know that the ratio of males who stutter to females who stutter increases with age. As a result, we might conclude that more females exhibit natural recovery when compared to males. A history of natural recovery in comparison to persistency of stuttering in families is another strong predictor for recovery. Children who have family members who recovered from stuttering have a 65% chance of natural recovery. In addition to biological factors influencing recovery, we also have a number of speech factors that influence recovery. The strongest speech predictor of recovery is the number of stutterings produced by the child during the first year post-stuttering onset. Yairi and his colleagues have noted that at about 7 months to 12 months after onset, those children who recover begin to show decreased numbers of stuttering until full recovery occurs and the child exhibits normal fluency. Children who tend to persist exhibit the same number of stutterings throughout their first year post-stuttering onset. In addition to the number of stutterings produced, other predictive factors include the type of stuttering, the length of stuttering, and the persistence of behaviors produced in association with the stuttering, although these predictors are not as strong as the number of stutterings produced.

Quiz on the Fly 10.1

1. Stuttered speech is composed of _____ and _____ repetitions and _____.
2. The percentage of the population who have stuttered at some point in their life is referred to as the _____ of stuttering, and the percentage of the population who presently exhibit the problem is referred to as the _____ of stuttering.
3. The onset of stuttering can be _____ or _____.
4. When a preschool child grows out of the problem of stuttering, this is referred to as _____ or _____ recovery.
5. By 5 years post-stuttering onset approximately _____% of the children who exhibited the problem are no longer stuttering.

THEORIES REGARDING THE CAUSES OF STUTTERING

In this section we will provide a brief description of some of the more popular explanations for the cause of stuttering. Examination of the literature reveals a wide range of explanations that range from breakdowns in the speech system to explanations blaming the parents and communicative environment. Given the vast number of attempts to explain this complex problem, we will only highlight a few of the more prominent hypotheses.

Organic Theories

Organic theories of stuttering focus on a biological or physiological explanation for the onset of the problem. For those who believe that stuttering occurs as a result of a breakdown within the speech system, it is believed that the child who stutters is born with some organic or biological deficit that puts the child at risk for the problem. As early as the 1920s, Samuel Orton and Lee Edward Travis (see Bloodstein & Ratner, 2008) at the University of Iowa suggested that, for most individuals, one cerebral hemisphere would become the dominant, or controlling, part of the brain, which would direct and control the other cerebral hemisphere. As most people develop a dominant side (i.e., right handed or left handed), this occurs as one cerebral hemisphere becomes dominant. Orton and Travis argued that for persons who stutter, cerebral dominance does not occur and, as a result, signals to the tongue and other parts of the speech system are sent by both cerebral hemispheres, resulting in muscle movements that are not synchronized, which causes stuttering. When individuals are placed in a communicative environment that places stress on the speech system, it is more likely that a breakdown will occur. Orton and Travis called their theory the *theory of cerebral dominance*. As this theory provided a concise and viable explanation for the cause of stuttering, it was initially well received. However, with further investigation and research, the theory could not be proven and was ultimately abandoned during the 1930s. However, more recent investigations of brain function have refocused attention back to this theory (e.g., Webster, 1997). Recent improvements in technology have enabled researchers to examine brain functioning in adults who stutter, resulting in suggestions for differences in functioning between speakers who are fluent and speakers who stutter. For example, DeNil, Kroll, Kapur, and Houle (2000) examined a group of adults who stutter using a special brain scan that reveals brain activity in a three-dimensional image. The results of this study suggested that persons who stutter exhibit greater activation in their right cerebral cortex when compared to normally fluent speakers. The authors suggested that their results provide limited support for the idea that differences with regard to how the brain manages speech and language exist between fluent speakers and speakers who stutter.

Behavioral Theories

In contrast to the theories suggesting that stuttering is a biological component of the child, or something the child is born with, behavioral theories suggest that stuttering is a learned behavior. The most influential person to promote this view of stuttering was Wendell Johnson and his colleagues and students at the University of Iowa. Johnson suggested that the speech of all young children was produced in a similar manner and was characterized by normal repetitions and hesitations. It was Johnson's idea that the parents of some of these children were more aware of and sensitive to these breakdowns in fluency. When these parents reacted to their child's speech by correcting the child, the child in turn would become more aware of his or her speech. As a result of the parental attention to the child's speech, the child would attempt to change their speech behavior or avoid producing those behaviors so that their parents would not react to their speech. For Johnson "stuttering begins not in the speaker's mouth, but in the listener's ear" (Johnson, 1955, p. 11). In addition, Johnson believed that it was the diagnosis of the problem by the

---

Quiz on the Fly 10.1 Answers

1. Stuttered speech is composed of **sound** and **syllable** repetitions and **sound prolongations**. **2.** The percentage of the population who have stuttered at some point in their life is referred to as the **incidence** of stuttering, and the percentage of the population who presently exhibit the problem is referred to as the **prevalence** of stuttering. **3.** The onset of stuttering can be **sudden** or **gradual**. **4.** When a preschool child grows out of the problem of stuttering, this is referred to as **spontaneous** or **natural** recovery. **5.** By 5 years post-stuttering onset approximately **65% to 80%** of the children who exhibited the problem are no longer stuttering.

parents that ultimately led to the problem developing. As a result, Johnson's hypothesis was termed the *diagnosogenic theory*, suggesting that the diagnosis of the problem was the cause of stuttering. It is interesting to note that Johnson's theory gained a lot of popularity during the 1950s and 1960s without any substantial data to support these suggestions. Johnson was particularly influential with his suggestions that labeling the problem of stuttering would make the problem worse. Even today parents are encouraged to not label the child's speech as stuttering, as if there is something magical about the word that would permanently affect the child. However, as more and more evidence was collected, it became clear that parents were not responsible for causing their child's stuttering.

Linguistic Theories

The *covert-repair hypothesis* received a lot of attention since it was introduced during the 1990s (Postma & Kolk, 1993). These authors suggested that during normal speech production, the speaker has an internal, subconscious monitor that enables the speech system to make corrections in the formulation of speech sounds to produce words. It was reported that this monitoring system is active as the individual is formulating words and sentences. However, according to Postma and Kolk, when a person stutters, the system for monitoring and repairing phonological errors is delayed, and as a result the person stutters as they cannot repair the error before it is actually produced. In this model, stuttering is seen as a typical reaction to a breakdown in the person's attempt to formulate sounds and words.

Biology Plus Environment

Another popular perspective regarding the development of stuttering was first proposed by Adams (1990) and later expanded upon by Starkweather and Gottwald (1990). This perspective was called the *demands and capacities model*. Starkweather noted that he was not attempting to explain the cause of stuttering, but rather wanted to consolidate the information that we knew about the problem to help to explain why a child's speech might break down. It was suggested that a child is born with a set of abilities or capacities related to motoric function, emotional development, cognitive development, and linguistic development. It was hypothesized that when the demands of the communicative environment or the internal demands of the child exceeded his or her capacities for dealing with the demand, stuttered speech would result. Although a superficial examination of this model appears to make a lot of sense, the model lacked specificity so that researchers had a difficult time specifying the exact nature of linguistic capacity or specific motor skills that might be affected. In addition, unlike other breakdown models, the demands and capacities model did not suggest that a biological deficit was present as a cause of the problem. Rather, the model just suggested that when the demands exceed the capacities, stuttering would result. This hypothesis remains controversial, and in its original forms was not able to be tested in a practical way. Numerous investigators (e.g., Siegel, 2000) have suggested that in order for this model to be valid, individual capacities need to be identified and environmental demands need to be specified.

EVALUATING STUTTERING

The results of a stuttering evaluation help the speech–language pathologist to make a decision regarding the presence of the problem, the need for intervention, and the nature of the intervention required. As a result, the evaluation will focus on the client's speech and language skills, the interaction between the client and his or her communicative environment, and the client's awareness and reactions to both his or her speech and the environment.

To examine the characteristics of the client's speech, the speech–language pathologist may observe an interaction between the client and another person (e.g., parent, spouse), in addition to the clinician's conversation with the client. During these interactions, the speech–language pathologist will record video or audio of the interaction so that detailed analysis can be completed following the evaluation. However, as the clinician will need to provide objective information to the client and/or parent following the evaluation, the clinician will be collecting data and calculating results throughout the evaluation. During the initial interaction, the clinician will focus on the client's frequency of stuttering, types of disfluencies being produced, and the number of unit repetitions produced by the client, all in an attempt to determine the presence of a stuttering problem. In addition, the clinician will also examine additional speech and language skills, vocal quality, and speech motor coordination.

Many clinicians recognize that communicative environments do not cause stuttering. However, communicative environments can often help to perpetuate the problem (Conture, 2001) and cause the client to react to his or her stuttering. As a result, the speech–language pathologist needs to determine the potential influence of the communicative environment upon the client. This can be accomplished by observing the child interacting with his or her parents, interviewing the parents, or using a more formal questionnaire to examine the adult client's reactions to various situations outside of the therapy room. Observing conversational interactions between the child and his or her parents enables the clinician to observe how the parents respond when the child stutters and how the child responds to the parents' responses. Although it has been demonstrated that parents of children who stutter are no different than parents of children who don't stutter, normal parent reactions like encouraging a child to slow down or take a deep breath can have a negative impact if a child reacts to the parents' responses. In addition, parents often exhibit behavioral reactions and are completely unaware of their responses. However, the child might be very aware and state, "I can see my mom holding her breath when I stutter." Observing parent and child interactions can provide extremely useful information regarding the role of the communicative environment in the perpetuation of the problem.

The interview with the parent of the child who stutters or the interview with the adult who stutters can provide valuable insights into the communicative environment in which the child or adult interacts. Parents will often share stories of difficulties faced by the child when talking with peers or relatives, and the adult may bring a detailed list to the evaluation to explain the ease with which he or she can order food at a fast-food restaurant and the significant difficulty experienced at a sit-down restaurant where ordering has to be done from the menu. In addition to the interview, questionnaires may be used to help the adult to identify and rate a variety of communicative situations so that the clinician will have a baseline of the client's perceptions regarding communication outside of the therapy room. It is not unusual during therapy to discover that an adult client can easily learn to make speech modifications within the therapy room, but any attempt to use his or her newly learned skills outside of therapy is extremely difficult. This difficulty is often associated with the client's emotional perceptions regarding communicating outside of the therapy sessions. Unless those perceptions are addressed, the client will have difficulty using the newly learned skills in a meaningful way.

During the entire evaluation process, the clinician obtains objective information regarding the nature of the client's stuttering problem and the influences of the communicative environment. Additionally, the clinician is also evaluating the degree to which the client is reacting to his or her stuttering and the communicative environment. A number of adults spend a lot of time trying to avoid stuttering and avoid situations in which they think they will stutter. However, if an individual is spending a good portion of the day trying not to stutter, this behavior is going to prevent a lot of other tasks from being completed. The amount of avoidance varies from individual to individual, so one goal of an adult evaluation is to determine the degree to which the person avoids. You should recognize that avoidance and behavior change are also concerns when working with children who stutter. It is not unusual to see young children substituting words, avoiding words, or even expressing to their parents "Why can't I say that?" and then giving up and walking away. As a result, in order to get a complete picture of the client's problem, the speech–language pathologist will need to examine the characteristics of the client's speech, the communicative environment and its potential impact upon the client, and, finally, the degree to which the client avoids and reacts to his or her speech and the communicative environment. When a decision is made that a client has a stuttering problem, the speech–language pathologist needs to develop a management and treatment program that will meet the needs of the individual client.

TREATING ADULTS WHO STUTTER

Traditionally, stuttering therapy has been classified into two schools of thought. These approaches have been referred to as *stuttering-modification therapy* and *fluency-shaping therapy*. Therapy programs that are classified as stuttering modification generally focus on the reduction of avoidance behaviors, with the ultimate goal being acceptance of stuttering, confronting fears and difficult communicative situations, and learning to stutter in an easier manner. Clients are taught that stuttering will always be a part of their lives and, in order to be successful, they have to address it and learn to deal with it. In contrast, therapy programs that focus on fluency shaping work with the client to replace stuttered speech with fluent speech. It is believed that the client is using a number of inappropriate strategies to produce speech and these result in stuttering. When a client produces fluent speech, he or she will receive verbal rewards and is encouraged to continue to use this same speech during progressively more difficult speaking situations.

TABLE 10.3
Van Riper's MIDVAS program

Motivation—client learns to be more accepting of his or her stuttering

Identification—aggressive program of self-analysis with an exploration of guilt, fear, anger, frustration, and anxiety

Desensitization—working toward increased tolerance for stuttering, and reducing avoidance behaviors

Variation—teaching client to vary stuttering and associated behaviors to gain feeling of control

Approximation—producing stuttering in a more acceptable manner

   Cancellations—repeating stuttered word fluently immediately after stuttering

   Pull Out—modifying the stuttering in the middle of a word in order to keep speech flowing

   Preparatory Set—client anticipates the production of a stuttering, and makes laryngeal and articulatory changes to modify speech

Stabilization—getting the client to accept responsibility for all changes

---

Source: Information from *The Treatment of Stuttering*, by C. Van Riper, 1973, Englewood Cliffs, NJ: Prentice Hall.

One of the more well-known proponents of stuttering-modification therapy is Charles Van Riper. Van Riper, a person who stuttered, developed a therapy program that encouraged the client to confront his or her fears and avoidances and then ultimately learn to modify their speech. Van Riper (1973) referred to his program by the acronym MIDVAS (see Table 10.3), where each letter stands for a stage of his program. As you can see from the table, the early stages of Van Riper's therapy program focus on the client confronting his or her fears regarding communication. Van Riper believed that before a client could be taught to modify his or her stuttering, the client first had to be willing to admit that he or she had a problem. Clients are often encouraged to enter into situations outside of the speech clinic and force themselves to communicate without avoiding or running away from the situation. At the same time, the client is asked to keep a log of the date, situation, emotional reaction, and how they stuttered. When the client returns to the therapy room, he or she can share the results with the clinician and discuss any progress. It is important to note that during this therapy there is no focus on achieving a level of fluency. The fact that a client was willing to enter into a communicative situation when in the past he or she would have avoided the situation was seen by Van Riper as progress. If the client complains that "I stuttered like crazy," the clinician points out to the client that the situation was probably not as bad as he or she thought it was, and when the client approaches the same situation during the next week, it is likely that his or her feelings about communicating will improve.

As the clients' emotional outlook improves regarding stuttering and their willingness to enter into previously avoided situations, therapy focuses on strategies for learning to modify stuttering. For Van Riper, this involved teaching the client to anticipate a stuttering and change the manner in which they used their articulators (e.g., preparatory sets), but other clinicians suggested easy onset of the stuttered word or light articulatory contacts as methods for maintaining the flow of speech

IN THE CLINIC

Jerry, a 37-year-old male, appeared to be fluent but reported that he had a bad stuttering problem that he worked very hard to hide. Jerry indicated that it was very important for him to not let people know that he stuttered. As Jerry had recently lost his job, he has started interviewing for jobs, which resulted in a lot of stress for him. Jerry noted that working and communicating with authority figures had always been difficult for him.

Until recently Jerry never thought of himself as a person who stutters. He had been spending time on the Internet and reading a lot about stuttering. He realized that all the things he did to avoid stuttering were tricks that just postponed dealing with the problem: He and he was indeed a person who stuttered, and this was a great shock to him.

Growing up, Jerry had never discussed his speech or stuttering with his mother or his siblings. He used to stutter badly when talking with his parents and in school. Jerry stated that his family did not admit to nor discuss any weaknesses that an individual might exhibit. Jerry's wife is a speech–language pathologist who works with autistic children. When he first got married he told his wife that he used to be a person who stuttered but grew out of it. It is only very recently that Jerry admitted to his wife that he had a stuttering problem.

Jerry appeared to be highly motivated to attend therapy despite the fact that he realized he was going to have to confront all of those fears that he had been working so hard to avoid. Although Jerry was not fluent during the early stages of therapy, he completed telephone tasks that required identification of both overt (stuttering on a word) and covert behaviours (avoiding a word so that his speech sounded fluent) associated with his problem. In order to decrease his avoidance behaviors, Jerry realized that he would have to use pseudostuttering, or fake stuttering, to let others know that he had a problem during progressively more difficult social situations. By "advertising" his stuttering, Jerry was learning to be more accepting of his stuttering when others were aware of his speech, and he was allowing more of his stuttering to be heard and recognized. This change in his behavior was viewed to be an achievement. He was making excellent progress and was clearly aware of what he had accomplished. Jerry decided to establish his own business and began to extend and explore new contacts and avenues while using techniques to let people know that he stuttered.

Within the therapy room, discussions focused on the nature of stuttering and Jerry's willingness to confront his stuttering and no longer avoid it. Jerry was enthusiastic about seeking answers to questions that he had about his problem. However, as therapy continued, Jerry was reluctant to do voluntary stuttering during certain threatening real-life situations. During a 4-hour drive with his mother, Jerry had intended to use voluntary stuttering but decided to not try this during conversations with his mom. He explained that all his life he had avoided stuttering

(continued)

with his family, his mother in particular, who tended to be a rather critical person. However, soon after this failed attempt, Jerry spoke with his mother and told her what his intentions had been and had several stints of voluntary stuttering with her.

About three quarters of the way through therapy, Jerry's wife accompanied him to a therapy session. She said she was "astounded" at the change in him, conveying that he had always tended to keep to himself, hide his feelings, and avoid his stuttering. At the present time he was now more willing to let others hear him stutter, more willing to communicate, and was more positive in general. "It's all wonderful."

During almost all work-related meetings and situations, including very important meetings where the stakes were large, Jerry used voluntary stuttering. He began to enjoy the relaxation he felt about his stutter and the control he believed that he had. There seemed to be little doubt that he had broken down practically all the negative reactions and attitudes about stuttering. Even if he was tired and had a bad period, his speech was not affected. Most importantly, Jerry had become more outgoing than ever. He no longer retreated to his emotional shell or avoided words or situations. Jerry continued to feel quite free and in fact felt that he had undergone a change in personality. A big part of therapy was spent on helping Jerry to develop a format that he could follow on his own to become his own therapist when he was no longer attending therapy on a regular basis. We also encouraged Jerry to continue to work on his speech and not take the tremendous improvements that he had made for granted. Jerry had become involved with a large stuttering association and had started manning their national telephone help line one night a week.

During the final therapy session and again in the review session some months later, Jerry indicated how profound the effect of therapy had been on him, especially his personality. His wife continued to refer to the remarkable changes he had made. Jerry was now seen as being more assertive. Four years later during a conversation, Jerry reported that he did not need to work on his speech any longer as he was totally unconscious of the way he spoke and it did not bother him in any way.

Contributed by Myrtle "Chookie" Aron, PhD, retired faculty member, Department of Speech Pathology and Audiology, University of the Witwatersrand.

and producing the stuttering in a different way. As clients become skilled at modifying their stutterings during conversations, therapy activities begin to focus outside of the therapy room, and clients are encouraged to use these newly learned skills during previously avoided situations. As clients gain confidence and continue to use their new skills outside of the therapy room, the number of sessions is gradually reduced as clients take on increased responsibility for their speech.

In contrast to stuttering-modification programs, clinicians who use fluency-shaping programs work with the client to replace stuttered speech with fluent speech.

Although there are a variety of ways of teaching the client to be fluent, the use of slow, prolonged speech has been demonstrated to be the most effective method for reducing stuttering and establishing fluency (Ingham, 2003). Clinicians who use fluency-shaping approaches in the most rigid manner believe that fluency is the focus of therapy and both fluency and stuttering can be manipulated by rewards and punishments. For this group of clinicians, fluency is the goal, with therapy sessions structured to address increasingly more complex speaking tasks (e.g., name single pictures to conversation). Ultimately, the client is expected to converse with the clinician while maintaining fluent speech. Unlike the clinicians who provide stuttering-modification therapy, this group of fluency-shaping clinicians target the production of fluent speech and set goals for their clients related to the degree of fluency produced by the client. Therapy is directed toward the reduction in the frequency of stuttering in the belief that as the client becomes more fluent his or her emotional reactions regarding stuttering will change because the client is not stuttering as often. This perspective continues to be controversial as many clients show positive changes in therapy but, after a period of time, the stuttering returns. This process is called *relapse.*

A third group of clinicians realized that any therapy provided in a rigid manner has the potential to not be as effective as a program of therapy that focuses on both the client's fluency and his or her emotional reactions associated with stuttering. These clinicians focus on a program that borrows the positive aspects of both fluency-shaping and stuttering-modification programs to provide a comprehensive treatment program that addresses the reduction in the frequency of stuttering and counsels the client regarding emotional perspectives associated with the problem. The clinician first takes a fluency focus to teach the client a set of skills for improving fluency. These clinicians recognize that clients can be less than 100% fluent and still be viewed as successful. For example, Schwartz (1999) described four speaking skills (see Figure 10.2) that will result in the production of fluent speech. Therapy techniques are often borrowed from existing programs but introduced in such a way as to describe success in terms other than 100% fluency. Success can also be measured as it relates to the client's pre-therapy and post-therapy responses to questions about avoidance behaviors, out-of-therapy participation during communicative activities, and willingness

---

1. Initiating speech in a slow, smooth manner—Clients are taught to start each phrase using "slow and smooth speech."

2. Phrasing—Clients are taught to break long sentences into chunks so that fluency skills are easier to apply.

3. Connecting across word boundaries—Clients are taught to blend their words together to achieve more fluent-sounding speech.

4. Increasing vowel duration—Clients are instructed to stretch their vowels as they connect their words during speech.

FIGURE 10.2

Fluency-enhancing skills.

Source: Based on information from *A Primer for Stuttering Therapy,* by H. D. Schwartz, 1999, Boston: Allyn & Bacon.

to verbally communicate. In contrast to the more rigid fluency-shaping programs, these hybrid programs also work to counsel clients, discuss avoidances and reactions to stuttering, and help to modify the client's emotional outlook associated with stuttering. When a client learns to modify his or her speech and at the same time learns to deal with the old fears and new fluency, the client has a much better chance at remaining fluent well after direct therapy has been discontinued.

TREATING CHILDREN WHO STUTTER

Therapy programs for children who stutter can be classified as indirect or direct treatment programs. Depending upon the time from stuttering onset, the changes observed in the child's stuttering, the communicative demands within the child's environment, and the child's reactions to his or her speech and the environment, the speech–language pathologist may choose an indirect form of therapy rather than a direct form of therapy.

Indirect therapy for children who stutter can range from suggestions for the parents to modify the communicative environment at home to more formal programs in which the parents are instructed in methods for facilitating communication at home. Most typically, indirect therapy is recommended for children who are close to stuttering onset, children who are producing more sound and syllable repetitions than sound prolongations, children with a family history of recovery, and children who do not appear to be reacting to the problem.

When a child has reached 6 months post-stuttering onset and has shown little to no positive changes in his stuttering, direct therapy is often recommended. One example of a very popular and successful program for children who stutter is called the Lidcombe program (Onslow, 2003). This program is named for a suburb of Sydney, Australia, and is a joint project of the Australian Stuttering Research Centre, the Discipline of Speech Pathology at The University of Sydney, and the Stuttering Unit, Bankstown Health Service, Sydney. The Lidcombe program is designed to be administered by the parents of a child who stutters. The program is divided into two sections: The first portion of the program involves the establishment of fluent speech and, according to the program developers, takes an average of 11 weeks. The second portion of the program focuses on maintaining speech fluency, and this takes at least 12 months to complete. As the parent is responsible for the daily practice sessions with the child, one or both parents receive weekly training from a speech–language pathologist regarding methods for facilitating and rewarding fluent speech in the home. Parents are taught to recognize both stuttered and fluent speech, and are encouraged to reward periods of fluency and provide negative feedback when a child stutters. Recognizing the benefits of rewards versus punishment, the program developers suggest that rewards be provided at a ratio of five rewards for each punishment. During weekly meetings between parent and clinician, the child's program is discussed in the form of a severity rating sheet that is filled in daily by the parent. By charting their child's behavior, the parents can share this information with the clinician and discuss methods for increasing speech fluency at home. The Lidcombe program has proven to be a very popular program, with 80% of the speech–language pathologists in Australia using the program and numerous clinicians in Europe, Canada, and the United States also using this program.

More traditional stuttering therapy programs with children generally take a fluency-shaping approach in which the child is taught to make speech modifications resulting in increased fluency. In a manner similar to adult therapy programs, direct therapy with a child will focus on teaching the child a set of fluency skills using vocabulary and descriptions that are appropriate to the child's chronological age. For example, to teach a child about stretching and connecting words, the clinician might bring silly putty to therapy and use the silly putty to demonstrate how to **s—t—r—e—t—c—h** out words, which makes them easier to say and helps eliminate stuttering. As part of this therapy program, parents will be asked to participate and learn the same fluency-enhancing skills. In this manner, parents can provide good communicative models at home and even model some of the fluency skills during practice sessions that are encouraged on a daily basis. Therapy is focused on helping the child to reduce his or her frequency of stuttering and take responsibility for the changes that occur so that the child can become more fluent outside of the therapy room.

In an attempt to compare the effectiveness of stuttering therapy for children, Franken, Kielstra-Van der Schalk, and Boelens (2005) compared the speech of children who participated in a Lidcombe program to children who participated in a traditional program based upon a demands and capacities model. The results of this investigation demonstrated that both programs were effective in reducing the child's frequency of stuttering. In addition, the parents of children in both programs were pleased with the results. It appears that at this time stuttering therapy for children might be conducted in a number of different ways depending upon available resources but still achieve similar outcomes.

Quiz on the Fly 10.2

1. According to Johnson, stuttering is caused by _____.
2. Replacing stuttered speech with fluent speech characterizes _____ therapy.
3. Teaching a client to decrease avoidance behaviors and face his or her stuttering characterizes _____ therapy.
4. Following therapy a client begins to stutter again. This is termed _____.
5. Therapy in the Lidcombe program is provided by the _____.

OTHER FLUENCY DISORDERS

Earlier in this chapter we indicated that, in addition to stuttering, there are other types of breakdowns in fluent speech production. Two additional problems are cluttering and neurogenic stuttering. Daly and Burnett (1996) described *cluttering* as a speech and language processing disorder characterized by rapid and dysrhythmic speech that is frequently unintelligible. It appears that a fast speaking rate is sometimes associated with the problem, but disfluencies in language formulation is always a characteristic of the disorder. These disfluencies often include interjections and revisions, as well as word and phrase repetitions. In addition, clients who clutter often exhibit articulation difficulty. This may be associated with their fast speaking rate, resulting in unintelligible speech. Therapy for cluttering often focuses on increasing the client's self-awareness regarding speech production and working on skills to modify the speaking rate. When the client has been instructed in methods for slowing down his or her speech, direct work can be undertaken to help the client learn to improve his or her speech articulation.

Neurogenic stuttering has been described as the gradual or sudden onset of stuttering-like disfluencies in adults. These disfluencies are typically associated with strokes, traumatic brain injuries, and diseases that affect the brain. It appears that lesions in a variety of different areas can result in neurogenic stuttering. For some patients, this breakdown in fluency is transient and resolves as the patient's condition improves; however, for other patients, the resulting speech is permanent. Depending upon the nature and location of the problem, disfluency types may be very different. Patients who have had strokes appear to produce repetitions of sounds and syllables and occasionally a longer word or phrase. It is interesting to note that although patients with head injuries also exhibit repetitions, these repetitions are often produced very rapidly in quick bursts and are sometimes unintelligible (Ludlow, Rosenberg, Salazar, Grafman, & Smutok, 1987). As brain injuries occur in a number of locations affecting a number of different areas of the brain, there is no specific pattern of disfluency that is associated with all brain damage. As a result, the speech–language pathologist must complete an evaluation to determine the nature of the adult client's fluency abilities and then devise a program that will help the patient to learn to compensate for these new speech difficulties.

SUMMARY AND REVIEW

The focus of this chapter was an examination of fluency disorders. We began our discussion by defining fluency and disfluency and then discussing both normal disfluency and stuttered disfluency. We continued by providing a definition of stuttering and looking at its onset and incidence, as well as the prevalence of genetics associated with the problem. Our next focus was an examination of the development of stuttering so that we have a better understanding of what the problem looks like at the onset and how the problem progresses. We then looked at stuttering from a historical point of view, noting a number of different perspectives for stuttering causation. Given that stuttering

---

Quiz on the Fly 10.2 Answers

1. According to Johnson, stuttering is caused by **the parents or the environment. 2.** Replacing stuttered speech with fluent speech characterizes **fluency-shaping** therapy. **3.** Teaching a client to decrease avoidance behaviors and face his or her stuttering characterizes **stuttering-modification** therapy. **4.** Following therapy a client begins to stutter again. This is termed **relapse. 5.** Therapy in the Lidcombe program is provided by the **parents**.

is a complex problem, we discussed the evaluation of the problem by suggesting that it is important to examine the client's speech, the communicative environment, and the client's awareness of and reactions to his or her speech and the environment. Following the assessment discussion, we identified two schools of thought regarding stuttering therapy. This was followed by a discussion regarding stuttering therapy for adults and stuttering therapy for children. We concluded the chapter with a short discussion of other fluency problems—cluttering and those breakdowns associated with neurological problems.

Fluency and Stuttering

What is the definition of stuttering?

Stuttering is a speech disorder in which sounds, syllables, or words are repeated or prolonged, disrupting the normal flow of speech. These speech disruptions may be accompanied by struggling behaviors, such as rapid eye blinks or tremors of the lips. Stuttering can make it difficult to communicate with other people, which often affects a person's quality of life.

The Onset of Stuttering

What do we know about stuttering onset?

Stuttering occurs more frequently in males than females, and as the client gets older the ratio of males to females gets larger. Stuttering runs in families; persons who stutter have more relatives who stutter when compared with other families where there is no person who stutters. Although many people believe that the onset of stuttering is a slow and gradual process, we now know that, for a number of children who stutter, the onset occurs in a relatively short period of time (from 1 to 3 days).

The Development of Stuttering

What is spontaneous or natural recovery?

Natural recovery refers to the fact that 65% to 80% of children who stutter as preschoolers will grow out of the problem by 3 to 5 years post-stuttering onset. This phenomenon has been related to biological recovery suggesting some type of maturational process and also modifications in the child's communicative environment.

Theories Regarding the Causes of Stuttering

What types of theories have been proposed regarding the cause of stuttering?

Early theories for the onset of stuttering suggested brain differences between persons who stutter and normally fluent people. Although many of the early studies could not be proven, more recent studies have suggested possible brain differences between persons who stutter and normally fluent speakers. Behavioral theories of stuttering have focused on the child's communicative environment and have suggested that the manner in which the parents interact with a child results in the child's stuttering. Some more recent theories have focused on language and speech formulation as the cause of stuttering, and others have suggested that stuttering is the result of some biological differences within the child that, when combined with the demands of the environment, result in stuttering.

Evaluating Stuttering

What do we need to examine during a stuttering evaluation?

Because of the complex nature of stuttering, it is important that an evaluation focuses on the child or adult's speech behavior, potential influence of the communicative environment, and the manner in which the client reacts to both the stuttering and the environment. By identifying the characteristics of the client's speech and the reactions associated with stuttering and communication in general, the speech–language pathologist is better able to develop a comprehensive treatment plan.

Treating Adults Who Stutter

What is the basic difference between stuttering modification and fluency shaping?

Stuttering modification focuses on reducing the client's avoidance behaviors and teaching the client to modify his or her stuttering. The client is taught that he or she will always have a problem and it is best to learn how to deal with the stuttering. In fluency shaping the client is taught a new set of speaking skills that attempts to eliminate the stuttering. There are two groups of clinicians who use fluency-shaping therapy. One group, who follows a rigid approach to therapy, focuses on fluency and believes that as the client becomes fluent, his or her emotional reactions associated with stuttering will change as a result of being more fluent. A second group of clinicians also focuses on teaching fluency skills but takes a more direct approach toward counseling and teaching the client to deal with their emotional reactions associated with their fluency and stuttering.

Treating Children Who Stutter

How is the Lidcombe program different from traditional stuttering therapy for children?

The Lidcombe program is administered by parents on a daily basis within the child's home. The program is monitored by a speech–language pathologist but the changes that occur are related to all of the activities that the parent completes with the child outside of the therapy room. In a traditional therapy program, the speech–language pathologist directs the therapy program, and works directly with the child to make modifications in his or her speech while at the same time working with parents to modify the communicative environment outside of the therapy room.

Other Fluency Disorders

What is neurogenic stuttering?

Neurogenic stuttering is a breakdown in fluent speech production that results from a head injury, stroke, or disease.

What is cluttering?

Cluttering is a speech and language processing disorder characterized by rapid and dysrhythmic speech that is frequently unintelligible.

WEB SITES OF INTEREST

The American Speech-Language-Hearing Association
http://www.asha.org/public/speech/disorders/stuttering.htm

National Institute on Deafness and Other Communication Disorders
http://www.nidcd.nih.gov/health/voice/stutter.html

Stuttering Foundation of America
http://www.stuttersfa.org/

Stuttering Home Page
http://www.mnsu.edu/comdis/kuster/stutter.html

11

Anatomy and Physiology of Hearing and Hearing Disorders

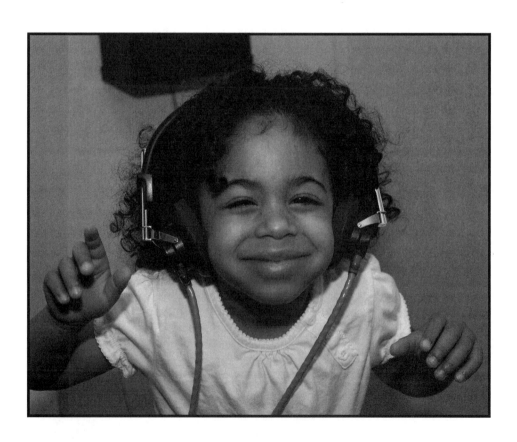

In order for you to understand the anatomy and physiology of hearing, you must first understand the nature of sound and how sound is transmitted. This chapter will begin with a discussion of sound transmission and the characteristics of sound. The chapter will then explore the anatomy and physiology of the hearing mechanism. This will include a discussion of how sound travels through the auditory system and is ultimately perceived by the brain. The final section of this chapter will be an examination of hearing disorders and hearing loss as they relate to the specific portions of the auditory system.

THE TRANSMISSION OF SOUND

The collection and transmission of sound occur within the specialized sensory system called the *auditory system*. We will begin our discussion by describing the characteristics of sound, and then explain how the sound travels through the ear, gets modified along the way, and ultimately is perceived by the brain. To begin the process, we need to examine the characteristics of sound.

Sound

Sound has been described as both a particle disturbance and a change in pressure in an elastic medium (Clark & Ohlemiller, 2008). When examining sound, the elastic medium is typically air within the environment. The disturbance of these particles results in a pressure variation among air molecules that can be detected by the ear. When a sound source such as a rubber band, guitar string, tuning fork, or the vocal folds begin their back-and-forth motion, the movement of these objects results in a collision of air molecules so that they collide with an adjacent molecule and then return to their previous resting state. However, as the adjacent air molecule was subsequently disturbed, we have a continuing disturbance of air molecules. As these air molecules continue to collide and then return to a resting state, we note areas of increased pressure resulting from a bunching of air molecules (*compressions*) and areas of decreased pressure where the molecules have returned to their resting state (*rarefactions*, see Figure 11.1). As sound is characterized by this back-and-forth motion, the transmission of sound is actually a transfer of energy across molecules rather than a transfer of matter. The movement of sound can be depicted as a waveform where the compressions are represented by

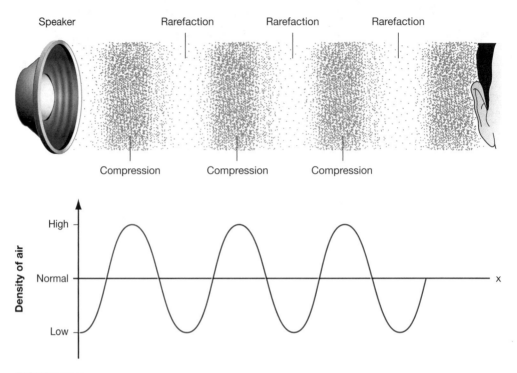

FIGURE 11.1
Transmission of sound: compressions and rarefactions.

the peak of the wave and the rarefactions are represented by the trough of the wave (Figure 11.1). If we consider one compression and one rarefaction, we have one complete cycle of vibration.

Frequency and Pitch

The number of back-and-forth movements of an air molecule that occur within 1 second is called the *frequency* of the sound. Frequency is measured in units called Hertz (abbreviated Hz), named for a German scientist. As the number of times an object vibrates per second increases or decreases, its frequency of vibration changes. Human hearing is often reported to range from 20 Hz to 20,000 Hz although the speech frequencies are reported to be 125 Hz to 8,000 Hz. However, my dog Teddy may exhibit a hearing range from 67 Hz to 45,000 Hz, and your pet porpoise Wally may exhibit a hearing range from 75 Hz to 150,000 Hz. Frequency is often described as a physical property of sound, a property that you can measure. If we look at a graph of two sound waves of different frequencies, we will note more peaks and valleys within the same time period for a higher frequency sound (see Figure 11.2). When we are interested in measuring the frequency of vibration, we can use a microphone, a computer, and specialized software to determine the frequency characteristics

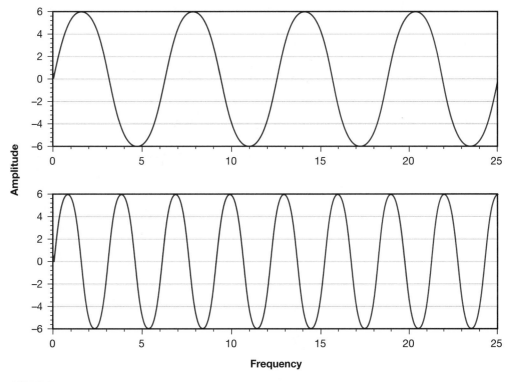

FIGURE 11.2
Waveforms of two different-frequency sounds.

of specific sounds. *Pitch*, on the other hand, has been described as the perceptual correlate of frequency. Pitch is associated with the sounds that we hear and is often based on our perceptual judgment. For example, a change in the frequency of vocal-fold vibration results in our perception of a pitch change.

Intensity and Loudness

A second physical property of sound is intensity. Intensity is associated with the amount of sound pressure that occurs as a result of the collision of air molecules. When we examine the back-and-forth motion of the air molecules, we note that the greater the displacement, the greater the collision of air molecules, resulting in the increased intensity of the sound signal. We previously reported that sound is the transfer of energy rather than the transfer of matter. As a result, when a greater force results in greater displacement of the air molecules, a more intense sound is produced. If we examine a graph of two sound signals of differing intensities, we will note that a more intense signal is represented by a larger wave, and the difference between the two signals is represented by the greater height, or *amplitude*, of the waveform (see Figure 11.3). When the intensity of sound increases, we perceive that change as an increase in *loudness*. As a result, intensity is a characteristic of sound

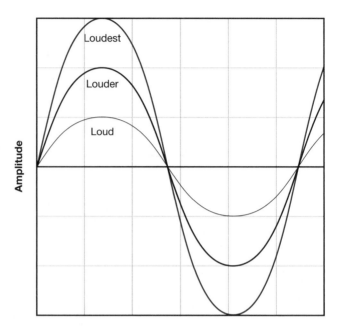

FIGURE 11.3
Waveforms of different amplitudes.

that we can measure, but loudness, like pitch, is the perceptual correlate that is determined by the listener.

As we previously noted, intensity is associated with the pressure produced when molecules collide. Sound pressure level (SPL) is measured using a decibel (dB) scale. The decibel is calculated using a logarithmic scale that relates the ratio of two sound pressure levels or intensities to one another. In the case of our auditory system, a fixed reference point is used that denotes the lowest intensity level at which a change in SPL can be detected. This point is identified as 0 db SPL and the dB scale is referenced to this level. Without the use of a logarithmic scale, the range of sound pressures would result in numbers that are much too large to deal with when examining sound intensity. As a result, by using the dB scale we are able to scale our measurements from 0 dB SPL to about 120 db SPL when measuring sounds within our environment. It is important to recognize that because of this logarithmic scale, a sound that is 30 dB SPL is not half as loud as a sound that is 60 db SPL. Using this relative scale, for every 3-dB increase in intensity, the perceived sound will actually be twice as loud. Examination of Figure 11.4 provides you with some insights into the relative intensities of sounds that are encountered within our day-to-day environment.

Given this background on the basics of sound, we will now explore the anatomy and physiology of the ear, the transmission of sound, and the energy conversions associated with sound transmission through the auditory system.

0 dB	Threshold of hearing
10 dB	Rustling leaves
20 dB	Whisper
30 dB	Library
40 dB	Refrigerator hum
50 dB	Light auto traffic
60 dB	Conversation
70 dB	Vacuum cleaner
80 dB	Tractor
90 dB	Concert orchestra
100 dB	Your iPod or MP3 player
110 dB	Chain saw
120 dB	Rock concert

FIGURE 11.4
Environmental sounds and their intensity levels.

EAR ANATOMY AND PHYSIOLOGY

In the discussion to follow we will examine the anatomy and physiology of the ear. The ear can be divided into three sections: the outer ear, middle ear, and inner ear. Each of these sections will be described in terms of the anatomy and physiology associated with that section. As each portion of this system is involved in the transmission of sound, we will also discuss the transfer of energy that occurs during each stage of sound transmission.

Outer Ear

The outer ear has been described as the acoustic portion of the auditory system. As speech is produced as an acoustic signal, the outer ear is that portion of the system that collects the sound. The outer ear is made up of the *auricle*, or *pinna*, and the *external auditory canal*, or *external auditory meatus* (see Figure 11.5). The auricle is that part of the ear where earrings are attached. The auricle serves a sound-gathering function and helps to funnel sounds toward the ear canal. It is interesting to note that persons who lack an auricle will typically not demonstrate any hearing loss, but it appears that the auricle is important for sound localization, or determining the direction of a sound and the sound source (Van Wanrooij & Van Opstal, 2004). Because of the shape of the auricle, it is more efficient at transferring high-frequency sounds than low-frequency sounds. As a result, speech signals that contain many of these high-frequency sounds are

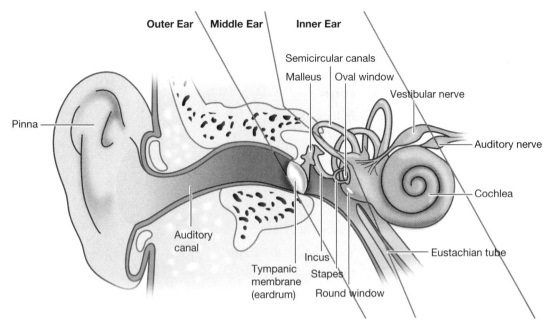

FIGURE 11.5
The outer, middle, and inner ear.

efficiently transferred to the external auditory canal. The external auditory canal is a closed-end tube, about 26 mm in length (1 inch), that helps in the transmission of sound from the external environment to the middle ear. The ear canal has two sections. The outer section is made of cartilage and the innermost section is bone. Within the outermost cartilaginous section of the ear canal, *cerumen*, or earwax, is produced. Cerumen helps to prevent dirt and foreign bodies (e.g., sand, insects) from reaching the bony portion of the ear canal. The earwax exits your ear in natural ways as you chew, move your jaw to speak, and through body movements. The skin lining the ear canal slowly travels toward the opening of the canal and drops out.

The external auditory canal helps to filter low-frequency sounds while maximizing the transmission of higher frequency sounds, particularly those within the speech range. In addition, as you have two external auditory canals, these function to help you to locate or localize sounds that are being transmitted. As sounds may arrive at each ear at different times, the external auditory canal helps you to determine the location and direction of the specific sound. For example, as you are crossing a street where you cannot see around a corner, you have the ability to hear an oncoming car and determine its direction. In this manner, you will turn your head to view the direction of the oncoming car and avoid any significant problems. As the sound travels down the external auditory canal, it encounters the *tympanic membrane*, or eardrum, that begins the middle ear.

Middle Ear

The middle ear is an air-filled space found within the hardest bone of the body, the *temporal bone*. The middle ear connects the outer ear to the inner ear by converting the acoustic energy of the sound pressure wave of the outer ear into mechanical vibrations.

The border between the outer ear and the middle ear occurs at the tympanic membrane. The tympanic membrane is composed of three layers, is about 0.07 mm thick, and is an efficient vibrator, helping to convert the energy of the acoustic signal to mechanical energy resulting from the movement of the three smallest bones within the body. These bones are collectively referred to as the *ossicles* and are individually known as the hammerlike *malleus*, the anvil-like *incus*, and the stirruplike *stapes* (see Figure 11.5). The malleus is embedded within the tympanic membrane. When the sound pressure wave moves down the auditory canal, it causes the tympanic membrane to vibrate. As the tympanic membrane vibrates, the malleus will vibrate in a similar manner. Because the ossicles are attached to the tympanic membrane, the movement of the tympanic membrane results in mechanical vibrations that transmit sound toward the inner ear.

In order for the tympanic membrane and ossicles to function properly, the air pressure within the middle ear must be consistent with the air pressure in the external auditory canal. To accomplish the equalization of air pressure, you will use your *eustachian tube*. The eustachian tube runs from your middle-ear cavity to the back of your throat, just above your soft palate. This tube generally remains closed but opens about one time per minute for adults. In contrast, the eustachian tube in children often remains open until about 6 months of age when it functions as the adult tube. If you remember the last time you rode in an elevator or flew in an airplane, you can remember how your "ears popped." This process is actually the equalization of pressure when you swallow, yawn, or widely open your mouth. By accomplishing this pressure equalization, you are able to keep your ears healthy and free from problems.

Returning to our discussion of the ossicles, we note that the stapes is attached to the *oval window* that serves as the boundary between the middle ear and inner ear. Further examination of the middle ear reveals the presence of two muscles whose function continues to be debated. One of these muscles attaches to the malleus and the second muscle attaches to the stapes. The muscle that attaches to the stapes responds to loud sounds by contracting in a manner that helps to reduce the movement of the stapes, which helps to reduce the transmission of mechanical energy through the oval window to the inner ear and serves to protect the inner ear from these loud sounds. In the discussion that follows, we will describe the results of movement of the stapes and its impact on the workings of the inner ear.

Inner Ear

The inner ear has two important components. The semicircular canals are responsible for balance, movement, and helping to determine the position of our body in space. As we are primarily concerned with communication, we will not explore the workings of the semicircular canals. The second component of the inner ear is the

FIGURE 11.6
The inner ear: semicircular canals
and the cochlea.

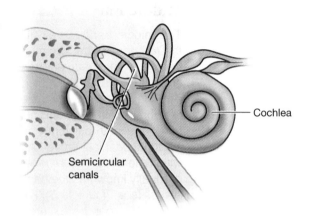

Cochlea

Semicircular
canals

cochlea, which we will explore in detail as it relates to our ability to hear. The cochlea has been described as a bony, snail shell-like structure (see Figure 11.6) that if uncoiled would be approximately 1.5 inches long (about 3.8 cm). In our discussion of the middle ear, we noted that the stapes rests upon the oval window of the cochlea and that the oval window serves as the border between the middle ear and the inner ear. As the cochlea is a closed system filled with fluid, when the stapes pushes inward on the oval window, this causes wavelike motion in the cochlea, and a second window, *the round window*, will move outward in response to the inward movement of the oval window.

While all cochlear activity takes place in this coiled shell, it is often easier to visualize the anatomy and physiology of the cochlea if we think about it as uncoiled. The bony shell of the cochlea is analogous to a piece of plumber's pipe. If we insert a long thin balloon into this pipe, we will have a hard outer shell protecting the flexible balloon within the middle of the pipe. The space between the bony shell and the membranous tube is called the *scala tympani* and *scala vestibuli*. This space is filled with *perilymph*, which is described as being about twice as thick as water. Within the bony shell of the cochlea we have a long, thin membranous structure that is flexible like the balloon and is called the *scala media*. Within the membranous tube we find a fluid called *endolymph*, which is described as being jellylike and quite thick.

Running along the entire length of the scala media is the *organ of Corti* (see Figure 11.7). The organ of Corti, described as the end organ of hearing, sits on the *basilar membrane* that forms the base of the scala media. The organ of Corti has thousands of hair cells that respond to different frequencies of sound. When the basilar membrane moves, these hair cells are bent or sheared, resulting in neural, or nerve, activity that sends a signal to the acoustic nerve. The wavelike movement caused by the stapes pushing against the oval window ultimately results in the movement of the basilar membrane, organ of Corti, and shearing of the hair cells. In this manner the mechanical energy of the ossicles is converted into hydraulic, or fluid, energy within the cochlea. It is this hydraulic energy that results in the movement of the hair cells and the final energy conversion to a neural signal, or bioelectrical energy, that is transmitted to the acoustic nerve.

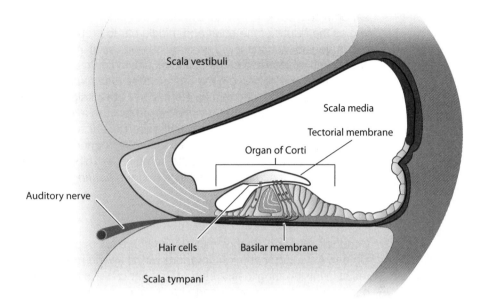

FIGURE 11.7
Cross section of the cochlea with the organ of Corti.

Quiz on the Fly 11.1

1. The perceptual correlate of intensity is _____.
2. A sound wave is made up of _____ and _____ of air molecules.
3. The acoustic portion of the auditory system is the _____ear.
4. The three smallest bones in the body make up the _____.
5. The bending of hair cells occurs on the _____ within the _____ ear.

DISORDERS OF HEARING

The typical pathway for hearing requires that the sound pass through the outer ear, middle ear, and inner ear. As previously described, this transmission of sound involves the conversion of the acoustic signal into a nerve impulse that is going to be recognized by the brain. As we know the normal pathway for hearing, it is important for us to understand where the system might break down and problems that might occur as a result of any breakdowns. A hearing loss that is associated with problems in the outer ear or middle ear is known as a *conductive hearing loss.* You might think of this problem as the failure of the outer and middle ear to properly conduct sound to the inner ear. In general, a conductive hearing loss will result in a decrease of the signal intensity but not a distortion of the sound signal. In contrast, hearing loss associated with the cochlea and acoustic nerve is called *sensorineural hearing loss.* A person may have an intact outer and middle ear and yet exhibit significant hearing problems with the inner ear. Sensorineural hearing losses result in a reduction of both the intensity of the signal and a distortion of various frequencies associated with the sound. In some cases, a person may exhibit both a conductive hearing loss associated with problems in the outer or middle ear and at the same time exhibit a sensorineural hearing loss. This person is described as exhibiting a *mixed hearing loss.*

Conductive Hearing Loss

Conductive hearing losses can occur as a result of problems with the outer or middle ear. Anything that might interfere with a sound moving through the system can result in this hearing loss. *Atresia* of the ear canal is a condition where the ear canal has failed to develop or damage has occurred to the ear canal as a result of some trauma (e.g., severe burns). Atresia is often associated with syndromes such as Treacher Collins syndrome (a collection of symptoms that include downward slanted eyes, small jaw, cleft palate, and no auricle or ear canal) and is one of many symptoms exhibited by the individual. Atresia of the external ear canal can cause problems with sound localization and hearing loss.

It is not unusual for some children to place toys, crayons, or food into their noses, mouths, and ears. Placing toys within the ear canal will block sounds and may cause additional swelling of the ear canal. In the best-case scenario, a physician will have easy access for removal; however, in the worst-case scenario, a child may require surgery to remove the foreign object. A condition known as *external otitis,* or *swimmer's ear,* may result in a mild conductive hearing loss and cause a lot of pain for the patient. External otitis can occur in people who have infected water trapped in their ears or infected water that enters any compromised skin in their ear canal. Because this condition is painful, it is often difficult to complete hearing testing as moving the auricle or placing earphones on the patient can result in pain. Treatment involves oral medications and medications directly applied to the infected area.

Some individuals produce larger amounts of cerumen than average and, in their attempts to clean out their ear canal, they actually push this earwax farther into the canal. At times the cerumen can form a small plug that will prevent sound transmission, and removal by a physician may be required.

Quiz on the Fly 11.1 Answers

1. The perceptual correlate of intensity is **loudness**. **2.** A sound wave is made up of **compressions** and **rarefactions** of air molecules. **3.** The acoustic portion of the auditory system is the **outer** ear. **4.** The three smallest bones in the body make up the **ossicles**. **5.** The bending of hair cells occurs on the **organ of Corti** within the **inner** ear.

IN THE CLINIC

Howie, a speech–language pathologist at a large midwestern university, has been wearing hearing aids for 2 years. On a number of occasions Howie's hearing aids have become blocked with cerumen, requiring him to replace the wax traps on his hearing aids. When visiting his family physician for a yearly checkup, the physician noted a large plug of cerumen within the external auditory canal. The physician placed ear drops in Howie's ears to soften the wax and then flushed out Howie's ear with water to remove the cerumen. The procedure was successful. However, during the following week, Howie noted some pain in his ear. Having access to audiologists within the university speech and hearing clinic enabled Howie to be examined. Upon inspection, the audiologist noted that Howie's ear canal was red and his tympanic membrane appeared to be inflamed. As audiologists are involved in the nonmedical treatment of hearing, Howie was referred back to his family physician who identified the problem as external otitis. During the irrigation of Howie's ear to remove the cerumen, the ear canal was apparently irritated in a manner that increased the possibility of infection. During the period from first seeing the physician to identifying external otitis, Howie developed an infection in his external ear canal. The physician prescribed a liquid medication to be directly placed within the ear canal and oral antibiotics to fight infection. The problem resolved within 2 weeks.

The most common cause of conductive hearing loss is a condition known as *otitis media*, or inflammation and fluid in the middle ear. We previously noted that the eustachian tube equalizes the pressure between the middle ear and the back of the throat. However, for individuals with upper respiratory infections, sinus infections, allergies, or enlarged adenoids, the eustachian tube may become swollen or blocked and unable to open to equalize the pressure. When this occurs, the air pressure within the middle-ear cavity will be less than the pressure in the patient's throat and outside environment. As a result, the tympanic membrane is retracted (pulled inward) and the patient reports that "my head feels full" or "I feel like I'm talking in a tunnel." As long as the eustachian tube remains closed, the negative pressures within the ear will result in fluid being drawn out of the cells lining the middle ear. Initially this fluid is sterile (germ free) but can still cause problems by making it difficult for the ossicles to move and transmit sound. At this point the person may notice that it is more difficult to hear conversations, the television, or a music player. If the problem persists and the eustachian tube fails to open, the lack of light and oxygen within the middle-ear space creates a perfect environment for growing bacteria. As the fluid within the middle ear becomes infected, the patient may experience pain in his or her ear and also exhibit a fever. As the problem progresses, the infected fluid within the ear continues to increase and push against the tympanic membrane. Ultimately, the tympanic membrane can perforate, or

---

1. Eustachian tube is blocked.

2. Pressure in the middle ear is less than atmospheric pressure.

3. Tympanic membrane retracts.

4. Fluid is drawn from tissues lining the middle ear.

5. Fluid becomes infected.

6. The infected fluid begins to push against the tympanic membrane.

7. Fluid pressure builds and causes perforation of the tympanic membrane.

FIGURE 11.8
Stages in the development of otitis media.

burst from this fluid pressure (see Figure 11.8). In some cases, the tympanic membrane will heal itself, but in other cases, surgical intervention is necessary.

It is interesting to note that in young children, the eustachian tube is relatively short and horizontal, which can result in more frequent problems associated with the middle ear. When a child experiences an upper respiratory infection, the horizontal position of the eustachian tube makes it more susceptible to infection, swelling, and closure. In adults, the eustachian tube is more vertical and is less likely to become swollen and remain closed.

Children and adults with otitis media are initially treated with medication. It is important for adults and those individuals working with children who experience otitis media to recognize that fluid in the ear is going to result in a hearing loss. As the ossicles attempt to transmit sound within this fluid-filled environment, the sound transmission will be less efficient, and the patient will require sounds of greater intensity in order to overcome sound transmission problems caused by the fluid.

When a physician prescribes medication for otitis media, the medication helps to fight the bacterial infection but does not help the body to reabsorb the fluid in the middle ear. In order for the fluid to be reabsorbed, the eustachian tube must open again to aerate the middle ear and equalize the pressure. For this reason a physician will encourage adults with otitis media and parents of children with otitis media to bring the child back for a follow-up examination approximately 6 weeks following the occurrence of the ear infection. If the eustachian tube fails to open even after the infection is gone, the fluid in the middle ear will remain, the child will continue to experience a hearing loss, and the infection may return. In cases where the otitis media is left untreated or is treated with home remedies, infection can spread to the bone behind the ear, the mastoid, and then to the brain, resulting in meningitis (inflammation of the covering of the brain) and sometimes death. It is well documented that a child who experiences frequent bouts of otitis media with persistent fluid in the ear will exhibit associated hearing loss. While this hearing loss has been related to both speech and language delays (Klein, 2001), there is some controversy as to whether these children actually experience any real problems with speech and language development (Roberts, Rosenfeld, & Zeisel, 2004). When multiple occurrences of otitis media continue, a physician might recommend the use of pressure-equalizing (PE) tubes.

FIGURE 11.9
Pressure-equalizing tubes.

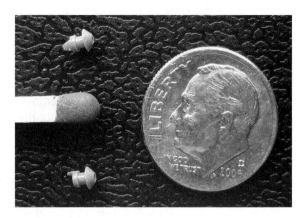

A procedure known as a *myringotomy* involves a small incision into the tympanic membrane. The physician is able to suction out the fluid from the middle ear and insert the PE tubes within the incision (see Figure 11.9). In this manner, the newly inserted tubes act in a manner similar to the eustachian tube, allowing for pressure equalization and reducing the risk of fluid buildup and further infection.

Otosclerosis is a disorder that occurs when spongy bone originating from the cochlea forms at the boundary of the stapes and oval window. This bony growth restricts the movement of the stapes, resulting in a conductive hearing loss. This problem typically occurs during adolescence and continues through adulthood. It is more common in females than males and often requires surgical intervention.

In summary, a conductive hearing loss occurs when sound cannot be completely transmitted through the outer or middle ear. We have discussed a number of conditions that can result in conductive hearing loss and identified some methods of remediation. In the section to follow, we will discuss sensorineural hearing loss.

Sensorineural Hearing Loss

Sensorineural hearing loss occurs when there is damage to the cochlea or any of the pathways from the cochlea to the acoustic nerve and the brain. Sensorineural hearing loss not only affects the loudness of the signal being received by the listener but also the person's ability to recognize and understand speech sounds and words being produced. For the purposes of our discussion, we will categorize sensorineural loss as either *congenital* (child was born with the problem) or *acquired* (problem occurred after birth).

Congenital Sensorineural Hearing Loss

Congenital hearing loss indicates that the child is born with the problem. These problems may be related to genetic issues or occur as a result of issues affecting the child in utero or at the time of birth. According to a report by ASHA (American Speech-Language-Hearing Association, 2010a), more than 50% of congenital hearing loss is related to genetic factors. These genetic factors are often associated with parents carrying a dominant or recessive gene for deafness. For example, a parent who is deaf may carry a dominant gene for deafness and there will be a 50% chance of the child being deaf. If both parents are deaf and carry the dominant gene, the chances will be higher that the child will be born deaf. When two normal-hearing parents carry a recessive gene for deafness, the child has a 25% chance of being deaf. In this example, as the parents have normal hearing, they would have no prior expectations that their child would have a hearing loss. It is interesting to note that 9 out of 10 children who are born deaf have parents who can hear (National Institute on Deafness and Other Communicative Disorders, 2010a). It is also interesting to note that hearing loss is often associated with various syndromes such as Down syndrome (the presence of an extra chromosome resulting in cognitive impairment, unique facial features, impaired physical growth) and Usher syndrome (one parent carries a recessive gene resulting in congenital deafness and blindness). Other congenital factors associated with sensorineural hearing loss include prematurity of the infant and diseases such as rubella (German measles), cytomegalovirus, and maternal diabetes.

Acquired Sensorineural Hearing Loss

Acquired sensorineural hearing loss appears anytime after birth and throughout the lifetime of the individual. Acquired sensorineural hearing loss in children can be related to viral disease processes such as chicken pox, mumps, or measles. Bacterial infections arising from untreated otitis media can lead to meningitis, or inflammation of the brain coverings, and associated hearing loss.

Acquired sensorineural hearing loss in older adults is the third-most prevalent chronic condition in the United States (Yueh, Shapiro, MacLean, & Shekelle, 2003). Hearing loss associated with aging is called *presbycusis* and the prevalence of this problem rises as the person gets older. Presbycusis occurs in both ears and usually begins to become evident in men in their early 60s, but women are a little older, showing problems in their late 60s. However, it is unusual for individuals to exhibit these age-related hearing problems earlier or later.

A second common cause of acquired hearing loss in adults is noise. Have you ever attended a rock concert only to find that your hearing has been affected? You find that you have to raise the intensity of your voice so you can hear yourself speaking while your friends are also talking more loudly so you can hear them. This phenomenon is said to be the result of a *temporary threshold shift* and usually results in a complete return of your hearing. Those individuals who encounter repeated exposure to high levels of noise often experience a *permanent threshold shift*.

The problem of *noise-induced hearing loss* has been associated with workers in factories, musicians in rock bands, persons in the military, and others repeatedly exposed to explosions and gunfire. It appears that noise has a detrimental effect on the cochlea, is often cumulative, and may be prevented by using external protective devices like headphones during noise exposure and pharmacological agents within a specific time period following noise exposure (LePrell, Yamashita, Minami, Yamasoba, & Miller, 2007). Individuals who have been repeatedly exposed to explosions and gunfire often exhibit *acoustic trauma*, a type of noise-induced hearing loss that affects specific hearing frequencies around 4,000 Hz. In general this type of hearing loss occurs in a similar manner in both ears. In contrast, rifle shooters often exhibit a greater hearing loss in the ear opposite the shoulder that supports their rifle.

There is now growing concern among professionals who work with the hearing impaired and deaf that our frequent use of portable music players and earphones has the potential to cause permanent hearing loss in the future. A number of newspaper reports have quoted audiologists regarding the potential detrimental impact on hearing of loud, portable music players, although it will only be through systematic, well-conducted research studies that we are able to identify the impact of this loud music. However, by the time we are able to identify the hearing loss, it may be too late to intervene.

Acquired sensorineural hearing losses in adults can also occur as a result of a number of different processes. An *acoustic neuroma* is a type of tumor that grows near the acoustic nerve and can affect a person's hearing. *Ototoxicity* is the damage to the inner ear that occurs as a result of medications that can cause hearing loss. It is not unusual for a patient to experience a severe medical condition for which the selection of an ototoxic drug is necessary. Recognizing the potential effects of these drugs, a physician will order the close monitoring of a patient's hearing in an effort to avoid hearing problems while at the same time improving the patient's health. *Ménière's disease* results in a sudden unilateral hearing loss with associated dizziness and vertigo. Patients often report a roaring noise in their ear called *tinnitus*. Ménière's disease has been related to problems within the cochlear duct; it is reported to be quite debilitating and appears suddenly, resolves, and often returns. Because of the sudden onset of the problem, it often affects a person's ability to complete routine daily activities like driving a car or going to work.

Quiz on the Fly 11.2

1. Hearing loss associated with the outer or middle ear is called

   _____.

2. Inability to open the eustachian tube to equalize pressure often results in _____.

3. Hearing loss associated with the inner ear is called _____.

4. Hearing loss associated with aging is called _____.

5. _____ is the damage caused to the inner ear by certain drugs.

Mixed Hearing Loss

You might have wondered about the patient who experiences presbycusis or some other sensorineural hearing loss while simultaneously experiencing a conductive hearing loss. A mixed hearing loss occurs when a person's hearing loss has a sensorineural component, the more permanent problem, while at the same time the person is experiencing a conductive hearing loss that further adds to the person's difficulties. These individuals might be treated medically to deal with the conductive component of their problem while also wearing hearing aids to assist with their sensorineural hearing loss.

SUMMARY AND REVIEW

The focus of this chapter has been an examination of the anatomy and physiology of the outer, middle, and inner ear as they relate to the transmission of sound from the environment to our brain. We began our discussion by explaining the components of sound and sound transmission as they relate to our ability to hear and process speech. We then examined the outer, middle, and inner ear with respect to energy transfers and sound transmission. We concluded the chapter with a discussion of various disorders that affect our ability to hear, their locations within the system, and the impacts of the disorders on sound and speech transmission.

The Transmission of Sound

What is sound and how is it transmitted?

Sounds are changes in pressure that occur when molecules of air collide. Through this collision, we have energy transferred from one molecule of air to the next while the actual molecule returns to its resting state. The sound wave is made up of compressions and rarefactions of air molecules. Frequency of sound has been described as the number of times an object vibrates during a given period of time. This physical property determines the pitch that we perceive. Intensity of sound relates to the force of the collision of the air molecules; we perceive this as loudness.

Ear Anatomy and Physiology

What are the three divisions of the auditory system and the important components of each system?

The ear is divided into the outer ear, the middle ear, and the inner ear. The outer ear is described as the acoustic portion of the system, and it is the part of the system that collects the sound. The middle ear is described as the mechanical portion of the system. When the sound travels down the external auditory canal and moves

---

Quiz on the Fly 11.2 Answers

1. Hearing loss associated with the outer or middle ear is called **conductive**. **2.** Inability to open the eustachian tube to equalize pressure often results in **otitis media**. **3.** Hearing loss associated with the inner ear is called **sensorineural**. **4.** Hearing loss associated with aging is called **presbycusis**. **5.** **Ototoxicity** is the damage caused to the inner ear by certain drugs.

the tympanic membrane, the sound energy traveling through the ossicles of the middle ear is converted to mechanical energy. When the mechanical energy reaches the oval window of the cochlea, the sound is converted into hydraulic energy that causes movement of the organ of Corti in the cochlea. The movements of the organ of Corti result in the final conversion of hydraulic energy into a neural signal, or bioelectric energy, that is transmitted to the acoustic nerve.

Disorders of Hearing

What are the two categories of hearing loss and what are the most prevalent examples of each?

Hearing losses associated with disorders of the outer ear or middle ear are called conductive hearing losses. These losses occur as a result of the ear's reduced ability to conduct sound. The most prevalent conductive hearing loss is associated with otitis media, which often results in fluid buildup in the middle ear. This type of conductive hearing loss has the potential to delay a child's speech and language development. Hearing disorders associated with the inner ear are called sensorineural hearing losses and can be congenital or acquired. Congenital hearing loss comes about as a result of heredity or as a result of issues affecting the child in utero or at the time of birth. The most prevalent acquired hearing loss, however, is a result of aging.

WEB SITES OF INTEREST

American Speech-Language-Hearing Association
http://asha.org/public/hearing/

InnerBody: Ear (Cut View)
http://www.innerbody.com/image/nerv13.html

University of Wisconsin Animations of Anatomy and Physiology of the Ear
http://www.neurophys.wisc.edu/h&b/auditory/animation/animationmain.html

Virtual Tour of the Ear (Augustana College, Sioux Falls, SD)
http://www.augie.edu/perry/ear/hearmech.htm

12

Hearing Testing and Management of Hearing Disorders

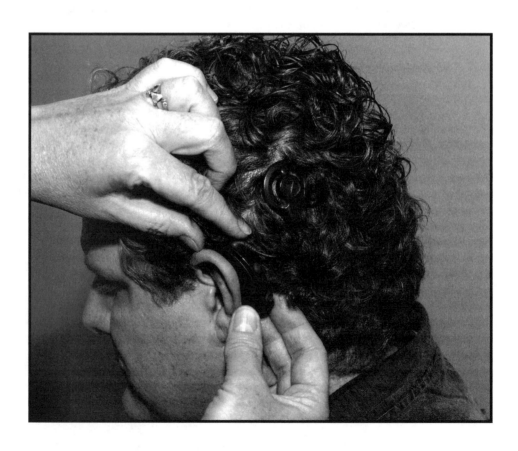

The focus of this chapter will be an exploration of hearing testing and the management and treatment of people with hearing disorders. We will examine the use of amplification and surgery to assist individuals with hearing loss and discuss auditory and communication training to assist the development of language skills. Finally we will explore how acoustics in the classroom can impact a child's ability to hear and grow academically. We will begin our discussion by focusing on the testing procedures used by audiologists to test hearing.

HEARING TESTING

Audiometers

A *pure tone* is defined as a tone produced at one frequency. A *pure-tone audiometer* is a device that generates acoustic signals at specific frequencies and is used to assess a person's hearing. Although the human ear is capable of hearing sounds from 20 Hz to 20,000 Hz, the primary frequencies associated with speech production range from 125 Hz to about 8,000 Hz. A pure-tone audiometer is designed to generate sounds within the speech range. In addition, the audiometer is designed to vary the intensity of the signal so that the audiologist can determine the lowest possible intensity level at which a patient can correctly respond to a tone 50% of the time. This is known as the *threshold* of hearing. Audiometers can be stationary pieces of equipment that are found in the audiology clinic (see Figure 12.1A) or portable devices that can be used by audiologists and speech–language pathologists to complete hearing screenings in locations away from a clinic (see Figure 12.1B). It would not be unusual for a school audiologist and speech–language pathologist to screen the hearing of kindergarten children using a portable audiometer.

As we are surrounded by noise in our day-to-day environment (e.g., car engines, people talking, machinery vibrating), it is important for the audiologist to be able to test a person's hearing in an environment that is relatively noise-free. Although it is nearly impossible to create a room that is totally noise-free, an audiologist will use a "sound proofed" booth, or audiometric suite, in an effort to minimize the effects of extraneous noise on testing the person's hearing. Typically, a patient will sit in one side of the booth and communicate with the audiologist on the other side of the partition. The walls of this suite are extremely thick and the entire suite is designed to minimize the effect of outside noise. When required to use a portable audiometer in a classroom or school setting, the tester recognizes the potential

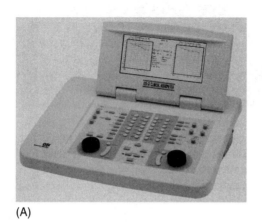
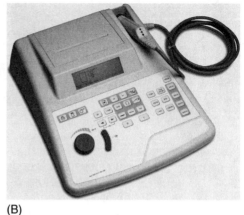

(A)   (B)

FIGURE 12.1
(A) Stationary audiometer for testing hearing in the clinic and (B) a portable audiometer.
(Reprinted with permission of Grason-Stadler)

impact of background noise on the child's ability to hear and makes some accommodation for the noisier environment. When it appears that a child may have a hearing loss within this school environment, a more complete hearing evaluation in a clinic with an audiometric suite will be recommended.

When participating in pure-tone testing, the patient is often seated facing the audiologist and instructed to "raise your hand or push the button when you hear the sound." When testing very young children, an audiologist may provide a bucket and blocks, with instructions to "place a block in the bucket when you hear the sound."

Air Conduction Audiometry

In the previous chapter, we described the typical pathway that sound travels through the outer ear, middle ear, and inner ear to the acoustic nerve. In order to assess the integrity of the hearing system, one of the first tests that will be completed by an audiologist will be air conduction testing. Air conduction testing typically involves the use of earphones or speakers to deliver the sound to one ear and then the other ear. A person having a hearing test will typically wear a set of earphones and receive instructions to "raise your hand or push the button when you think that you hear the sound" (see Figure 12.2). As the intensity of the sound will continually decrease, the patient is encouraged to respond even when the signal is barely perceptible. The audiologist will assess the patient's hearing in each ear across the speech frequencies. When the patient's threshold for a specific frequency is determined, the audiologist will plot the results of the air conduction testing on an *audiogram* (see Figure 12.3). As you will note, an audiogram depicts the tested frequencies along the x-axis (horizontal axis) of the graph and the hearing level, or intensity, measured in decibels on the y-axis (vertical axis).

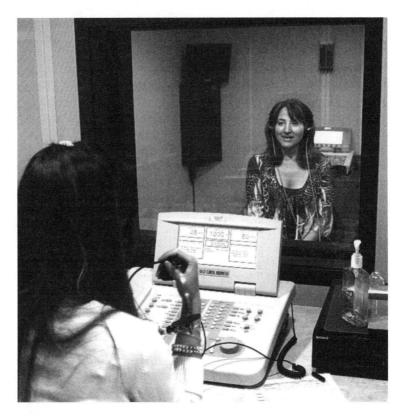

FIGURE 12.2
Hearing testing.

The results of air conduction testing can reveal the presence or absence of problems within the auditory system. However, upon completion of air conduction testing, the audiologist may know that a hearing loss is present but the type of hearing loss remains a mystery. As a result, the next step in the process is to determine the integrity of the inner ear using a process that bypasses the outer ear and middle ear and directly assesses the sensitivity of the inner ear.

Bone Conduction Audiometry

Bone conduction audiometry, like air conduction audiometry, uses pure tones to assess the functioning of the ear. However, unlike air conduction audiometry, bone conduction audiometry bypasses the structures of the outer and middle ear to only assess the functioning of the inner ear. In this manner, a person who may only be experiencing a conductive hearing problem affecting either the outer or middle ear should exhibit normal hearing sensitivity during bone conduction testing. Bone conduction testing involves the placement of a bone vibrator on the patient's forehead or mastoid bone (behind the ear). When the bone vibrator is placed on the

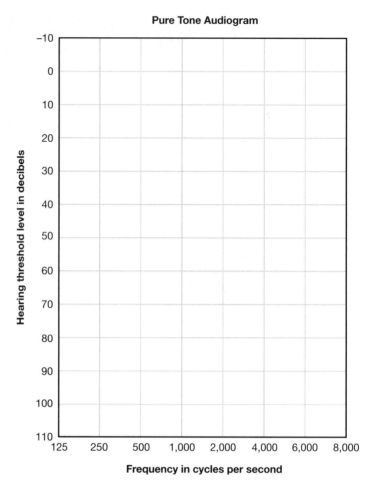

FIGURE 12.3
Audiogram.

skull and a pure-tone signal is generated, the patient's skull helps to transmit the signal directly to the cochlea. As the pure-tone signal will travel to both ears through the skull, it is necessary to mask or cover up the nontest ear so that each ear can be tested independently. *Masking* is a process by which noise is introduced into the nontest ear through an earphone to remove it from testing so that only one ear is tested at a time. When the results of air conduction testing reveal a hearing loss and bone conduction testing is normal, it is likely that the patient is experiencing a conductive hearing loss affecting either the outer or middle ear. When a patient exhibits a hearing loss during air conduction testing and also exhibits a hearing loss during bone conduction testing, that patient may be exhibiting a mixed hearing loss (conductive and sensorineural hearing loss) or solely a sensorineural hearing loss.

Speech Audiometry

Although the results of both air conduction and bone conduction testing are extremely valuable at helping an audiologist determine a level and type of hearing loss, it is important to recognize that we don't go to the grocery store or movie theater and listen for pure tones. In reality, the average person must recognize and understand spoken language so that effective communication can transpire. To determine a person's ability to understand speech, an audiologist will complete two different speech tests. These are the *speech reception threshold* (SRT) test and the *speech or word recognition test*.

As we discussed in the section on audiometers, a threshold is determined when a patient correctly responds 50% of the time to the signal being provided. During the SRT test, the audiologist is also interested in determining a threshold for the reception of speech. During this task, a group of two-syllable words called *spondees* are presented to the patient through earphones. These words are presented via tape, compact disc, or verbally by the audiologist, making sure to put equal emphasis on both syllables. The patient will hear words like *hotdog*, *baseball*, or *cowboy* and will be asked to repeat each word as the intensity level of the signal is lowered. The intensity level where the patient is able to repeat half of the words is determined to be that patient's SRT.

The second speech test that is completed by the audiologist is the *speech or word recognition test*. As each sound occurs with greater or lesser frequency in English, this recognition test uses a list of words reflecting the frequency of speech sound occurrence in English. These one-syllable words may be presented at a conversational speech intensity, a most comfortable intensity level, in a quiet area or with competing noise in an attempt to determine whether there are sound confusions and distortions associated with a patient's hearing loss. For example, the word *pew* might be presented and the patient might repeat the word *few*. In another example, the word *deaf* is presented and the repeated word is *dead*. When all of the words are presented from these word lists, the audiologist will compute a percentage of total correct words and this will reflect a patient's ability to hear speech within a functional environment. This information will be used along with the other test results to determine a patient's functional ability to understand speech and determine whether a hearing aid might benefit the patient.

Acoustic Immittance

In addition to the previously described tests, an audiologist is interested in assessing the functioning of the middle ear. As we previously described, the middle ear, beginning at the tympanic membrane, is involved in the transfer of acoustic energy to mechanical energy. The transmission of this energy can be examined as a function of the resistance present within the middle ear (*acoustic impedance*) or the ability of the middle ear to allow sound to pass (*acoustic admittance*). As you might imagine, the presence of fluid in the middle ear or a perforated tympanic membrane is going to restrict the middle ear's ability to transmit sound.

To assess middle-ear functioning, an audiologist will use a *tympanometer*, or *immittance meter*, to determine sound-transmission characteristics of the middle ear. The test is referred to as *tympanometry*. An airtight probe is placed in the ear canal and the pressure in the ear canal is modified while a tone is introduced. The tympanic membrane responds to the tone and changes in ear canal pressure, and these results are plotted on a graph, or *tympanogram*, representing the ability of the middle ear to transmit sound.

In addition to examining the movement of the tympanic membrane, an audiologist will assess the ability of the middle ear to respond to an intense sound. Using the immittance meter, the audiologist will introduce a loud tone into the test ear and examine the response of the middle ear as a function of the stiffness of the tympanic membrane. The response of the system and subsequent stiffening of the tympanic membrane is known as the *acoustic reflex*. It is important to note that when a patient demonstrates decreased air conduction thresholds and normal bone conduction thresholds, tympanometry and acoustic-reflex testing can help the audiologist to confirm the presence of a conductive hearing loss and differentiate the cause of this hearing loss.

Quiz on the Fly 12.1

1. Air conduction testing assesses the functioning of the _____, _____, and _____ ear.
2. You graph the results of a hearing test on an _____.
3. Testing inner-ear functioning by bypassing the outer and middle ear is called _____ testing.
4. The point at which a patient correctly responds to a tone 50% of the time is called the _____.
5. A test that assesses the functioning of the tympanic membrane is called _____.

Otoacoustic Emissions

Kemp (1978) reported that the cochlea is capable of producing sounds that can be detected in the external auditory canal. Researchers investigating this phenomenon discovered that in addition to the spontaneous sounds produced by the cochlea, sounds could be evoked from the cochlea following acoustic stimulation. These sounds have been called *evoked otoacoustic emissions*. To assess otoacoustic emissions (OEAs), a probe is placed in the patient's ear. This probe contains both a speaker for producing a rapid series of audible clicks and a microphone to capture the signal produced by the cochlea. Because of the low intensity of the signal produced by the cochlea and the presence of noise within the system, the signal received by the microphone has to be processed by a sophisticated computer

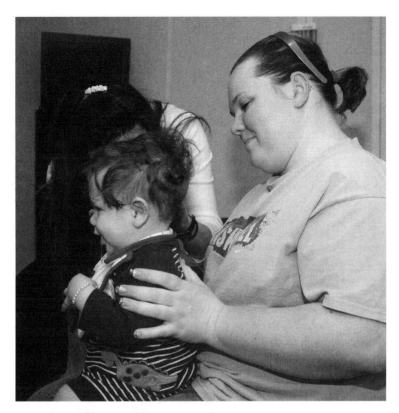

FIGURE 12.4
A child who has failed an otoacoustic emission screening is retested sitting on his mother's lap.

that helps to amplify the signal and minimize the noise. An audiologist is able to use the results of this test to determine whether the cochlea of a child or adult is functioning normally. These results are very helpful when monitoring the effects of ototoxic drugs on the cochlea and for screening newborn infants. Because of the ease with which this test can be completed and the fact that it does not require the active participation of the client, it is now routinely used as one component of a universal newborn hearing screening process in many hospitals throughout the United States and the world (see Figure 12.4). In fact, De Boer, Brennan, Lineton, Stevens, and Thornton (2007) reported reliable measurements of OEAs in newborns 6 to 13 hours following birth. It is important to recognize that this test focuses on cochlea functioning and does not assess the functioning of the acoustic nerve or pathways to the brain. Finally, the testing of OEAs has proved to be a significant innovation toward the early identification of hearing loss in children.

Auditory Evoked Potentials

In our discussion of cochlear anatomy, we discussed the shearing of hair cells in the organ of Corti, resulting in the creation of a bioelectric signal from the organ of Corti to the eighth cranial nerve, the acoustic nerve. Although OEAs can provide information regarding the functioning of the cochlea, we are also interested in measuring the electrical activity that occurs when the signal reaches the acoustic nerve and travels to the brain. When an auditory stimulus is presented and we measure the electrical activity of the acoustic nerve and brain, we are measuring *auditory evoked potentials*. The auditory signal is presented and, using surface electrodes that are attached to a patient's scalp, the electrical signals from the auditory pathway are recorded using a special computer program that helps to sort out electrical activity of interest from the noise and other signals that might be present. As this testing process doesn't require the active participation of the client, it is a useful measure for assessing difficult-to-test patients, patients in comas, and newborns.

Quiz on the Fly 12.1 Answers

1. Air conduction testing assesses the functioning of the **outer**, **middle**, and **inner** ear. **2.** You graph the results of a hearing test on an **audiogram**. **3.** Testing inner-ear functioning by bypassing the outer and middle ear is called **bone conduction** testing. **4.** The point at which a patient correctly responds to a tone 50% of the time is called the **threshold**. **5.** A test that assesses the functioning of the tympanic membrane is called **tympanometry**.

I CAN'T DO THIS ALONE

All states now have an Early Hearing Detection and Intervention (EHDI) program to help connect families with follow-up services for children who do not pass newborn hearing screening. An important component of EHDI is collaborating with other professionals because for children and families to benefit from the early screening process, diagnostic testing and intervention must be accessed in a timely fashion. Indeed, the goals of EHDI are to have screening completed before 1 month, diagnostic testing by 3 months, and intervention initiated by 6 months. I have found that I achieve the EHDI goals more easily and earlier when I work with a team of professionals. In other words, "I can't do it alone."

As an audiologist involved in working with newborn hearing screening and follow-up, I have come to recognize the importance of teamwork. Families interact with a wide range of professionals in their journey from hearing screening to intervention. If those professionals do not work together and communicate, the family runs the risk of receiving inadequate, delayed, or no services. My concern led me to contact other professionals both inside and outside of my practice setting in order to create a network that could provide timely and comprehensive services.

Baby Mary was born full-term with no complications before, during, or after birth except that Mary did not pass her newborn hearing screening. Mary's pediatrician was not familiar with follow-up for hearing screening and did not know where to send the family for additional hearing testing. If the parents had not pursued this follow-up, there could have been long-lasting implications for Mary. Through discussions with a friend, the family learned about Early Intervention (EI) services (i.e., each state has federal funding to support testing and intervention for children 0 to 3 years of age suspected of a delay or at risk of being delayed, through Part C of the Individuals with Disabilities Education Act). It turned out that the family friend had a child in the EI system and she contacted her case coordinator (i.e., the professional that coordinates testing and services for families). The case coordinator was familiar with my work as an EI provider so she contacted me to find out what to do next. Because time was of the essence, Mary and her family were scheduled for hearing testing within the week and completed diagnostic hearing testing at 2 weeks of age.

Mary was found to have a moderate to severe sensorineural hearing loss in each ear. This was distressing and difficult news for Mary's parents. It was important for me to be sensitive to the parents' emotional state and to help them navigate the steps they needed to take after receiving the diagnosis. Without the cooperation of Mary's pediatrician and case coordinator, this process would have taken a lot longer.

The next step was for Mary and her parents to schedule an appointment with an otolaryngologist who specialized in pediatrics. Because I have previously worked with this physician, I phoned him and provided background information prior to Mary's appointment. The doctor was aware of the need for the timeliness of an appointment and scheduled them within the week, setting the appointment to occur at the end of his day. In this manner, the doctor could spend as much time with the family as needed to examine Mary and answer all of their questions. During the appointment, the physician reviewed the child's history and recommended further medical tests in an attempt to identify the etiology of Mary's hearing loss. He also provided medical clearance for use of hearing aids (required for children less than 18 years of age). Because of the timely and sensitive collaboration with the pediatric otolaryngologist, Mary's parents were able to get information about the cause of her hearing loss and there were no delays in obtaining Mary's new hearing aids; Mary was fit with hearing aids at 5 weeks of age. When Mary was 8 weeks of age and used to her hearing aids, a developmental team evaluation was completed. This team included a speech–language pathologist and a developmental therapist, along with her case coordinator and me. In addition to a speech, hearing and developmental evaluation, the case coordinator also participated and an Individual Family Service Plan (IFSP) was completed. The IFSP is a document that outlines the family's goals for intervention and describes the nature of the needed services. Progress is formally reviewed every 6 months. Mary's parents chose to receive center-based services to take advantage of team services that included audiology. Team services facilitated communication between providers and the family, reduced the number of appointments, and through monitoring, enabled changes to be implemented as needed.

Mary's journey demonstrates the many points throughout the process where a breakdown in services can occur. Each family and child is unique and has different needs, and services should be individualized to reflect those needs. It is essential that professionals understand how their role impacts other services and ultimately the child's progress. Delays and inadequate services reduce the benefits that can be achieved by having newborn hearing screening. Helping children reach their potential takes "a village."

Contributed by Karen Munoz, EdD, assistant professor, Utah State University.

As part of a routine universal newborn hearing screening process, a specific evoked potential called the *auditory brain stem response* (ABR) is assessed. The ABR equipment is portable and often used by technicians under an audiologist's supervision within a hospital as part of the routine newborn screening process. When an infant fails this screening, additional hearing tests may be warranted.

Hearing Testing Summary

Hearing testing involves a number of specific diagnostic procedures that enable the clinical audiologist to determine the nature of a patient's hearing problem. Air conduction testing provides information regarding the patient's ability to hear sound through the outer-, middle-, and inner-ear pathway. Should the audiologist determine that a hearing loss is present, bone conduction testing can help to bypass the outer and middle ear to assess the functioning of the cochlea. Speech audiometry enables the audiologist to assess a person's ability to perceive speech in addition to pure tones and make a practical evaluation regarding the patient's ability to hear speech and language within the real world. Acoustic immittance testing will help the audiologist determine the nature of a conductive hearing loss, and OEAs testing and auditory brain stem response testing are two very important tests to further assess the auditory system and are used to assess the hearing of newborns. Although these descriptions are not an exhaustive explanation of all of the tests and procedures available to the audiologist, we believe that we have provided a comprehensive view for the beginning student. For additional information you are encouraged to examine the reference list at the end of the book.

Hearing Testing Results and Definitions

One method of classifying the results of hearing testing is to classify the results according to the degree of hearing loss exhibited by the patient. As you will note in Figure 12.5, normal hearing ranges from −10 dB HL to about 15 dB HL. You will observe that this classification system progresses from slight to mild and ends with a profound hearing loss being greater than 91 dB HL.

During practical discussions among speech–language pathologists and audiologists, additional classification discussions occur. While all individuals who exhibit hearing loss could be classified as exhibiting some degree of deafness, it is typical to refer to those individuals with severe-to-profound hearing losses as deaf, while all others with hearing loss would be considered hearing impaired, or hard of hearing. According to the Alexander Graham Bell Association for the Deaf and Hard of Hearing (2010), deaf is defined as "hearing loss, which is severe enough to make it hard for a person to understand speech through listening with or without hearing aids or cochlear implants."

When discussing hearing loss, we can also look at the time when the hearing loss occurred. As we discussed in the previous chapter, congenital hearing loss is related to genetic factors or other issues that affect the child before and during birth. Genetic testing and newborn screenings can help the parents to become aware of this issue so that management strategies can be implemented as soon as

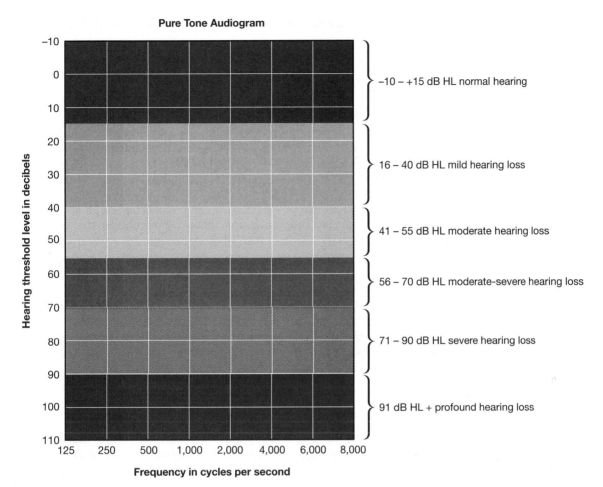

FIGURE 12.5
Degree of hearing loss.

possible following the birth of the child. When an individual loses his or her hearing any time after birth, this is referred to as *adventitious deafness*. Adventitious deafness can be related to a child's learning of language. Deafness that occurs before a child has learned language is called *prelingual* deafness, and deafness that occurs after a child has learned language, typically after 6 years of age, is called *postlingual* deafness. When adventitious deafness occurs in individuals 13 years of age or older, often because of disease or trauma, the disorder is referred to as *deafened* or *late deafened*. As these individuals have grown up relating to the hearing world, the loss of their hearing can be quite traumatic and requires much adjustment and learning new methods for communication. These individuals can no longer understand speech and must use all means possible (assistive devices, speech reading, and sign language) to assist their communication. The Chicago chapter of the Association for Late-Deafened Adults makes the point succinctly: "Whatever Works."

HABILITATION/REHABILITATION

Rehabilitation has been defined as "the physical restoration of a sick or disabled person by therapeutic measures and reeducation to participation in the activities of a normal life within the limitations of the person's physical disability" (*Merriam-Webster's Medical Dictionary*). If we think about providing therapy for children who are born deaf, we recognize that these children have not lost their hearing ability but in fact were born without it. As a result, the correct term for therapy with children who are born deaf should be *habilitation*, as they will be taught speech and language skills for the first time. However, while we recognize the difference between habilitation and rehabilitation, it is generally accepted that when we discuss therapy for children who are born deaf or adults who have lost their hearing, we will use the term *rehabilitation* to discuss management approaches.

The following section on rehabilitation will examine the management of hearing loss with a focus on amplification (e.g., hearing aids, FM systems) and cochlear implants. This will be followed by a discussion of auditory training, communication training, and will conclude with an examination of classroom issues that can affect a child's ability to maximize his or her hearing abilities.

Amplification

Hearing Aids

For most patients with sensorineural hearing loss, an audiologist will consider amplification as the first method of treatment. Amplification means that the sound signal is made louder. For persons with a hearing loss, this process is typically accomplished with a hearing aid. Most people today get fitted with a digital hearing aid. These hearing aids have five basic components: a microphone, analog-to-digital converter, signal processor, digital-to-analog converter, and receiver. The microphone will receive the acoustic signal and convert the sound signal to an electrical signal. The electrical signal passes through the analog-to-digital converter where the signal is converted to a series of 0s and 1s that is modified by the signal processor to meet the hearing needs of the person receiving the hearing aid. The modified signal then passes through the digital-to-analog converter and is sent to the receiver that changes the signal to an acoustic signal that the listener can hear.

Hearing aids come in a number of different styles. Body-type hearing aids, while frequently used in the past, are rarely used today. Because of their relatively large size, body-type aids were able to produce a more powerful signal and benefit those individuals with severe-to-profound hearing loss. The downside to these devices was that they were large and cumbersome and often attached to a body strap. With the advent of new technology, smaller, less cumbersome devices were developed that provide the same amount of amplification as the larger device.

A very common type of hearing aid that most readers will recognize is the *behind-the-ear* (BTE) hearing aid (see Figure 12.6A). A hard plastic case contains the hearing aid components and connects to an ear mold that fits into the patient's external auditory canal. A second type of BTE hearing aid, the Open Fit BTE hearing aid (see Figure 12.6B), does not use the ear mold and just uses a tube from the hearing aid to the ear canal to transmit the sound. The use of this tube enables the patient to hear the amplified signal without having the "full" feeling associated with an ear mold. These hearing aids are worn by children and adults with mild-to-profound hearing losses. A third type of hearing aid is called an *in-the-ear* (ITE) hearing aid (see Figure 12.6C). The ITE fits completely in the outer ear and all of the components are contained within the small plastic case. These hearing aids are used for mild-to-severe hearing losses. As these hearing aids are made to fit the size of the opening of the external canal, they are typically not used with children who are continually growing and would require frequent changes to their hearing aids. The fourth and fifth types of hearing aids are the *in-the-canal* (see Figure 12.6D) and *completely-in-the-canal hearing aids* (see Figure 12.6E). These are small devices that fit within the ear canal and are barely visible to another person. Because of their size, these devices are not recommended for children. In addition, the small size of these devices limits their power and they are typically not recommended for persons with severe-to-profound hearing loss.

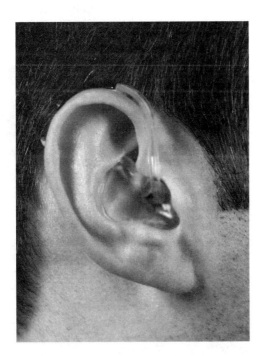

FIGURE 12.6A
Behind-the-ear hearing aid.

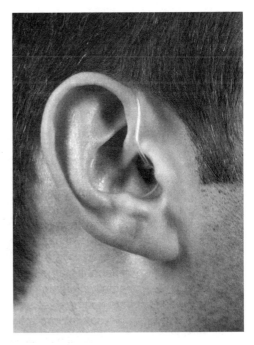

FIGURE 12.6B
Behind-the-ear Open Fit hearing aid.

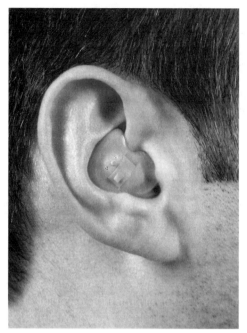

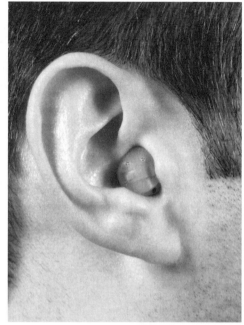

FIGURE 12.6C
In-the-ear hearing aid.

FIGURE 12.6D
In-the-canal hearing aid.

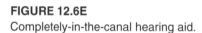
FIGURE 12.6E
Completely-in-the-canal hearing aid.

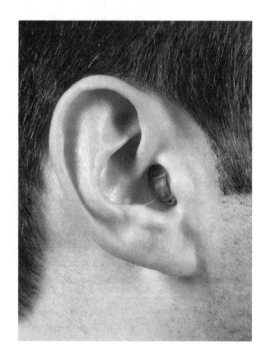

(Figure 12.6 images reprinted with
permission of Widex Hearing Aid
Company)

In addition to the different styles of hearing aids, there are two types of hearing aids available to the consumer. These are analog and digital hearing aids. It is important to recognize that many hearing aid manufacturers no longer make analog hearing aids and the discussion that follows will focus on the digital hearing aid. The digital hearing aid may be programmed by the audiologist to meet the needs of the patient in multiple acoustic settings. The patient may access a number of different program settings by pressing a button on the hearing aid so that the amplified signal may be adjusted according to the environment. These may include a setting for a quiet room at home, a school cafeteria, or a large movie theater. A digital hearing aid provides the audiologist with flexibility to program the hearing aid according to the specific nature of the patient's hearing loss. In addition, this flexibility enables the audiologist to amplify specific sound frequencies or program the device to meet the listening needs of the patient. In the case of the author, my digital hearing aids have been programmed to maximize my hearing when delivering a lecture in a large auditorium, and upon completion, I am able to push a button and put the hearing aid back into an "auto" mode. This auto mode will automatically adjust the loudness level and programming choice according to level of noise and activity within the environment. Decisions regarding hearing aids are best made by the patient working closely with an audiologist who has tested the person's hearing and has provided a number of options to meet the person's needs.

MAKING A DIFFERENCE

Diane Schecklong, AuD, a clinical audiologist and faculty member at Northern Illinois University, shares one of her experiences:

In the course of a typical day at a busy university speech-language-hearing clinic, an audiologist may see clients that range in age from infants to centenarians. In my current position I see all ages, but I work primarily with the geriatric population. I love to share in the rich lives of these mature people. While I am able to help them with their hearing problems, I also have the opportunity to hear their unique stories that reflect their insight and the wisdom that they've accumulated throughout their lifetime. A success story to me is when I can truly make a difference in someone's life. The following is one such story.

Two months ago, a couple in their mid 70s, Mr. and Mrs. Walter, came into my office so that Mr. Walter could have his hearing evaluated. Mrs. Walter strongly encouraged Mr. Walter to get some help so that he could once again participate in the world around him. Mrs. Walter noticed that Mr. Walter was no longer interested in going to movies, plays, or concerts. He declined invitations to dine with family and friends, saying that he preferred to eat at home. Mr. Walter was no longer a regular for morning coffee with the guys in town. Weekly bridge games at the senior center became once a month before they stopped altogether. Mr. Walter was withdrawing from all activities that used to be enjoyable for him and his wife

(continued)

was genuinely worried. Mr. Walter often downplayed his hearing difficulties. He was skeptical, hesitant, and clearly not motivated to wear hearing aids. To please his wife, he went along with my recommendations and purchased two hearing aids in spite of his utter disinterest in the entire process. The first week or two with the new hearing aids was challenging. Mr. Walter was distracted by all of the everyday noises: the crinkling of the newspaper as he turned the pages, the thunderous roar when he flushed the toilet, and the clatter of dishes and cups carelessly thrown into the bus pan at the coffee shop. At his recheck appointment during week 3, I adjusted the hearing aids and spent some time discussing realistic expectations. I encouraged Mr. Walter to keep wearing the hearing aids full-time to speed along the adjustment process. Mr. Walter and Mrs. Walter enrolled in our 4-week aural rehabilitation classes in which several new hearing aid users and their spouses meet with me once a week to discuss their experiences and learn how to best manage their hearing loss. We have interactive discussions about listening strategies, assertiveness training, and controlling environmental factors that can affect hearing. By the last week of class when I invited all the participants to share some of their positive experiences with their new hearing aids, the man who was once a skeptic was quick to volunteer.

Mr. Walter reported that "I can now sit on my deck and hear the birds in the morning. I can actually hear the different calls they make. My wife is so much happier not having to repeat things to me all the time. Sure, they're not perfect, but I can follow conversations more easily now. But let me tell you, my granddaughter Emily is 6 years old. When she hops up onto my lap and starts to tell me about something that happened at school, usually, I nod my head in approval, laugh with her, but I can never follow her little voice talking a mile a minute. Just yesterday, she came by my chair to give me a hello kiss, and I said, 'Come here and sit on my lap and tell me what's going on. I haven't seen you for a whole month.' She sort of looked down and said, 'Grampa, I felt really sad the last time when you laughed when I told you about the dead bird I found in the grass. I don't know why you thought that was funny.' It hit me like a thunderbolt! I probably laughed and brushed off what she said because I never really heard her. You can really get yourself into trouble by faking it! I'm so grateful that I went ahead and invested in these hearing aids. They have really made a difference in my life."

And that is the beauty of my job.

FM Systems and Assistive Listening Devices

A second type of amplification system uses a broadcast signal similar to those produced in your radio. These systems use a frequency modulated (FM) wave to deliver the signal from a microphone to a receiver. For many hearing-impaired children in classroom settings, children with attention problems, and children easily distracted by classroom noises, an FM system can be used to maximize the child's ability to hear the information being presented and remain on task. An FM system usually has a microphone that is often worn by the teacher in the classroom. The teacher will also wear a transmitter that sends the signal to the students (see Figure 12.7). Depending upon the classroom setup, a child will wear a receiver or have a receiver on his or her desk so that the signal can be routed to the hearing aid, headphones, or speaker on the desk. By using an FM system, the classroom

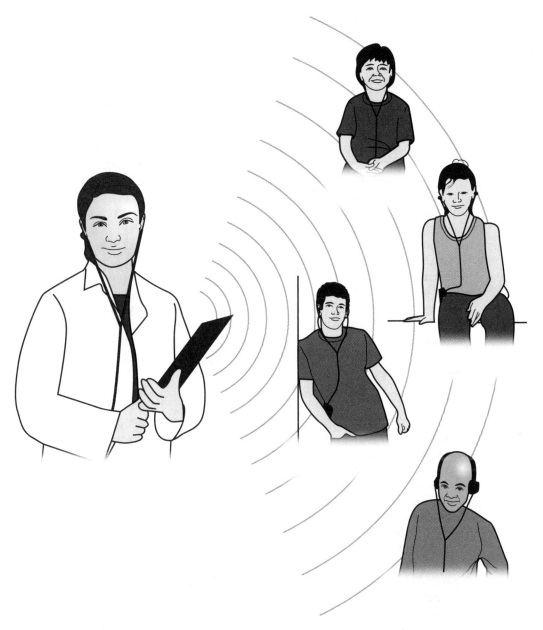

FIGURE 12.7
FM system.

teacher can directly provide an auditory signal to the child without the distractions of classroom noise. As the teacher is wearing a microphone, he or she is able to move around the classroom and still have the sound delivered directly to the child. By using an FM system, there is a greater opportunity to keep the child's attention and minimize the impact of extraneous classroom noise.

For adults with a hearing loss, there are a number of *assistive listening devices* that have been developed to improve their hearing abilities within their day-to-day environments where they must communicate. In a manner similar to that previously described, some adults will be active in environments where an FM system might be in place. These might include a theater, convention center, or even a church, mosque, or synagogue. If the FM system is in place, adult listeners will attach an FM receiver to their hearing aid or wear a headset to improve their ability to hear. At home, adults might purchase an infrared system that plugs into a television set and sends a signal directly to a set of headphones. In this manner, family members can watch the television at a comfortable loudness level while the person with a hearing loss can adjust the volume on their headphones so that they can hear at a comfortable level and not disturb the other viewers. In addition, there are a variety of devices that are available to make hearing activities at home less troublesome. These include amplifiers for telephones (mobile, cordless, etc.) and amplified computers and wake-up alarms.

In addition, for those individuals with severe-to-profound hearing loss for whom amplification will not meet their needs, there are a variety of alerting devices that can assist them within their environment. Many of these alerting devices use a strobe light or typical light bulb to signal the individual. These signals might be used for fire or smoke alarms, baby monitors, door bells, or alarm clocks. Other devices use a vibrating mechanism, as in alarm clocks (put it under the pillow), watch alarms, pagers, or text-messaging devices. For additional information about assistive devices, you are encouraged to look at the Web site listings at the end of the chapter.

Cochlear Implants

For a number of severely to profoundly deaf individuals, hearing aids and amplification provide little to no benefit. Improvements in hearing technology have led to the development of a device known as a *cochlear implant.* Whereas a hearing aid will make a sound louder, the cochlear implant is a small electronic device that helps to deliver an acoustic signal converted to an electrical signal directly to the acoustic nerve in the cochlea.

The cochlear implant is made up of a number of components. The external components (see Figure 12.8A) include an ear-level microphone that detects the sounds from the environment, a speech processor that transforms the signal, and a transmitter that sends the signal. Very often the microphone and speech processor are housed in a BTE case that looks like a hearing aid. The internal device components (see Figure 12.8B) are surgically implanted and include a receiver that is placed behind the pinna under the skin and an electrode array that will distribute the signal throughout the cochlea and stimulate the acoustic nerve.

When a child or adult is fitted with a cochlear implant, the device will be turned on anywhere from 2 to 6 weeks following surgery. It is not uncommon for the patient to initially experience headaches and follow-up with the otolaryngologist usually takes place 1 week following the procedure.

It is important to recognize that the cochlear implant is not a switch that when turned on automatically results in a patient hearing and understanding speech. Because the acoustic nerve and the brain are receiving signals in a manner that is not familiar, the patient will require extensive training and therapy to maximize the

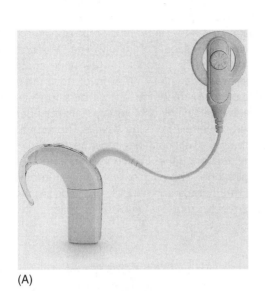

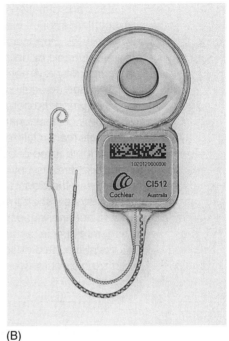

(A)   (B)

FIGURE 12.8

(A) External components of a cochlear implant and (B) internal components of a cochlear implant. (Reprinted with permission of Cochlear™ Americas, © 2009 Cochlear Americas)

potential of the device. A procedure known as *mapping* is used to fine-tune the patient's ability to use the implant. During the first year following the implant, the patient may return on multiple occasions so that the signals being delivered via the electrode array within the cochlea can be adjusted to maximize the patient's hearing.

At the present time, cochlear implants are being completed with children as young as 12 months of age and with many adults. As the critical periods for speech and language development occur in most children prior to age 6, cochlear implants have enabled many children to develop speech, language, and social skills. Once again it is important to note that learning these skills is not the same automatic process as in a normally developing hearing child. Skill development comes about as a result of the surgical procedure and the postsurgical therapy. Additionally, cochlear implants along with postsurgical therapy have enabled some children with postlingual deafness and late-deafened adults to regain some of their lost hearing, speech, and language skills (Gyo, Hato, Hakuba, Takahashi, & Takahashi, 2006; Hearing Loss Association of America, 2007).

For many hearing parents with congenitally deaf children and adults who are late-deafened, the cochlear implant seems to be a miracle of modern technology. The children are able to develop speech and language skills, parents are able to communicate with their children, and adults are able to be more functional in a hearing society. However, for individuals in the Deaf community (noted with a capital *D*), there are questions and concerns associated with the cochlear implants. Is the cochlear implant really the miracle device that will change all deaf people? Persons within the Deaf community see their deafness as an integral part of who they are, rather than a disability that needs to be overcome. The primary language of the Deaf community is American Sign Language (ASL) and these individuals celebrate their language and cultural history. As a result, there is some question regarding the fate of ASL and the perpetuation of the Deaf community. The Deaf community has tried to provide cautionary information for parents that although cochlear implants will benefit many children, there is still a lot of therapy involved in the process. Additionally, the degree of benefit of the cochlear implant will be a function of the individual rather than the device. Individuals with cochlear implants may derive limited benefits from the device or a lot of benefit from the device. The situation is not a black-and-white issue as many persons with cochlear implants may have both deaf friends and hearing friends, learn sign language, function within a traditional classroom, or require special services at school. The cochlear implant is merely a device that can assist the child or adult. With therapy and support, the individual will learn to maximize his or her hearing, speech, language, and social skills.

Auditory Training

Auditory training is a process that is typically begun after an individual has been fitted with a hearing aid or cochlear implant so that they can learn to maximize their abilities to use their residual hearing. Auditory training is going to be directed toward the amount of residual hearing that a person has and their ability to use that hearing in a meaningful way. It is not uncommon to work with a person whose audiogram shows a greater degree of hearing loss but has better functional speech and language skills than a person with a less severe hearing loss. There are many factors involved in a person's ability to learn or relearn speech and language.

Older therapy programs often focused on lip reading, more commonly referred to at the present time as *speech reading*. Speech reading is a method of encouraging the client to focus on the visible movements of the lips, jaw, and tongue in addition to body language and facial expression so that these added visual clues can help to assist the person's perception of the message being conveyed. However, in English only about 30% of the sounds are visible, so this form of therapy is limited in the amount of help that can be provided to the client.

A functional approach toward auditory training will focus on teaching the client to discriminate sounds that are confused, words that might be easily confused, speech versus nonspeech sounds, speech versus noise, or speech within a noisy environment. Although many of us take our hearing and speech skills for granted, when we examine the process of teaching or reteaching hearing skills, we recognize that normal-hearing people use a number of modalities to assist their ability to hear. As a result, in therapy a teacher, speech–language pathologist, or audiologist providing auditory training encourages the use of visual clues (e.g., videotape, mirrors, pictures) and sensory clues (e.g., forming the sounds in the mouth, feeling laryngeal vibration) to assist in the learning of the specific sounds and words.

Communication Training

It is a generally accepted fact that the early acquisition of language for a deaf child is a key step toward this child's ability to successfully communicate as an adult. This communication may take a number of forms and historically has been a major point of debate among advocates for the various approaches. On one side of this debate we have a group of people who believe that deaf and hard-of-hearing children must learn to function within a traditional society, and in order to accomplish this, the children must be taught to make maximum use of their residual hearing abilities and language skills. These individuals strongly promote the teaching of oral speech and language skills and are often referred to as *oralists*. In contrast, there is a group of individuals who believe that many deaf children will never attain the necessary oral speech and spoken language skills to make them functional. As a result, this group believes that it is better to focus on the teaching of sign language so that these children will be able to immediately learn language skills that will help prepare them for future success and also be able to function within a nonhearing community. These individuals are referred to as *manualists*. In the following section we will examine a number of different programs that focus on oral and manual communication.

Oral Communication

In general, oral approaches emphasize the use of speech skills while discouraging the use of any type of signing program. Oral approaches require that the child wears his or her hearing aid on a regular basis and work at teaching the child to maximize use of residual hearing. Visual and written cues are also components of some oral programs. The *aural/oral* approach emphasizes auditory training, speech reading, and written prompts to encourage the development of speech and language skills. Like most therapy programs, the key to success in the aural/oral program is consistency of practice. In order for a child to be successful, there has to be a strong commitment on the part of the family and school personnel toward the development of oral speech and language.

Manual Communication

For many severe-to-profound deaf individuals, learning to orally communicate may not be a reasonable option given the nature of their hearing loss. As a result, a number of manual communication systems have been developed. ASL is a complex language system used by many deaf individuals. ASL is the primary language for many deaf individuals and English is learned as a second language. ASL is a symbol-based system that uses hand-shape gestures, hand movements, body movements, and facial expression to effect communication. Acceptance into the Deaf community is often related to the individual's ability to sign rather than their loss of hearing. As many deaf individuals must also function within a typical hearing society, children are often taught another sign system that is based on the rules of the English language. *Signed English* (SE) follows the rules of English grammar and uses finger spelling (hand gestures that represent the letters of the English alphabet) to fill in when no sign exists for a specific word. When using SE, an individual will use typical ASL signs and follow the rules of English grammar.

Total Communication

Historically we have noted that individual groups have strongly advocated for one method of communication versus another for deaf individuals. However, educators, speech–language pathologists, and audiologists have come to recognize that a multimodality approach toward communication might be most beneficial toward helping the child develop speech and language skills. As a result, many programs for children with sensorineural hearing loss will now use a *total communication* approach for teaching speech and language skills. Total communication uses sign language, finger spelling, oral speech, speech reading, amplification, writing, gestures, and any other method available to enable the child to communicate. As these programs are often part of an academic curriculum with the goal of improving English language skills, the signing component of these programs is often based on English grammar as described in SE. It is important to note that like many other programs, total communication will be dependent in part on the sign language skills and oral language abilities of the teacher providing the instruction. Some individuals who advocate for mastery of sign skills question whether total communication can provide the necessary training that will enable a child to sign, but others argue that the goal of total communication is improved language skills and anything that can be done to improve a child's language is going to have a positive benefit toward the child's academic development.

Quiz on the Fly 12.2

1. Deafness that occurs after birth is called _____.
2. Two hearing tests conducted on newborn infants are _____ and _____.
3. Five basic components of a hearing aid are _____, _____, _____, _____, and _____.
4. The procedure that is used to fine-tune the functioning of a cochlear implant is called _____.
5. Three approaches toward communication for the deaf are _____, _____, and _____ communication.

ACOUSTICS IN THE CLASSROOM

It is not unusual for a teacher, speech–language pathologist, or audiologist to forget one of the most critical issues associated with learning in the classroom. This is the acoustic environment that will foster or hinder the educational process. When we think about this acoustic environment, we typically think about the deaf child who must function within a hearing environment. However, we must also recognize that many of the children within this classroom may experience transient conductive hearing losses and other children may experience attention issues. In addition, even the hearing abilities of a normal-hearing child are going to be affected by the acoustic environment within the classroom. Although our focus in this chapter has been the deaf and hearing-impaired child, all children can benefit from our understanding of how the acoustic environment can be modified to best meet the needs of children in a classroom environment. The two basic concepts associated with classroom acoustics are the signal-to-noise ratio (SNR) and the reverberation within the room.

Signal-to-Noise Ratio

For the purposes of our discussion, the SNR is the relationship between the speech signal and the amount of noise within the environment. Each component of the ratio is measured in decibels. The ideal ratio is +15 db HL where the speech signal is 15 dB HL louder than the noise within the environment. A classroom example may be the best method of illustrating the problem. A teacher is talking to her class and a sound engineer in the back of the room is measuring both the loudness of her voice and the amount of noise within the classroom. This noise is produced by the blowers in the air conditioner, student conversations within the classroom, and the humming of the fluorescent lights. The engineer measures the teacher's vocal intensity as 50 dB HL and the noise at 35 dB HL. In this case we have a SNR of +15 (SNR 50:35 = +15), which is our target and will enable most students to hear the teacher's message. In some cases the SNR may vary according to the environmental conditions within and outside of the classroom. Increased noise levels come about when air conditioning systems are running within the classroom, maintenance crews are mowing the lawn, or when the entire class is talking at the same time. For those individuals with hearing loss or attention problems, a change in the SNR from +15 to 0 (e.g., teacher's voice at 50 dB HL: noise in classroom at 50 dB HL = 0 SNR) can have a significant impact on the information received by the student. Likewise, in some classroom situations where the teacher is trying to give suggestions to all of the students working on group projects, the SNR may be in the negative range (e.g., speech signal 50 dB HL: noise at 65 dB HL = −15) where the noise is considerably louder than the signal, making it very difficult for the typical student to understand the instructions and nearly impossible for the deaf student or other students with auditory impairments to receive the information. Crandell (1993) compared the speech recognition ability of students with mild hearing losses with normal-hearing children, and reported that in a room with a +6 SNR, the children with hearing loss were 13% poorer at speech recognition than their normal-hearing counterparts, and at −6 SNR these hearing-impaired children were 33% poorer at speech recognition. It is not hard to imagine that as a child's hearing loss increases or the SNR in the classroom decreases, the amount of information that is lost between the teacher and student is quite significant.

Reverberation

When an individual is speaking in a large classroom, a portion of the speech signal travels directly to the listener. However, another portion of that signal bounces off of the walls and ceilings and reaches the listener at a later time. This echo of sound is also known as *reverberation*. As you might imagine, large rooms with high ceilings and hard walls often result in a lot of reverberation, but in other smaller rooms, the speech signal travels more directly to the listener. The reverberation time, or time it takes for the signal to be perceived by the listener, is an important factor when related to classroom acoustics and a student's perception of speech. The longer the reverberation time, the greater the chance for missed information within the classroom. When reverberation is present, the student will perceive the reverberant speech signal at a somewhat later time than the direct speech signal. The later arriving reverberant signal may cancel out some of the direct signal frequencies or result in a "smearing or masking of the direct signal" (Crandell & Smaldino, 2000, p. 365) that will ultimately affect the child's ability to perceive the original.

What Can Be Done?

When an educator or school administrator is able to recognize the potential difficulties associated with noise and reverberation within a classroom, the question arises as to what types of modifications are available to improve this learning environment. A teacher can visually inspect a classroom and note the presence of high ceilings, hard walls, large distances between the front and back of the classroom, and then investigate potential modifications that can have a positive impact on the acoustics in the classroom. Sound-absorbing ceiling tiles, suspended ceilings, and sound-absorbing wall panels are all possible remedies for excessive sound reverberation. Noise in the classroom may come from air conditioning fans, gaps between the doors and door frames, gaps between the window and frame, and furniture scraping across an uncarpeted floor. Although it may be cost prohibitive to make all of these modifications, when a classroom teacher is aware of these issues, some modifications may be possible. Teachers may also recognize that some additional modifications may help to facilitate communication without added expenses. It may be possible to position chairs and desks within the room so that the sound signal will reach the students in a more direct manner with less reverberation. The teacher can be positioned within the room so that more of the students will receive the teacher's instructions without the effect of noise or reverberation. Finally, as previously discussed, classroom amplification systems may be used: The teacher wears a microphone and the speech signal is received via a loudspeaker in the room, or in some cases an FM system may be used to deliver the speech signal directly to each student within the classroom.

Quiz on the Fly 12.2 Answers

1. Deafness that occurs after birth is called **adventitious deafness**. **2.** Two hearing tests conducted on newborn infants are **otoacoustic emissions** and **auditory brain stem response**. **3.** Five basic components of a hearing aid are **microphone, analog-to-digital converter, signal processor, digital-to-analog converter,** and **receiver**. **4.** The procedure that is used to fine-tune the functioning of a cochlear implant is called **mapping**. **5.** Three approaches toward communication for the deaf are **oral, manual,** and **total** communication.

SUMMARY AND REVIEW

The focus of this chapter was hearing testing and the management of hearing loss in children and adults. Our discussion began with an exploration of hearing testing through the traditional pathway from the environment to the inner ear. We continued by discussing specific tests that help us to measure the functioning of the middle ear and the cochlea. Our next large discussion focused on the management of hearing loss, including a discussion of methods for amplifying the speech signal and a surgical procedure that involves the implantation of a device that can result in improved hearing through extensive rehabilitation. We also discussed auditory and communication training for individuals with hearing loss and concluded our discussion with an exploration of classroom acoustics and their impact on the learning abilities of all children.

Hearing Testing

What are the typical tests that are completed to test a person's hearing?

When a child or adult is seen for a hearing evaluation, it typically begins with air conduction testing, which assesses the general integrity of the system from the outer ear to the middle ear to the inner ear. A sound is introduced into the ear and the patient is asked to respond when he or she hears the sound. If a hearing problem is noted, an audiologist will complete bone conduction testing in a effort to determine whether the problem is in the inner ear (bone conduction scores are decreased) or middle ear (bone conduction scores are normal). The next test that may be done is speech audiometry, in which the patient is asked to repeat real words in an effort to determine how a person's hearing loss affects their perception of speech. Assessing the functioning of the middle ear focuses on the functioning of the tympanic membrane by using tympanometry and measuring the acoustic reflex.

What are two hearing tests that are routinely completed with newborns?

Otoacoustic emissions are sounds produced by the cochlea and indicate normal cochlear functioning. As these emissions can be evaluated without the active participation of the patient, this test is routinely completed with most newborns in the hospital to identify potential hearing problems. A second test called the auditory brain stem response does not require the active participation of the client and is also used to assess newborns. This test measures the electrical signal from the acoustic nerve to the brain.

Habilitation/Rehabilitation

What are hearing aids and what do they do?

A hearing aid is a device that amplifies sound and typically has five components. These are a microphone, an analog-to-digital converter, a signal processor, a digital-to-analog converter, and a receiver. The microphone will receive the acoustic signal and convert the sound signal to an electrical signal. The electrical signal passes through the analog-to-digital converter where the signal is converted to a series of 0s and 1s that is modified by the signal processor to meet the hearing needs of the person receiving the hearing aid. The modified signal then passes through the digital-to-analog converter and is sent to the receiver that changes the signal to an acoustic signal that the listener can hear. There are two types of hearing aids, analog and digital, with digital hearing aids becoming more and more popular given that they contain a miniature computer that can automatically adjust the volume and automatically select a program to meet the hearing needs of individuals. Hearing aids may be placed behind the ear, in the ear, or in the ear canal.

Will a cochlear implant guarantee that a deaf individual will hear and understand speech?

A cochlear implant is a device that is surgically inserted into the cochlea so that it can deliver a sound signal directly to the acoustic nerve. Although individuals with cochlear implants can now receive sounds, it takes extensive therapy for the individuals to learn to identify and use these sounds in a meaningful way. It is important to recognize that many patients benefit from a cochlear implant but a smaller percentage do not. Cochlear implants do not guarantee that a person will hear and understand speech.

What are the three approaches to communication training?

Communication training involves oral approaches, manual approaches, and total communication. Oral approaches work to maximize the client's residual hearing and focus on the client's aural (hearing) and oral (verbal) skills. Manual approaches may teach sign language based upon the English grammatical rules (Signed English) or the more universal symbol-based system, American Sign Language. Total communication advocates a philosophy of using both oral and manual approaches in an attempt to maximize the individual's language development.

Acoustics in the Classroom

What two factors need to be examined to improve classroom acoustics?

The two factors that need to be examined by the classroom teacher, audiologist, and school speech–language pathologist are the signal-to-noise ratio and reverberation within the classroom. The signal-to-noise ratio is a measure that is made to determine whether the speech signals reaching the child are loud enough to be understood when compared to the background noise within the classroom. The ideal ratio is +15. Sound reverberation relates to the direct and indirect transmission of sound in the classroom. Large, high-ceiling, hard-walled classrooms produce a lot of echoes caused by sounds reverberating and arriving later to the listener when compared with the direct signal. These later arriving sounds may cancel out frequencies in the direct signal and often provide confusing information to the listener.

WEB SITES OF INTEREST

Alexander Graham Bell Association for the Deaf and Hard of Hearing
http://nc.agbell.org/netcommunity/page.aspx?pid=348

Assistive Listening Devices
http://www.betterhearing.org/hearing_solutions/listeningDevices.cfm

Association of Late-Deafened Adults
http://www.alda.org/

Center for Hearing and Communication
http://www.chchearing.org/
http://www.lhh.org/about_hearing_loss/images/Audiogram-REV.4.gif

Hearing Loss Association of America
http://www.hearingloss.org/

REFERENCES

Adamovich, B. L. B. (2005). Traumatic brain injury. In L. L. LaPointe (Ed.), *Aphasia and related neurogenic language disorders* (pp. 225–236). New York: Thieme.

Adams, M. R. (1990). The demands and capacities model I: Theoretical elaborations. *Journal of Fluency Disorders, 15*(3), 135–141.

Alexander Graham Bell Association for the Deaf and Hard of Hearing (2010). Deaf. Retrieved from http://nc.agbell.org/NetCommunity/Page.aspx?pid=598#D

Allen, G. (2006). Cerebellar contributions to autistic spectrum disorders. *Clinical Neuroscience Research, 6*, 195–207.

American Psychiatric Association. (2000). *Diagnostic and statistical manual of mental disorders* (4th ed., text revision). Washington, DC: Author.

American Speech-Language-Hearing Association. (1985). Clinical management of communicatively handicapped minority language populations [Position statement]. Retrieved from http://www.asha.org/docs/html/PS1985-00219.html

American Speech-Language-Hearing Association. (1993). Definitions of communication disorders and variations. Retrieved from http://www.asha.org/docs/html/RP1993-00208.html

American Speech-Language-Hearing Association. (1998). Students and professionals who speak English with accents and nonstandard dialects: Issues and recommendations [Position statement]. Retrieved from http://www.asha.org/docs/html/PS1998-00117.html

American Speech-Language-Hearing Association. (2003). American English dialects [Technical report]. Retrieved from http://www.asha.org/docs/html/TR2003-00044.html

American Speech-Language-Hearing Association. (2010a). Causes of hearing loss in children. Retrieved from http://www.asha.org/public/hearing/disorders/causes.htm

American Speech-Language-Hearing Association. (2010b). Code of ethics. Retrieved July 6, 2010, from http://www.asha.org/docs/html/ET2010-00309.html

American Speech-Language-Hearing Association. (2010c). Multicultural affairs and resources. Retrieved from http://www.asha.org/practice/multicultural

American Speech-Language-Hearing Association Committee on Language. (1983). Definition of language. *ASHA, 25*(6), 44.

Aronson, A. E. (1985). *Clinical voice disorders: An interdisciplinary approach* (2nd ed.). New York: Thieme.

Bankson, N., & Bernthal, J. E. (2004a). Etiology/factors related to phonological disorders. In J. E. Bernthal & N. W. Bankson (Eds.), *Articulation and phonological disorders* (5th ed., pp. 139–200). Boston: Pearson/Allyn & Bacon.

Bankson, N., & Bernthal, J. E. (2004b). Phonological assessment procedures. In J. E. Bernthal & N. W. Bankson (Eds.), *Articulation and phonological disorders* (5th ed., pp. 201–267). Boston: Pearson/Allyn & Bacon.

Bankson, N., & Bernthal, J. E. (2004c). Treatment approaches. In J. E. Bernthal & N. W. Bankson (Eds.), *Articulation and phonological disorders* (5th ed., pp. 292–347). Boston: Pearson/Allyn & Bacon.

Baron-Cohen, S., Baldwin, D. A., & Crowson, M. (1997). Do children with autism use the speaker's direction of gaze strategy to crack the code of language? *Child Development, 68*, 48–57.

Baron-Cohen, S., Tager-Flusberg, H., & Cohen, D. J. (1993). *Understanding other minds: Perspectives from autism.* Oxford, England: Oxford University Press.

Battle, D. E. (2002). *Communication disorders in multicultural populations* (3rd ed.). Boston: Butterworth-Heinemann.

Blake, M. L. (2005). Right hemisphere syndrome. In L. L. LaPointe (Ed.), *Aphasia and related neurogenic language disorders* (pp. 213–224). New York: Thieme.

Bloodstein, O. (1960). The development of stuttering. II. Developmental phases. *Journal of Speech and Hearing Disorders, 25*, 366–376.

Bloodstein, O., & Ratner, N. (2008). *A handbook on stuttering* (6th ed.). Clifton Park, NY, Thomson Delmar Learning.

Bloom, L., & Lahey, M. (1978). *Language development and language disorders.* New York: Wiley.

Bloom, P., & Markson, L. (1998). Capacities underlying word learning. *Trends in Cognitive Sciences, 2*, 67–73.

Bluemel, C. (1932). Primary and secondary stammering. *Quarterly Journal of Speech, 18*, 187–200.

Boone, D. R., McFarlane, S. C., & Von Berg, S. L. (2005). *The voice and voice therapy.* Boston: Pearson/Allyn & Bacon.

Bransford, J. D., Brown, A. L., & Cocking, R. R. (Eds.). (2000). *How people learn: Brain, mind, experience, and school.* Washington, DC: National Academy Press.

Brown, R. (1973). *A first language: The early stages.* Cambridge, MA: Harvard University Press.

Bureau of Labor Statistics, U.S. Department of Labor. (2010a). *Occupational outlook handbook, 2010–11 edition.* Retrieved July 5, 2010, from http://www.bls.gov/oco/ocos085.htm

Bureau of Labor Statistics, U.S. Department of Labor. (2010b). *Occupational outlook handbook, 2010–11 edition (Speech-language pathologists).* Retrieved July 5, 2010, from http://www.bls.gov/oco/ocos099.htm

Capone, N. C., & McGregor, K. K. (2004). Gesture development: A review for clinical and research practices. *Journal of Speech, Language, and Hearing Research, 47*, 173–186.

Carey, S., & Bartlett, E. (1978). Acquiring a single new word. *Papers and Reports on Child Language Development, 15*, 17–29.

Catts, H. W., & Kamhi, A. G. (2005). *Language and reading disabilities* (2nd ed.). Boston: Pearson/Allyn & Bacon.

Chomsky, N. (1965). *Aspects of the theory of syntax.* Cambridge, MA: MIT Press.

Clark, J. G. (1981). Uses and abuses of hearing loss classification. *ASHA, 23*, 493–500.

Clark, W. W., & Ohlemiller, K. K. (2008). *Anatomy and physiology of hearing for audiologists.* Clifton Park, NY: Thomson Delmar Learning.

Cole, L. (1989). *E pluribus pluribus*: Multicultural imperatives for the 1990s and beyond. *ASHA, 31*(9), 65–70.

Colton, R. H., Casper, J. K., & Leonard, R. (2006). *Understanding voice problems.* Philadelphia: Lippincott Williams & Wilkins.

Communication. (2010). In *Merriam-Webster Online Dictionary.* Retrieved from http://www.merriam-webster.com/dictionary/communication

Conboy, B. T., Sommerville, J. A., & Kuhl, P. K. (2008). Cognitive control factors in speech perception at 11 months. *Developmental Psychology, 44*, 1505–1512.

Conture, E. G. (1990). *Stuttering* (2nd ed.). Englewood Cliffs, NJ: Prentice Hall.

Conture, E. G. (2001). *Stuttering: Its nature, diagnosis and treatment.* Boston: Allyn & Bacon.

Crandell, C. CX. (1993). Noise effect on the speech recognition of children with minimal hearing loss. *Ear & Hearing, 14*, 210–216.

Crandell, C. C., & Smaldino, J. J. (2000). Classroom acoustics for children with normal hearing and with hearing impairment. *Language, Speech, and Hearing Services in Schools, 31*, 362–370.

Crandell, C. C., & Smaldino, J. J. (Eds). (2001). Classroom acoustics: Understanding barriers to learning. *Volta Review, 101*, 5.

Cummins, J. (1984). *Bilingualism and special education: Issues in assessment and pedagogy.* San Diego, CA: College-Hill.

Daly, D. A., & Burnett, M. L. (1996). Cluttering: assessment, treatment planning, and case study illustration, *Journal of Fluency Disorders, 21*, 239–248.

Darley, F., Aronson, A. E., & Brown, J. (1969). Differential diagnostic patterns of dysarthria. *Journal of Speech and Hearing Research, 12*, 246–269.

De Boer, J., Brennan, S., Lineton, B., Stevens, J., & Thornton, A. R.D. Click-evoked otoacoustic emissions (CEOAEs) recorded from neonates under 13 hours old using and maximum length sequence (MLS) conventional stimulation. *Hearing Research 2007; 233(1–2):* 86–96.

DeNil, L., Kroll, R., Kapur, S., & Houle, S. (2000). A positron emission tomography study of silent oral single word reading in stuttering and nonstuttering adults. *Journal of Speech, Language, and Hearing Research, 43*, 1038–1053.

Deveney, C. W., Benner, K., & Cohen, J. (1993). Gastroesophageal reflux and laryngeal disease. *Archives of Surgery, 128*, 1021–1027.

de Villiers, J., & de Villiers, P. (1973). A cross sectional study of the acquisition of grammatical morphemes. *Journal of Psycholinguistic Research, 2*, 267–278.

Dore, J. (1974). A pragmatic description of early language development. *Journal of Psycholinguistic Research, 4*, 343–350.

Dore, J. (1978). Variation in preschool children's conversational performances. In K. Nelson (Ed.), *Children's language: Vol. 1* (pp. 397–444). New York: Gardner.

Ebbels, S. H., van der Lely, H. K. J., & Dockrell, J. E. (2007). Intervention for verb argument structure in children with persistent SLI: A randomized control trial. *Journal of Speech, Language, and Hearing Research, 50*, 1330–1349.

Eimas, P. D., Siqueland, E. R., Jusczyk, P. W., & Vigorito, J. (1971). Speech perception in infants. *Science, 171*, 303–306.

Ekman, P., & Friesen, W. V. (1978). *Facial action coding system: A technique for the measurement of facial movement.* Palo Alto, CA: Consulting Psychologists.

Facts About TBI in the USA. (n.d.). Retrieved July 6, 2010, from Brain Trauma Foundation, https://www.braintrauma.org/tbi-faqs/tbi-statistics/

Fernald, A. (1994). Human maternal vocalizations to infants as biologically relevant signals: An evolutionary perspective. In P. Bloom (Ed.), *Language acquisition: Core reading* (pp. 51–94). Cambridge, MA: MIT Press.

Fox, L., Long, S. H., & Langlois, A. (1988). Patterns of language comprehension deficit in abused and neglected children. *Journal of Speech and Hearing Disorders, 53*, 239–244.

Franco, F., Perucchini, P., & March, B. (2009). Is infant initiation of joint attention by pointing affected by type of interaction? *Social Development, 18*, 51–76.

Franken, M. C. J., Kielstra-Van der Schalk, C. J., & Boelens, H. (2005). Experimental treatment of early stuttering: A preliminary study. *Journal of Fluency Disorders, 30*, 189–199.

Gauger, L. M., Lombardino, L. J., & Leonard, C. M. (1997). Brain morphology in children with specific language impairment. *Journal of Speech, Language, and Hearing Research, 40*, 1272–1284.

Gillon, G. (2004). *Phonological awareness: From research to practice.* New York: Guilford.

Gleitman, L. (1990). The structural sources of verb meanings. *Language Acquisition, 1,* 3–55.

Goldstein, B., & Iglesias, A. (2002). Issues of cultural and linguistic diversity. In R. Paul (Ed.), *Introduction to clinical methods in communication disorders* (pp. 261–279). Baltimore: Brookes.

Goodglass, H., Kaplan, E., & Barresi, B. (2001). *The assessment of aphasia and related disorders* (3rd ed.). Baltimore: Lippincott Williams and Wilkins.

Gyo, K., Hato, N., Hakuba, N., Takahashi, M., & Takahashi, N., (2006). Late hearing recovery of postmeningitic deafness in a child after cochlear implantation. *International Journal of Pediatric Otorhinolaryngology Extra,* 1(2) 160–163.

Hammer, C., & Rodriguez, B. (2009). Individual differences in bilingual children's language competencies. In A. Weiss (Ed.), *Perspectives on individual differences affecting therapeutic change in communication disorders.* New York: Taylor & Francis.

Hammer, C., & Weiss, A. (1999). Guiding language development: How African American mothers and their infants structure play interactions. *Journal of Speech, Language, and Hearing Research, 42,* 1219–1233.

Hammer, C., & Weiss, A. (2000). African American mothers' views of their infants' language development and language-learning environment. *American Journal of Speech-Language Pathology, 9,* 126–140.

Hanson, M. (2004). Ethnic, cultural, and language diversity in service settings. In E. Lynch & M. Hanson (Eds.), *Developing cross-cultural competence: A guide for working with children and their families* (3rd ed., pp. 3–18). Baltimore: Brookes.

Hart, B., & Risley, T. (1995). *Meaningful differences in the everyday experience of young American children.* Baltimore: Brookes.

Hearing Loss Association of America. (2007). Cochlear implants [Position paper]. Retrieved from http://www.shhh.org/advocacy/cochlearimplantposition.asp

Hirano, M. (1974). Morphological structure of the vocal cord as a vibrator and its variations. *Folia Phoniatrica, 26,* 89–94.

Hobbs, F., & Stoops, N. (2002). *Demographic trends in the 20th century* (U.S. Census Bureau, Census 2000 Special Reports, Series CENSR-4). Washington, DC: U.S. Government Printing Office.

Hodson, B. W. (1989). Phonological remediation: A cycles approach. In N. Creaghead, P. Newman, & W. Secord (Eds.), *Assessment and remediation of articulatory and phonological disorders.* Columbus, OH: Charles E. Merrill.

Hodson, B. W., & Paden, E. (1991). *Targeting intelligible speech: A phonological approach to remediation* (2nd ed). Austin, TX: PRO-ED.

Howie, P. M. (1981). Concordance for stuttering in monozygotic and dizygotic twin pairs. *Journal of Speech and Hearing Research, 24,* 317–321.

Ingham, J. C. (2003). Evidence-based treatment of stuttering: I. Definition and application. *Journal of Fluency Disorders, 28,* 197–207.

Ingham, R. J., Fox, P. T., Ingham, J. C., Xiong, J., Zamarripa, F., Hardies, L. J., et al. (2004). Brain correlates of stuttering and syllable production: Gender comparison and replication. *Journal of Speech, Language, and Hearing Research, 47,* 321–341.

Johnson, W. (1955). A study of the onset and development of stuttering. In W. Johnson & R. Leutenegger (Eds.), *Stuttering in children and adults.* Minneapolis: University of Minnesota Press.

Johnson, W., & Associates (1959). *The onset of stuttering: Research findings and implications.* Minneapolis: University of Minnesota Press.

Jusczyk, P. W. (1997). *The discovery of spoken language.* Cambridge, MA: MIT Press.

Jusczyk, P. W. (2003). Chunking language input to find patterns. In D. H. Rakison & L. M. Oakes (Eds.), *Early category and concept development: Making sense of the blooming, buzzing confusion* (pp. 27–49). New York: Oxford University Press.

Jusczyk, P. W., Friederici, A. D., Wessels, J. M., Svenkerud, V. Y., & Jusczyk, A. M. (1993). Infants' sensitivity to the sound patterns of native language words. *Journal of Memory and Language, 32,* 402–420.

Kemp, D. T. (1978). Stimulated acoustic emissions from within the human auditory system. *Journal of the Acoustical Society of America, 64,* 1386–1391.

Kent, R. (2004). Normal aspects of articulation. In J. E. Bernthal & N. W. Bankson (Eds.), *Articulation and phonological disorders* (5th ed., pp. 1–62). Boston: Pearson/Allyn & Bacon.

Kent, R. D. (1997). *The speech sciences.* San Diego: Singular.

Kertesz, A. (1982). *Western aphasia battery.* New York: Grune & Stratton.

Kidd, K. K., Kidd, J. R., & Records, M. (1978). The possible causes of the sex ratio in stuttering and its implications. *Journal of Fluency Disorders, 3,* 13–23.

Klein, J. O. (2001). The burden of otitis media. *Vaccine, 19,* s2–s8.

Klerman, L. V. (1991). The health of poor children: Problems and programs. In A. C. Huston (Ed.), *Children in poverty* (pp. 136–157). New York: Cambridge University Press.

Knect, S., Drager, B., Deppe, M., Bobe, L., Lohman, H., Floel, A., et al. (2000). Handedness and hemispheric language dominance in healthy humans. *Brain, 123*(12), 2512–2518.

Langdon, H. (2008). *Assessment and intervention for communication disorders in culturally and linguistically diverse populations.* Clifton Park, NY: Thomson Delmar Learning.

LePrell, C. G., Yamashita, D., Minami, S. B., Yamasoba, T., & Miller, J. M. (2007). Mechanisms of noise-induced hearing loss indicate multiple methods of prevention. *Hearing Research, 226*, 22–43.

Liles, B. (1993). Narrative discourse in children with language disorders and children with normal language: A critical review of language. *Journal of Speech and Hearing Research, 36*, 868–882.

Logemann, J. A. (1998). *Evaluation and treatment of swallowing disorders.* Austin, TX: PRO-ED.

Ludlow, C. L., Rosenberg, J., Salazar, A., Grafman, J., & Smutok, M. (1987). Site of penetrating brain lesions causing chronic acquired stuttering. *Annals of Neurology, 22*, 60–66.

Lynch, E. (2004). Developing cross-cultural competence. In E. Lynch & M. Hanson (Eds.), *Developing cross-cultural competence: A guide for working with children and their families* (3rd ed., pp. 41–75). Baltimore: Brookes.

Månsson, H. (2000). Childhood stuttering: Incidence and development. *Journal of Fluency Disorders, 25*, 47–57.

McDonald, E. (1964). *A deep test of articulation.* Pittsburgh, PA: Stanwix House.

McGregor, K. K. (2008). Semantic deficits associated with developmental language disorders. In R. G. Schwartz (Ed.), *The handbook of child language disorders* (pp. 365–387). New York: Psychology.

McGregor, K. K., & Capone, N. C. (2004). Genetic and environmental interactions in determining the early lexicon: Evidence from a set of tri-zygotic quadruplets. *Journal of Child Language, 31*, 311–337.

McGregor, K. K., Newman, R. M., Reilly, R. M., & Capone, N. C. (2002). Semantic representation and naming in children with specific language impairment. *Journal of Speech, Language, and Hearing Research, 45*, 998–1014.

McLeod, S. (Ed.). (2007). *The international guide to speech acquisition.* Clifton Park, NY: Thomson Delmar Learning.

McMahon, S., & Dodd, B. (1997). A comparison of the expressive communication skills of triplet, twin and singleton children. *European Journal of Disorders of Communication, 32*, 328–345.

Miles, S., & Chapman, R. S. (2002). Narrative content as described by individuals with Down syndrome and typically developing children. *Journal of Speech, Language, and Hearing Research, 45*, 175–189.

Minshew, N., Sweeney, J., Bauman, B., & Webb, S. (2005). Neurologic aspects of autism. In F. Vokmar, R. Paul, A. Klin, & D. Cohen (Eds.), *Handbook of autism and pervasive developmental disorders: Vol. 1* (pp. 473–514). New York: Wiley.

Mirak, J., & Rescorla, L. (1998). Phonetic skills and vocabulary size in late talkers: Concurrent and predictive relationships. *Applied Psycholinguistics, 19*, 1–17.

Models of vocal fold vibration (n.d.). Retrieved from *Tutorials—Voice production*, National Center for Voice and Speech, http://www.ncvs.org/ncvs/tutorials/voiceprod/tutorial/model.html

Mundy, P., Kasari, C., Sigman, M., & Ruskin, E. (1995). Early language acquisition in children with Down syndrome and in normally developing children. *Journal of Speech and Hearing Research, 38*, 157–167.

Murry, T., & Carrau, R. L. (2006). *Clinical management of swallowing disorders* (2nd ed). San Diego, CA: Plural.

National Dysphagia Diet Task Force. (2002). *The National Dysphagia Diet: Standardization for optimal care.* Chicago, IL: American Dietetic Association.

National Institute on Deafness and Other Communication Disorders. (2010a). Statistics about hearing, balance, ear infections, and deafness. Retrieved from http://www.nidcd.nih.gov/health/statistics/hearing.asp

National Institute on Deafness and Other Communication Disorders. (2010b). Stuttering. Retrieved from http://www.nidcd.nih.gov/health/voice/stutter.html

Nelson, K. (1973). Structure and strategy in learning to talk. *Monographs of the Society of Research in Child Development, 38*, 1–2.

Newcomer, P. L., & Hammil, D. D. (1997). *Test of language development—Primary* (TOLD-P:3). Austin, TX: PRO-ED.

Newman, R. M., & McGregor, K. K. (2006). Teachers and lay persons discern quality difference between narratives produced by children with or without SLI. *Journal of Speech, Language, and Hearing Research, 49*, 1022–1036.

Nicolosi, L., Harryman, E., & Kresheck, J. (2004). *Terminology of communication disorders* (4th ed.). Baltimore: Williams & Wilkins.

Nippold, M. A. (2007). Later language development: School-age children, adolescents, and young adults (3rd ed.). Austin, TX: PRO-ED.

Office of the Surgeon General. (2004). The health consequences of smoking: A report of the Surgeon General. Retrieved from http://www.surgeongeneral.gov/library/smokingconsequences/

Oller, D. K. (1980). The emergence of the sounds of speech in infancy. In G. H. Yeni-Komshian, J. F. Kavanagh, & C. A. Ferguson (Eds.), *Child phonology: Vol. 1, Production.* New York: Academic.

Oller, D. K., Eilers, R. E., Neal, A. R., & Schwartz, H. K. (1999). Precursors to speech in infancy: the prediction of speech and language disorders. *Journal of Communication Disorders, 32, 4*, 223–246.

Onslow, M. (2003). *The Lidcombe program of early stuttering intervention: A clinician's guide.* Austin, TX: PRO-ED.

Pannbacker, M. (1999). Treatment of vocal nodules: Options and outcomes. *American Journal of Speech-Language Pathology, 8*, 209–217.

Paul, R. (1996). Clinical implications of the natural history of slow expressive language development. *American Journal of Speech-Language Pathology, 5*, 5–21.

Paul, R. (2007). *Language disorders from infancy through adolescence: Assessment and intervention* (3rd ed.). St. Louis, MO: Mosby Elsevier.

Peterson-Falzone, S. J., Hardin-Jones, M. A., & Karnell, M. P. (2001). *Cleft palate speech* (3rd ed.). St. Louis, MO: Mosby.

Petinou, K. C., Schwartz, R. G., Gravel, J. S., & Raphael, L. J. (2001). A preliminary account of phonological and morphophonological perception in young children with and without otitis media. *International Journal of Language and Communication Disorders, 36*(1), 21–42.

Phelps-Terasaki, D., & Phelps-Gunn, T. (1992). *Test of pragmatic language.* Austin, TX: PRO-ED.

Piaget, J. (1970). *Structuralism.* New York: Basic Books.

Pinker, S. (1989). *Learnability and cognition: The acquisition of argument structure.* Cambridge, MA: MIT Press.

Porter, J. H., & Hodson, B. W. (2001). Collaborating to obtain phonological acquisition data for local schools. *Language, Speech, and Hearing Services in Schools, 32*(3), 65–171.

Postma, A., & Kolk, H. (1993). The covert repair hypothesis: Prearticulatory repair processes in normal and stuttered disfluencies. *Journal of Speech and Hearing Research, 36,* 472–487.

Prather, E. M., Hedrick, D. L., & Kern, C. A. (1975). Articulation development in children aged two to four years. *Journal of Speech and Hearing Disorders, 40,* 179–191.

Ramig, L. O., & Verdolini, K. (1998). Treatment efficacy: Voice disorders. *Journal of Speech, Language, and Hearing Research, 41,* 101–116.

Rehabilitation. (n.d.). *Merriam-Webster's Medical Dictionary.* Retrieved November 1, 2010, from Dictionary.com website: http://dictionary.reference.com/browse/rehabilitation

Rescorla, L. (1989). The language development survey: A screening tool for delayed language in toddlers. *Journal of Speech and Hearing Disorders, 54,* 587–599.

Rescorla, L., & Lee, E. (2001). Language impairment in young children. In T. Layton, E. Crais, & L. Watson (Eds.), *Handbook of early language impairment in children: Nature* (pp. 1–55). Albany, NY: Delmar.

Rescorla, L., Roberts, J. E., & Dahlsgaard, K. (1997). Late talkers at 2: Outcome at age 3. *Journal of Speech and Hearing Research, 40,* 556–566.

Rescorla, L., & Schwartz, E. (1990). Outcome of toddlers with expressive language delay. *Applied Psycholinguistics, 11,* 393–407.

Researchers discover first genes for stuttering [Press release]. (2010, February 10). Retrieved from http://www.nidcd.nih.gov/news/releases/10/02_10_10.htm

Rice, M. L., Warren, S., & Betz, S. (2005). Language symptoms of developmental language disorders: An overview of autism, Down syndrome, fragile X, specific language impairment and Williams syndrome. *Applied Psycholinguistics, 26,* 7–27.

Rice, M. L., & Bode, J. (1993). GAPs in the lexicon of children with specific language impairment. *First Language, 13,* 113–132.

Rice, M. L., Wexler, K., & Hershberger, S. (1998). Tense over time: The longitudinal course of tense acquisition in children with specific language impairment. *Journal of Speech, Language, and Hearing Research, 41,* 1412–1431.

Roberts, J. E., Rosenfeld, R. M., & Zeisel, S. A. (2004). Otitis media and speech and language: A meta-analysis of prospective studies. *Pediatrics, 113*(3), e238–e248.

Roizen, N. J. (2002). Down syndrome. In Mark L. Batshaw (Ed.), *Children with disabilities* (5th ed., pp. 307–320). Washington, DC: Brookes.

Roy, N., Merrill, R. M., Thibeault, S., Parsa, R. A., & Smith, E. M. (2004). Prevalence of voice disorders in teachers and the general population, *Journal of Speech, Language, and Hearing Research, 47,* 281–293.

Rustad, M. (2007). Measuring the intensity of sound—Decibels explained. Retrieved June 26, 2009, from http://www.articlesbase.com/science-articles/measuring-the-intensity-of-sound-decibels-explained-252817.html

Rutter, M. (2005). Genetic influences and autism. In F. Vokmar, R. Paul, A. Klin, & D. Cohen (Eds.), *Handbook of autism and pervasive developmental disorders: Vol.1* (pp. 425–452). New York: Wiley.

Sander, E. (1972). When are speech sounds learned? *Journal of Speech and Hearing Disorders, 37,* 55–63.

Savic, S. (1980). *How twins learn to talk.* London: Academic.

Schwartz, H. D. (1999). *A primer for stuttering therapy.* Boston: Allyn & Bacon.

Siegel, G. (2000). Demands and capacities or demands and performance? *Journal of Fluency Disorders, 25,* 321–327.

Sinal, S. H., & Woods, C. R. (2005). Human papillomavirus infections of the genital and respiratory tracts in young children. *Seminars in Pediatric Infectious Diseases, 16*(4), 306–316.

Skinner, B. F. (1957). *Verbal behavior.* East Norwalk, CT: Appleton-Century-Crofts.

Smit, A. B., Hand, L., Frelinger, J. J., Bernthal, J. E., & Bird, A. (1990). The Iowa articulation norms project and its Nebraska replication. *Journal of Speech and Hearing Disorders, 55,* 779–798.

Smith, V., Mirenda, P., & Zaidman-Zait, A. (2007). Predictors of expressive vocabulary growth in children with autism. *Journal of Speech, Language, and Hearing Research, 50,* 149–160.

Splaingard, M., Hutchins B., Sulton L., & Chaudhuri, G. (1988). Aspiration in rehabilitation patients: Videofluoroscopic vs. bedside clinical assessment. *Archives of Physical Medicine and Rehabilitation, 69,* 637–640.

Stanton-Chapman, T. L., Chapman, D. A., Kaiser, A. P., & Hancock, T. B. (2004). Cumulative risk and low-income children's language development. *Topics in Early Childhood Special Education, 24*(4), 227–237.

Stark, R. E. (1980). Stages of speech development in the first year of life. In G. H. Yeni-Komshian, J. F. Kavanagh, & C. A. Ferguson (Eds.), *Child phonology: Vol. 1, Production.* New York: Academic.

Starkweather, C. W., & Gottwald, S. R. (1990). The demands and capacities model II: Clinical applications. *Journal of Fluency Disorders, 15*(3), 143–157.

Surgeon General's Report—Fact Sheets—The Health Consequences of Smoking. (2004). Retrieved from http://www.surgeongeneral.gov/library/smokingconsequences/

Tager-Flusberg, H., Paul, R., & Lord, C. E. (2005). Language and communication in autism. In F. Volkmar, R. Paul, A. Klin, & D. J. Cohen (Eds.), *Handbook of autism and pervasive developmental disorder: Volume 1* (3rd ed., pp. 335–364). New York: Wiley.

Taylor, O. (1986). Teaching standard English as a second dialect. In O. Taylor (Ed.), *Treatment of communication disorders in culturally and linguistically diverse populations* (pp. 153–178). Boston: Little, Brown.

Templin, M. C. (1957). *Certain language skills in children, their development and interrelationships* (Institute of Child Welfare, Monograph Series, No. 26). Minneapolis: University of Minnesota Press.

Terrell, S., & Terrell, F. (1983). Distinguishing linguistic differences from disorders: The past, present, and future of nonbiased assessment. *Topics in Language Disorders, 3*, 1–7.

Thal, D., Tobias, S., & Morrison, D. (1991). Language and gesture in late talkers: A 1-year follow-up. *Journal of Speech and Hearing Research, 34*, 604–612.

Thal, D. J., & Tobias, S. (1992). Communicative gestures in children with delayed onset of oral expressive language use. *Journal of Speech and Hearing Research, 35*, 1281–1289.

Titze, I. (n.d.). Models of vocal fold vibration. From *Tutorials—Voice production*. National Center for Voice and Speech. Retrieved from http://www.ncvs.org/ncvs/tutorials/voiceprod/tutorial/model.html

Tomasello, M. (1995). Joint attention as social cognition. In C. Moore & P. J. Dunhan (Eds.), *Joint attention: Its origins and role in development* (pp. 103–130). Hillsdale, NJ: Erlbaum.

Tomasello, M. (2003). *Constructing a language.* Cambridge, MA: Harvard University Press.

Tomblin, J. B., Smith, E., & Zhang, X. (1997). Epidemiology of specific language impairment: Prenatal and perinatal risk factors. *Journal of Communication Disorders, 30*, 325–344.

Torgeson, J. K., Al Otaiba, S., & Grek, M. L. (2005). Assessment and instruction for phonemic awareness and word recognition skills. In H. W. Catts & A. G. Kamhi (Eds.), *Language and reading disabilities* (2nd ed., pp. 127–156). Boston: Pearson.

Tsybina, I., & Eriks-Brophy, A. (2007). Issues in research on children with early language delay. *Contemporary Issues in Communication Science and Disorders, 34*, 118–133.

U.S. Census Bureau. (2006). Language spoken at home by ability to speak English for the population 5 years and over (American Community Survey; Table B16001). Retrieved January 2008 from http://factfinder.census.gov/

Van Kleeck, A. (1994). Potential cultural bias in training parents as conversational partners with their children who have delays in language development. *American Journal of Speech-Language Pathology, 3*, 67–78.

Van Riper, C. (1954). *Speech correction: Principles and methods* (3rd ed.). New York: Prentice Hall.

Van Riper, C. (1973). *The treatment of stuttering.* Englewood Cliffs, NJ: Prentice Hall.

Van Wanrooij, M. M., & Van Opstal, A. J. (2004). Contribution of head shadow and pinna cues to chronic monaural sound localization. *The Journal of Neuroscience, 24*(17), 4163–4171.

Verdolini, K. (1999). Critical analysis of common terminology in voice therapy. *Phonoscope, 2*, 1–8.

Vihman, M. M. (2004). Later phonological development. In J. E. Bernthal & N. W. Bankson (Eds.), *Articulation and phonological disorders* (5th ed.). Boston: Pearson/Allyn & Bacon.

Vygotsky, L. S. (1978). *Mind in society: The development of higher psychological processes.* Cambridge, MA: Harvard University Press.

Webster, R. I., Erdos, C., Evans, K., Majnemer, A., Kehayia, E., Thordardottir, E., et al. (2006). The clinical spectrum of developmental language impairment in school-aged children: Language, cognitive, and motor findings. *Pediatrics, 118*, 1541–1549.

Webster, W. G. (1997). Principles of brain organization related to lateralization of language and speech motor functions in normal speakers and stutterers. In W. Hulstijn, H. F. M. Peters, & P. H. H. M. v. Lieshout (Eds.), *Speech production: Motor control, brain research and fluency disorders* (pp. 119–139). Amsterdam: Elsevier.

Wellman, B. L., Case, I. M., Mengert, I. G., & Bradbury, D. E. (1931). *Speech sounds of young children* (University of Iowa Studies in Child Welfare, 5). Iowa City: University of Iowa Press.

Westby, C. E. (2009). Social-emotional bases of communication development. In B. B. Shulman & N. C. Capone (Eds.), *Language development: Foundations, processes, and clinical applications.* Boston: Jones and Bartlett.

Whitehurst, G., Fischel, J., Lonigan, C., Valdez-Menchaca, M., Arnold, D., & Smith, M. (1991). Treatment of early expressive language delay: If, when, and how. *Topics in Language Disorders, 11*, 55–68.

Williams, K. (1997). *Expressive vocabulary test.* Circle Pines, MN: American Guidance Services.

Willis, W. (2004). Families with African American roots. In E. Lynch & M. Hanson (Eds.), *Developing cross-cultural competence: A guide for working with children and their families* (3rd ed., pp. 141–177). Baltimore: Brookes.

Wolfram, W. (1991). *Dialects and American English.* Englewood Cliffs, NJ: Prentice Hall.

Wyatt, T. (1998). Assessment issues with multicultural populations. In D. Battle (Ed.), *Communication disorders in multicultural populations* (pp. 379–425). Boston: Butterworth-Heinemann.

Yairi, E. (2004). The formative years of stuttering: A changing portrait. *Contemporary Issues in Communication Science and Disorders, 31*, 92–104.

Yairi, E., & Ambrose, N. G. (1992). Onset of stuttering in preschool children: Selected actors. *Journal of Speech, Language, and Hearing Research, 35*, 782–788.

Yairi, E., & Ambrose, N. G. (2005). Early childhood stuttering for clinicians. Austin, TX: PRO-ED.

Yairi, E., & Seery, C. H. (2011). *Stuttering: Foundations and clinical applications.* Upper Saddle River, NJ: Pearson.

Yueh, B., Shapiro, N., MacLean, C. H., & Shekelle, P. G. (2003). Screening and management of adult hearing loss in primary care. *Journal of the American Medical Association, 289*, 1976–1985.

INDEX